Parental Stress and Early Child Development

Kirby Deater-Deckard · Robin Panneton
Editors

Parental Stress and Early Child Development

Adaptive and Maladaptive Outcomes

Springer

Editors
Kirby Deater-Deckard
Department of Psychological and Brain Sciences
University of Massachusetts Amherst
Amherst, MA
USA

Robin Panneton
Department of Psychology
Virginia Tech
Blacksburg, VA
USA

ISBN 978-3-319-55374-0 ISBN 978-3-319-55376-4 (eBook)
DOI 10.1007/978-3-319-55376-4

Library of Congress Control Number: 2017934313

Printed on acid-free paper

This Springer imprint is published by Springer Nature
The registered company is Springer International Publishing AG
The registered company address is: Gewerbestrasse 11, 6330 Cham, Switzerland

Kirby Deater-Deckard *would like to dedicate this volume to Keirsten, Anna and Elly Deater-Deckard, with my gratitude and love.*

Robin Panneton *would like to dedicate this volume to her identical twin sons (Sam and Jack) and her husband (Lee) for collectively challenging and sculpting the parenting system that has enveloped her for the past 26 years (including pregnancy!). Parenting twins was transformative on almost every level imaginable. We were stressed—all of us, because none of us "knew" what we were doing. We allowed ourselves to be both teacher and student on a continual basis, earning our successes as well as our failures as we went along. It was wonderful and frightening at all times, and allowed me to fully appreciate the power of bio/psycho/socio/cultural dynamics in affecting our family, all families.*

Preface

In scientific scholarship, knowledge is constructed as a *social enterprise*, in relationships between the scholar and others (Nelkin & Lindee 2004). This is what makes scholarship fun and engaging (even though it may not always feel that way) and makes human inquiry unique when compared to every other type of knowledge system in the universe. To say that scientific scholarship is socially constructed is not to say that science is not real—it most certainly is real in the sense that our knowledge of the mechanisms and processes of all that surrounds us depends completely on our collective abilities to see, hear, feel, and touch that which we aim to understand. But ultimately, our understanding emerges from social action. We observe, explain, debate, reason, defend, debunk, and/or rationalize our understanding of the world with each other. We socially negotiate the "truth" by agreeing with each other, anchoring our agreements to sets of standards that work well for delimited periods of time and space. But occasionally assumptions get challenged, standards fall, and intellectual revolutions ensue. This is the fun part.

The story of this scholarly edited book is a case in point. The seed for this book was planted in the late winter of 2005, when we first met. Kirby had come to Virginia Tech for a faculty interview in developmental science. At that time, his work was focused on applying statistical modeling approaches to partitioning variance into "pockets" of genetic, shared environmental, and non-shared environmental influences on individual difference attributes—and, whether these effects were additive or interactive. Robin's empirical work was centered on infants' perception of aspects of adult communicative action that lead to successful language learning. But her teaching was often focused on issues and controversies within the domains of genetic and epigenetic contributions to developmental outcomes (largely due to the influence of Gilbert Gottlieb, Timothy Johnston, and Robert Lickliter during her graduate training). On the surface, it was unlikely that Kirby and Robin were headed into any social negotiations of their science!

Like all academic job interviews, Kirby's itinerary was packed with meetings and the job talk was stressful. However, his memory of dinner with Robin and their department chair is clear as a bell. While he consumed sea scallops and a very dry martini, Robin confessed that she had reservations about his statistical interactionist method and view of genes and environments as separable and quantifiable; nonetheless, she would be a willing and true colleague who would engage him in debate and inquiry. She could not have known it at the time, but that was precisely the kind of "look in the eye and hand in the hand" that Kirby was looking for in a new collaboration and friendship. We were on our way to social negotiation of science after all.

In the true spirit of collaborative scholarship, we eventually co-taught an integrated graduate/undergraduate seminar on "genetics and epigenetics in development." Each week, we would meet with a group of 10 graduate students for an hour, then 2 hours with an additional 40 undergraduate seniors (overlapping with the graduate students), and a final hour with just the undergraduates. Throughout this time, we worked collectively and intensively to understand important readings concerning gene and non-gene processes that affect developmental outcomes and trajectories (with the graduate students serving as mentors to the undergraduates).

This "seminar-fest" was exhausting but also exhilarating. It made us realize how hungry we were, and our students were, for this different kind of discourse. The seed had been planted years before, and the seminar watered it well. Still, it took us five more years before we converged on the idea to co-edit this book. (Development is hard, and it takes time.) The opportunity arose to bring together voices of a broad range of scientists who could speak to our emerging collaborative perspective on stress, parenting, intergenerational transmission, and developmental systems. With excitement and considerable anxiety, we forged ahead with our invitations to authors and were simply astonished by how receptive our colleagues were to the ideas for the book. We purposefully approached scholars who not only examine various aspects of parenting stress as it relates to developmental processes, but do so from a dynamic, organic, and multidirectional perspective. The end product is a book that fully embodies the perspective to which we are committed, and that we feel is the most likely to generate fruitful discussions and inspire future thinking about this very complex web of relationships. We are grateful to these authors for capturing our enthusiasm and bringing it to each page of their contributions.

Amherst, USA — Kirby Deater-Deckard
Blacksburg, USA — Robin Panneton

Reference

Nelkin, D., & Lindee, M.S. (2004). *The DNA mystique: The gene as a cultural icon.* Ann Arbor, MI: University of Michigan Press.

Contents

Editors and Contributors

About the Editors

Kirby Deater-Deckard, Ph.D. is a professor of psychological and brain sciences at the University of Massachusetts Amherst, and a fellow of the Association for Psychological Science. Dr. Deater-Deckard conducts research and teaches courses on biological and environmental influences on individual differences in social-emotional and cognitive development in childhood and adolescence. The emphasis in this work is on intergenerational transmission, gene–environment mechanisms, and home and school environments. His publications span developmental and family sciences and developmental psychopathology areas, with research currently and previously funded by NSF and NIH. Applications focus on parenting stress: identifying its antecedents and consequences, its adaptive and maladaptive features, and implications for parenting prevention and intervention programs. In his current collaborative work on parenting, he is examining maternal cognitive and physiological self-regulation and its role in parenting stress and harsh caregiving, in the face of challenging child behavior and contextual stressors.

Robin Panneton, Ph.D. is an associate professor of psychology, member of the Faculty of Health Sciences, and an affiliated member of the School of Neuroscience at Virginia Tech. Dr. Panneton conducts research on the processes and mechanisms of how infants learn to communicate in the first two years after birth. Predominantly, she is interested in how information available from caretakers is attended to, processed, and remembered by infants as they begin their pathways to being language users. With the support of funding from NICHD and the James S. McDonnell Foundation, she has looked at voice recognition, processing of intonational contours, integration of information across facial and vocal displays, attention modulation via emotional information in speaker's faces and voices, and early indicators of individual differences in learning styles as they relate to emerging language skills in low- and high-risk infants. In her teaching, she has concentrated on dynamic systems view of development, epigenetics, pre- and postnatal contributions to early human development, language learning, and the development of attention in infancy and early childhood.

Contributors

John E. Bates Department of Psychological and Brain Sciences, Indiana University, Bloomington, IN, USA

Clancy Blair Department of Applied Psychology, New York University, New York, NY, USA

Rochelle C. Cassells Department of Human Development, Cornell University, Ithaca, NY, USA

Neilson Chan Department of Psychology, Loma Linda University, Loma Linda, CA, USA

Keith Crnic Department of Psychology, Arizona State University, Tempe, AZ, USA

Kirby Deater-Deckard Department of Psychological and Brain Sciences, University of Massachusetts Amherst, Amherst, MA, USA

Gary W. Evans Department of Design and Environment Analysis, Cornell University, Ithaca, NY, USA; Department of Human Development, Cornell University, Ithaca, NY, USA

Eric D. Finegood Department of Applied Psychology, New York University, New York, NY, USA

Alison S. Fleming Department of Psychology, University of Toronto, Toronto, Canada

Sophie Havighurst Department of Psychiatry, Mindful: Centre for Training and Research in Developmental Health, University of Melbourne, Melbourne, VI, Australia

Marinus H. Van IJzendoorn Centre for Child and Family Studies, Leiden University, Leiden, The Netherlands; School of Pedagogical and Educational Sciences, Erasmus University Rotterdam, Rotterdam, The Netherlands

Christiane Kehoe Department of Psychiatry, Mindful: Centre for Training and Research in Developmental Health, University of Melbourne, Melbourne, VI, Australia

Brian T. Leitzke University of Wisconsin—Madison, Madison, USA

Maureen E. McQuillan Department of Psychological and Brain Sciences, Indiana University, Bloomington, IN, USA

Viara R. Mileva-Seitz Department of Psychology, University of Toronto, Toronto, Canada

Melissa A. Milkie Department of Sociology, University of Toronto, Toronto, ON, Canada

Rosa H. Mulder Centre for Child and Family Studies, Leiden University, Leiden, The Netherlands

Cameron L. Neece Department of Psychology, Loma Linda University, Loma Linda, CA, USA

Regula Neuenschwander Department of Pediatrics, BC Children's Hospital Research Institute, University of British Columbia, Vancouver, BC, Canada

Kei Nomaguchi Department of Sociology, Bowling Green State University, Bowling Green, OH, USA

Timothy F. Oberlander Department of Pediatrics, BC Children's Hospital Research Institute, University of British Columbia, Vancouver, BC, Canada

Robin Panneton Department of Psychology, Virginia Tech, Blacksburg, VA, USA

Seth D. Pollak University of Wisconsin—Madison, Madison, USA

Jolien Rijlaarsdam Centre for Child and Family Studies, Leiden University, Leiden, The Netherlands

Emily Ross Department of Psychology, Arizona State University, Tempe, AZ, USA

Chapter 1
Unearthing the Developmental and Intergenerational Dynamics of Stress in Parent and Child Functioning

Kirby Deater-Deckard and Robin Panneton

No doubt, life is stressful. In this modern time, we associate our stress with work commitments, financial obligations, relationship tensions, and meeting biological needs, to name but a few of its sources. Most of all young- and middle-aged adult humans are in positions to somehow manage and/or balance their levels of stress emanating from these sources on a daily basis. For many of these same individuals, an additional and potent source of stress enters their lives when they become parents. Stress associated with parenting reflects "a set of processes that lead to aversive psychological and physiological reactions arising from attempts to adapt to the demands of parenthood" (Deater-Deckard, 2004, p. 6). Parenting stress is not the exception—it is the rule. Being responsible for the care and well-being (both psychologically and physically) of infants, toddlers, children, adolescents, and/or young adults is challenging, and at times, overwhelming. Furthermore, it arises not only from more extreme acute and chronic stressors that are unique to the parenting role, but is part and parcel of the ongoing experience of daily stressors over which we have only limited control (Crnic, Gaze, & Hoffman, 2005).

So what is "stress" and is it always toxic? For important reasons, stress is best defined as a "state of mind" involving both the brains and bodies of those experiencing adverse, negative, and/or threatening conditions (McEwen et al., 2012). Whether or not any given event is "stressful" depends critically on the perceiver of the event, their history with respect to the event, their current state of psychological and physiological well-being, and their intentions, goals, and aspirations. Often, short-term stress promotes plasticity and resilience (e.g., physical exercise and its

K. Deater-Deckard (✉)
Department of Psychological and Brain Sciences,
University of Massachusetts Amherst, Amherst, MA, USA
e-mail: kdeaterdeck@umass.edu

R. Panneton
Department of Psychology, Virginia Tech, Blacksburg, VA, USA
e-mail: panneton@vt.edu

K. Deater-Deckard and R. Panneton (eds.), *Parental Stress and Early Child Development*, DOI 10.1007/978-3-319-55376-4_1

benefits for immunoprotection; Dhabhar, 2014). Periodic exposure to stressors operates by keeping us "tuned up," so that our bodies and minds are able to respond nimbly and effectively (most of the time) when stressors are acute—and maintain resources for prolonged periods of time if stressors are chronic (e.g., coping; Compas, 1987; Holahan, Moos, & Schaefer, 2006).

Thus, keys to healthy development of individuals in general and parent–child relationships in particular include a certain degree of plasticity or flexibility in stress processes, along with some exposure to acute and occasional chronic stressors. However, longer-term chronic stress is a major contributor to disease, impairment, and psychological risk (e.g., allostasis; Lupien et al., 2006; but see also Ellis & Del Giudice, 2014). The scientific evidence is clear with respect to pervasive deleterious effects of chronic stress on developing systems of the body over the entire lifespan (Danese & McEwen, 2012).

One of the most powerful sources of broad deleterious allostatic effects is poverty and its covarying factors such as ethnicity and social capital (Evans, 2004; Kawachi, 1999). These sources carry with them a host of other covarying factors, ranging from family and neighborhood structures and processes, to security of income, food, and shelter. Their effects accumulate, and over time create changes in individual's bodies and minds, as well as in their social relationships. In the longer run, it becomes more and more difficult to repair damage to cells and selves (Evans, Li, & Whipple, 2013). However, the very same stress reactivity and self-regulation process, even within chronically stressful environments, is the very same "natural experiment" that evolution may be using to produce novel and highly adaptive phenotypes (Blair & Raver, 2012). Stress is probably one of the crucibles in which evolutionarily conserved adaptations are forged.

As mentioned in the preface, as editors of this volume we were specifically keen to invite perspectives that would clearly flesh out the complex, bidirectional, and multifaceted nature of parental stress and its effect on children's developmental trajectories that begin at conception, and for some processes even prior to that. Beginning with the parent prior to becoming a parent, the individual's stress reactivity and regulation already has potential influence on the future child's own stress reactivity and regulation, via epigenetic modifications of DNA—in ova and sperm cells, and prenatally for the child's own somatic and germ cells. These epigenetic modifications also can occur postnatally, as a result of the child's exposure to a distressed and harsh parenting environment. As the postnatal relationship unfolds, the parent's and child's own stress reactivity and regulation influence parent and child behavior directly. Furthermore, each partner in the dyad—the parent and the child—and her or his own stress reactivity and regulation—is influenced by the partner's behavior that serves to socialize reactivity and regulation while also serving as a stressor itself. Finally, these developmental and interpersonal processes can be altered by transient and temporally stable contextual factors, such as poverty, cultural beliefs and practices, social statuses, and physical environments.

Thus, acquisition and execution of adaptive responses to stress develops throughout our lifetimes and extends to the next generation. This includes aspects of our experiences prenatally, during infancy and childhood, during our adolescence, as young adults, and the effects we have on the next generation as we become parents ourselves (Archer & Kostrezewa, 2013; Radley, Morilak, Viau, & Campeau, 2015). Accordingly, we have organized the volume into three major sections: Part I (Chaps. 2–5) explores important sources of parenting stress, including sociocultural factors, such as poverty, ethnicity, gender, and parenting ideology, and child characteristics, such as temperament and disability. Part II (Chaps. 6–10) focuses on the consequences of parenting stress for children's neurological, physiological, cognitive, affective, and behavioral development as well as their own parenting behavior. Part III (Chaps. 11–12) examines pathways to managing parenting stress via parental self-regulation of social cognition and emotions. As readers will realize over the course of the three sections of the book, the intergenerational transmission of stress reactivity and self-regulated coping involves biological *and* psychosocial processes, *within* and *between* the parent and child in each family, but also *within* and *between* adjacent and lagged generations in families, groups of families, and even broader communities of people (e.g., cultural practices and beliefs, Boyd & Richerson, 1988; self-regulation, Bridgett, Burt, Edwards, & Deater-Deckard, 2015; depression, Goodman & Gotlib, 1999).

Part I: Common Sources of Parenting Stress

Adaptive functioning in the face of stressors requires capacities to accurately perceive stressors and behave in ways that effectively reduce and or eliminate stress before it registers negative effects on health and well-being. Although the stress process is dynamic, there are a number of sources of stress common to most parents who are exposed to them. The first section of the volume brings to the forefront current theory and compiled empirical evidence regarding some of the most powerful and common of these sources. These factors include, but are not limited to, poverty and restriction or lack of access to socioeconomic resources, social contexts surrounding the parents such as race-ethnicity, marital status, gender and sexuality, welfare-state regime, embodied psychological tendencies represented in temperament and personality, and the extra demands placed on caregivers of children with special developmental and health needs.

The sociocultural and physical environment in which the parent and child are embedded sets the stage for many aspects of the stress and coping parents will experience—and the effects of stress on the child's development. At the time of publication of the current volume, the USA and most other developed economies in the world were still experiencing the aftermath of a deep global economic recession spanning 2007–2010. This downturn was part of a much longer, ongoing trend of underemployment, flat wages and growing economic inequality—processes that disproportionately affect ethnic minority families and children living in poverty (Bell & Blanchflower, 2011; Shapiro, Meschede, & Osoro, 2013). Cassells and Evans (Chap. 2) consider the effects of both actual and perceived lack of access on to basic necessities for poor parents. These authors systematically examine several of the most powerful factors that account for the effects of poverty and minority status on parenting function (e.g., neighborhood features, household composition or structure, and family members' chronic depression) via the family stress model. At its core, this model makes clear the reciprocal and negative effects of poverty on parenting as mothers and fathers face expanding failure in meeting the basic needs of their children. Cassells and Evans also address many current challenges to the health and well-being of families, such as the plight of parents who have emigrated due to geopolitical or economic forces and the stressors that arise from that experience. In keeping with a theme that is covered by Nomaguchi and Milkie in Chap. 3, Cassells and Evans also discuss how poverty appears to differentially manifest in parental stress depending on racial and ethnic context and contingencies (e.g., the relationship between parenting stress and parenting behavior appears to differ between low-income Black and Hispanic mothers). They conclude with specific recommendations for how researchers and policy makers can reconsider the contexts of poverty in ways that more accurately reflect the daily lives and experiences of children and parents.

Nomaguchi and Milkie (Chap. 3) turn a sociological lens on parenting stress and its effects, with an emphasis on social structures, statuses, and culture (e.g., socioeconomic status and social class, race, ethnicity, gender). Some of these factors are stable over time and contribute in powerful ways to shaping parenting stress within families and among groups of families in similar socioecological niches. Other factors are emergent, forcing modern-day parents to reorganize and adapt to stress in new and productive ways (e.g., increases in mothers' participation in the labor force; increased incarceration rates among modern parents). Importantly, this chapter also addresses the associations between parenting strain and racial/ethnic disparities, not only emanating from socioeconomic challenge, but also from differences in cultural ideology and structural resources that carry across generations. Nomaguchi and Milkie also emphasize the sources of family and individual resilience that are supported by the broader extra-familial context. Their chapter serves to remind us that prevention and intervention efforts that do not address the causes and consequences of parenting stress at the community and regional level are less likely to have sustaining effects on the next generation of parents growing up in that community.

Another important source of parenting stress arises from relatively stable individual differences in parents' and children's temperament-based emotions and behaviors that pertain to stress reactivity and regulation. McQuillan and Bates (Chap. 4) present theory and empirical evidence for internal state influences on parenting stress, bringing to the fore the novel yet growing emphasis in the literature on parents' and children's sleep problems and their connections with temperament. Although the responsibilities of childrearing convey some of the stress that is unique to the parenting role, the experience of coping with the stresses of parenthood is made all the more challenging with children who are high in negative emotionality and lack self-regulation (e.g., increased feelings of parental incompetence and lack of control). McQuillan and Bates present evidence that these hard-to-manage behaviors in children impact parenting stress and harsh reactive parenting, which only serves to elicit and reinforce these challenging behavioral and emotional problems in the child. This dyadic stress process is further enhanced when one or both partners experience chronic sleep problems, with sleep deprivation itself influenced by other factors within and beyond the immediate family context. At a more conceptual level, this emphasis on the dyadic nature of stress management (and dysfunction) between parents and children supports a critique of the family stress model by Cassells and Evans (Chap. 2); they call for a revision to the model to include a more child-as-active force in the research on stress and parenting dynamics. McQuillan and Bates' chapter contributes to this revision by emphasizing a "coercive" family stress model, bringing to light the importance of considering temperament in both parent and child, the importance of considering chaos in the home, and the importance of the cognitive skills of both parents and children in emotion regulation and cognitive functioning.

Another manifestation of the bidirectional, dynamic interplay between parents, parenting, and stress is made exceptionally clear when considering the various challenges of caring for a child with an intellectual or developmental disability (IDD). Neece and Chan (Chap. 5) highlight the experience of parenting a child with IDD and summarize evidence that the impact of the child's functioning and health on parenting stress varies widely. Consistent with McQuillan and Bates' discussion on temperament in typically developing children (Chap. 4), Neece and Chan note that it is the child's level of behavioral and emotional problems that most consistently and strongly predicts the levels of parenting stress in families raising a child with an IDD. The literature on IDD and parenting stress also provides evidence that chronic parenting stress in the face of these challenging child behaviors serves to increase harsh reactive parenting which further exacerbates child and behavioral problems. Like the previous chapters, Neece and Chan emphasize the importance of developing interventions for families that address parent and child stress and coping, given the dyadic transactional nature of the family stress process (which also dovetails nicely with (Chap. 12) by Havighurst and Kehoe on remediation strategies).

Part II: Consequences of Parenting Stress for Children

The goal of the prior section was to highlight common sources of parenting stress, and for these chapters to serve as models for future review and theory chapters and papers that can highlight other common sources not captured in the current volume (e.g., work–family role conflict, parental mental and physical health problems). Though common, these and other exogenous factors and forces can push typical parenting stress and coping processes into the realm of chronic stress and failure of coping. If not mitigated, this chronic stressful state becomes instantiated in parenting and child developmental trajectories that are maladaptive. Parenting stress transpires within parent–child dyads, but there is a need to focus specifically on the consequences of chronic parenting stress on the developing child. The chapters in this section of the book examine prenatal and postnatal maternal stress and its effects on child health and functioning via neurobiological and socialization mechanisms.

The bulk of the extant literature explicitly or implicitly implies that the effects of parenting stress on children begin in infancy. However, parenting stress exists before birth—as does its effects on fetal neurobehavioral organization. The largest body of human research evidence is from prospective and retrospective longitudinal studies across the birth of the child. These show that the largest and most consistent predictors of postnatal maternal and paternal depression, anxiety, and stress are their own symptoms during the pregnancy (O'Hara & Swain, 1996; Paulson & Bazemore, 2010). Neuenschwander and Oberlander (Chap. 6) describe mounting evidence from human prenatal studies that certain fetal adaptations that increase vigilance to the environment or response to stress could be maladaptive in one context but adaptive in another; thus, prenatal exposure to maternal stress can shape developmental outcomes for better *and* worse. Neuenschwander and Oberlander detail studies that emphasize how the prenatal environment plays a crucial role in subsequent (i.e., postnatal) neurocognitive regulation of stress reactivity. For those pregnant women who experience high levels of acute or chronic stressors, and those who have sustained depressive or anxious symptoms during pregnancy, the mother's bodily stress response exposes the fetus to high levels of hormones that can fundamentally alter the developing child's own stress response system. Neuenschwander and Oberlander focus on the particular example of women's antidepressant use during pregnancy and its potential lasting effects (via epigenetic modifications) on infants' serotonin regulation—a neurotransmitter that is critical to adaptive regulation of reactions to stressors. They emphasize that this entire system of prenatal stress exposure and its lasting effects have evolved to increase the flexibility and adaptability of the child's developing homeostatic self-regulation—a system that instead yields maladaptive outcomes when the prenatal exposures to stress hormones or serotonin disruptors are too extreme.

The epigenetic pathways to consider are many and varied. Much of the research to date has examined selective site methylation that alters gene expression by silencing genes or causing other changes in a complex system of neurotransmitters. Mulder, Rijlaarsdam, and Van IJzendoorn (Chap. 7) offer a comprehensive review of parental stress effects on children's development via these kinds of epigenetic changes. Findings are complex, and results are mixed, in these early and exciting days of longitudinal epigenetic research with humans. As the authors point out, ultimately our field will need to complete more definitive human and animal studies that explicitly test the mediating effects of epigenetic changes pre- and postnatally that bridge early acute and chronic parental stress exposure in the infant and its lasting effects on the growing child's neurobiological, cognitive, affective, and behavioral functioning. The research that needs to be done will challenge many current methods used in molecular biology and developmental science. The future work also will require changes in prevailing theories of what genes and phenotypes are and how they work, within a constantly evolving landscape of organisms, environments, and their ongoing transactional cascades (Pigliucci, 2007).

As hotly debated as contemporary theory may be regarding the status of evolutionary explanations for developmental processes, there is by comparison something akin to consensus (if not real consensus) that the frontal and prefrontal cortex is one of the most recently evolved regions of the brain. Furthermore, the growth and change in neocortex in evolutionary time may have brought with it the emergence of inhibitory cognitive processes that served to dampen reactive responses to the environment, while also providing novel skills involving theory of mind and planning that coevolved in humans and perhaps other higher primates (Dunbar, 2003).

One domain of these phylogenetically recent neural functions and cognitive capacities is executive function (EF). In their chapter, Finegood and Blair (Chap. 8) focus on stress and its effects on the developing system of EFs in childhood that serve self-regulation of thought, emotion, and behavior. EFs are complex, effortful cognitive capacities that develop rapidly over early childhood. It is during this same period of development that early exposure to chronic parenting stress is likely to instantiate lasting alterations to neurobiological and psychosocial factors that contribute to deficits in executive functions development. Finegood and Blair review the emerging empirical evidence and theories on the role of early social relationships with parents and other caregivers, with emphasis on the deleterious effects of poverty on children's executive function that are mediated by harsher and more reactive parenting behavior that is most prevalent in impoverished contexts. This chapter calls our attention to the importance of applying intervention experiments to refine our understanding of caregiving processes that can mitigate the deleterious consequences of chronic poverty on parents and children alike.

Continuing on the theme of caregiving as the postnatal mediator of parenting stress effects on children, Leitzke and Pollack (Chap. 9) focus specifically on parenting that is chronic and extreme in its harshness, unpredictability, or negligence. Child maltreatment comprises a variety of caregiving behaviors spanning physical and psychosocial forms of severe punishment to chronic neglect. The etiology of maltreatment is complex, but elevated parenting stress and insufficient coping play crucial roles. Leitzke and Pollack provide an overview of the growing literature on some of the ways in which parenting stress and maltreating behaviors perturb the child's developing systems of cognitive, social-emotional, and physical functioning. Consistent with several of the prior chapters' authors, they emphasize that the effects of maltreatment operate via alterations to children's learned behaviors, cognitions, emotions, and neurobiological systems. As these developmental processes become more clearly articulated, the hope is that our field will develop and refine prevention and intervention tools that effectively reduce the risk of maltreatment and mitigate its effects when it occurs.

Ontogenetic development and transgenerational transmission of parenting stress also operates "under the skin," and is codified at multiple levels of dynamic psychobiological function. Epigenetic and other prenatal and early postnatal environmental influences on gene expression have effects on the next generation through prenatal biological transmission at and after fertilization, and via that child's own caregiving behavior once she has reached sexual maturity and becomes a parent.

Mileva-Seitz and Fleming (Chap. 10) highlight foundational animal studies, as well as more recent studies with humans, that indicate that the wide variation seen between individuals in their stress reactivity and self-regulation is transmitted to the next generation. Capitalizing on the wealth of studies using the female rodent as a model for mothering dynamics, Mileva-Seitz and Fleming unpack many critical factors that influence complex interactions between chronic and acute stressors at key points in prenatal and postnatal development, as well as genomic and early postnatal caregiving differences. What becomes clear is that parental abuse, neglect, and/or deprivation not only have serious consequences for the health and well-being of immediate offspring, but on that of subsequent generations as well. Through these intergenerational processes, parenting stress is functionally "inherited" by subsequent generations in terms of increased probabilities that parenting stress will manifest in their own lives. This kind of inheritance is not purely through "simple" socialization and/or genetic transmission, but through complex interactions that produce lasting changes in neurological structures and functions that influence parenting behavior. Importantly, this chapter also deals with important neurobiological and neurophysiological factors that seem to increase resilience and buffer individuals from otherwise dire negative outcomes of negative parenting (see also Chap. 7 by Mulder, Rijlaarsdam, and Van IJzendoorn).

Part III: Pathways to Managing Parental Stress

Parenting stress is ubiquitous, but effective management of that stress and its effects on parenting and children's functioning is not. Some of the variability in parenting stress arises from individual differences in parents' self-regulation of thoughts, emotions, and behaviors in the face of acute and chronic stressors. For most parents most of the time, managing the stressors arising from the parenting role is a manageable challenge most of the time. However, sometimes the stress process overwhelms parents—and for a sub-group of parents, difficulties with stress reactivity and self-regulation chronically constrain effective management of stress. The book ends with an emphasis on stress management and self-regulation, because of their importance for prevention and intervention efforts that seek to create lasting change in parenting environments and children's developmental outcomes.

Crnic and Ross (Chap. 11) tackle the complex transactional associations between stress and self-relevant social cognitions, with particular emphasis on self-efficacy in the parenting role. Parenting is hard but rewarding work, and yet, it is sometimes even harder and less rewarding than anticipated. Crnic and Ross make the case for why and how the parent's own sense of competence and effectiveness as a caregiver and socializer can become deflected or impaired in the face of chronic parenting stress—and, how lower self-efficacy can itself increase exposure to parenting stress. Furthermore, an individual's own thoughts and feelings around parenting self-efficacy intersect with the parenting partner's self-efficacy as part of a broader family system. These coparenting social cognitive processes may differ systematically by parent's gender. Crnic and Ross integrate these ideas into a conceptual model that emphasizes parenting stress and its effects as part of a system that changes as the child develops and parenting demands and stressors evolve in the family's lifespan.

Bringing us full circle to where the volume began on transgenerational mechanisms, Havighurst and Kehoe (Chap. 12) examine emotion regulation and its role in emotion socialization, with implications for the next generation's own emotion and stress regulation. As complex social beings, humans have evolved embodied affective states (e.g., anger, fear) and motivational stances (e.g., to approach a potential reward or withdraw from a potential risk). Affect and motivation enhance survival and well-being through children's social worlds by enhancing communication and social bonding with caregivers and other members of their social worlds. However, these very same emotions and motives tend to occur as reactive responses to the environment and need to be regulated in order to provide appropriate and timely responses to the environment. Havighurst and Kehoe emphasize the instrumental role that parents play in the socialization of children's regulation and expression of emotion—and how normative emotion socialization processes can be impeded or even become deleterious in their effects, for parents who are chronically stressed and struggle to regulate their own emotions and behaviors. Their chapter also is unique to the volume, in its presentation of a specific example of the development and testing of a parenting intervention, *Tuning into Kids*, as a potentially fruitful approach to enhancing parents' own emotion regulation and psychological well-being in ways that reduce stress and enhance parental emotion socialization of children.

Parenting Stress and Children's Development

In sum, our hope is that the current collection of chapters will convey to readers that stress is a process that is continuous throughout development, and that it operates within each of us and between us in our social relationships including the parent–child dyad. Our bodies and social systems have evolved to respond rapidly to avoid potential dangers that threaten and approach opportunities that enhance the well-being of our children and ourselves (Elliot, 2006; Taylor, 2006). With regard to the processes "under our skin," scientists have focused primarily on the autonomic nervous system with its sympathetic and parasympathetic branches, and the more recently evolved neocortex brain regions that regulate reactivity (Harrell, Hall, & Taliaferro, 2003; Thayer & Lane, 2009). But "under the skin" is also "outside the skin"—the space between the faces and voices of caregivers and children. The evolution of these neurophysiological systems for reactivity and self-regulation has coevolved with changes in social and family groups and social communicative behavior (Porges, 2011). The development of these embodied internal and social external processes occurs in tandem for better or worse, wherein each can compensate for damage or limitations in the other, as seen in the literature on resilience in the face of severe chronic stressors (Cicchetti & Rogosch, 2009).

In the spirit of the dynamic systems' approach that runs throughout the excellent contributions to this volume, we end our introduction with another hope. We hope that the science that is represented in these chapters will challenge and inspire current and future investigators of human development and family sciences to continually evaluate the rigor of our methods, interpretations of data, and the processes we use to make inferences and translate those conclusions into practice. All fields of science continue to adopt the newest technologies that improve the precision of measurement of their phenomena of interest. In doing so, scientists find themselves confronting new levels of complexity of the systems they study and their need to recruit diverse research teams to describe and explain them (Ledford, 2015). Most who study families, and who develop and deliver prevention and intervention tools to improve their lives, will not become biological scientists or anthropologists—but increasingly, they will read work from a broader range of disciplines in order to wisely consume the science of parenting stress and children's development. The current collection of chapters demonstrates that this is not only feasible, but that it sharpens the eye and the mind of inquiry. There could be no more important subject for such efforts than the development of healthy and happy families—past, current, and future.

References

Archer, T., & Kostrezewa, R. M. (2013). The inductive agency of stress: From perinatal to adolescent induction. In G. Laviola & S. Macri (Eds.), *Adaptive and maladaptive aspects of developmental stress* (pp. 23–44, 1–20). New York, NY: Springer.

Bell, D. N., & Blanchflower, D. G. (2011). Young people and the Great Recession. *Oxford Review of Economic Policy, 27*(2), 241–267. http://nbn-resolving.de/urn:nbn:de:101:1-201105173104

Blair, C., & Raver, C. (2012). Individual development and evolution: Experiential canalization of self-regulation. *Developmental Psychology, 48*(3), 647–657. doi:10.1037/a0026472

Boyd, R., & Richerson, P. J. (1988). *Culture and the evolutionary process*. Chicago, IL: University of Chicago Press.

Bridgett, D. J., Burt, N. M., Edwards, E. S., & Deater-Deckard, K. (2015). Intergenerational transmission of self-regulation: A multidisciplinary review and integrative conceptual framework. *Psychological Bulletin, 141,* 602–654. doi:10.1037/a0038662.

Cicchetti, D., & Rogosch, F. A. (2009). Adaptive coping under conditions of extreme stress: Multilevel influences on the determinants of resilience in maltreated children. *New Directions for Child and Adolescent Development, 2009*(124), 47–59. doi:10.1002/cd.242

Compas, B. E. (1987). Coping with stress during childhood and adolescence. *Psychological Bulletin, 101*(3), 393–403.

Crnic, K. A., Gaze, C., & Hoffman, C. (2005). Cumulative parenting stress across the preschool period: Relations to maternal parenting and child behaviour at age 5. *Infant and Child Development, 14*(2), 117–132. doi:10.1002/icd.384

Danese, A., & McEwen, B. S. (2012). Adverse childhood experiences, allostasis, allostatic load, and age-related disease. *Physiology & Behavior, 106*(1), 29–39. doi:10.1016/j.physbeh.2011.08.019.

Deater-Deckard, K. (2004). *Parenting stress*. New Haven, CT: Yale University Press.

Dhabhar, F. S. (2014). Effects of stress on immune function: the good, the bad, the beautiful. *Immunological Research, 58,* 193–210. doi:10.1007/s12026-014-8517-0.

Dunbar, R. I. (2003). The social brain: Mind, language, and society in evolutionary perspective. *Annual Review of Anthropology, 32,* 163–181. doi:10.1146/annurev.anthro.32.061002.093158

Elliot, A. J. (2006). The hierarchical model of approach-avoidance motivation. *Motivation and Emotion, 30*(2), 111–116. doi:10.1007/s11031-006-9028-7

Ellis, B. J., & Del Giudice, M. (2014). Beyond allostatic load: Rethinking the role of stress in regulating human development. *Development and Psychopathology, 26,* 1–20. doi:10.1017/S0954579413000849.

Evans, G. W. (2004). The environment of childhood poverty. *American Psychologist, 59*(2), 77–92. doi:10.1037/0003-066X.59.2.77

Evans, G. W., Li, D., & Whipple, S. (2013). Cumulative risk and child development. *Psychological Bulletin, 139*(6), 1342–1396. doi:10.1037/a0031808

Goodman, S. H., & Gotlib, I. H. (1999). Risk for psychopathology in the children of depressed mothers: A developmental model for understanding mechanisms of transmission. *Psychological Review, 106*(3), 458–490.

Harrell, J. P., Hall, S., & Taliaferro, J. (2003). Physiological responses to racism and discrimination: An assessment of the evidence. *American Journal of Public Health, 93,* 243–248.

Holahan, C. J., Moos, R. H., & Schaefer, J. A. (2006). Coping, stress resistance, and growth: Conceptualizing adaptive functioning. In M. Zeidner & N. S. Endler (Eds.), *Handbook of coping: Theory, research, applications* (pp. 24–43). Oxford, UK: Wiley.

Kawachi, I. (1999). Social capital and community effects on population and individual health. *Annals of the New York Academy of Sciences, 896*(1), 120–130.

Ledford, H. (2015). How to solve the world's biggest problems. *Nature, 525*(7569), 308–311. doi:10.1038/525308a

Lupien, S. J., Ouellet-Morin, I., Hupbach, A., Tu, M. T., Buss, C., Walker, D., et al. (2006). Beyond the stress concept: Allostatic load: A developmental biological and cognitive perspective. In D. Cicchetti & D. J. Cohen (Eds.), Developmental psychopathology: Vol. 2. Developmental neuroscience (2nd ed., pp. 578–628). Hoboken, NJ: Wiley.

McEwen, B., Eiland, L., Hunter, R. G., & Miller, M. M. (2012). Stress and anxiety: Structural plasticity and epigenetic regulation as a consequence of stress. *Neuropharmacology, 62,* 3–12. doi:10.1016/j.neuropharm.2011.07.014.

O'Hara, M. W., & Swain, A. M. (1996). Rates and risk of postpartum depression—a meta-analysis. *International Review of Psychiatry, 8*(1), 37–54.

Paulson, J. F., & Bazemore, S. D. (2010). Prenatal and postpartum depression in fathers and its association with maternal depression: A meta-analysis. *JAMA, 303*(19), 1961–1969.

Pigliucci, M. (2007). Do we need an extended evolutionary synthesis? *Evolution, 61*(12), 2743–2749. doi:http://dx.doi.org/10.1111/j.1558-5646.2007.00246.x

Porges, S. W. (2011). *The polyvagal theory: Neurophysiological foundations of emotions, attachment, communication, and self-regulation.* New York, NY: WW Norton & Company.

Radley, J., Morilak, D., Viau, V., & Campeau, S. (2015). Chronic stress and brain plasticity: Mechanisms underlying adaptive and maladaptive changes and implications for stress-related CNS disorders. *Neuroscience and Biobehavioral Reviews, 58,* 79–91. doi:10.1016/j.neubiorev.2015.06.018.

Shapiro, T., Meschede, T., & Osoro, S. (2013). The roots of the widening racial wealth gap: Explaining the Black-White economic divide. *Institute on Assets and Social Policy Research and Policy Briefs, February 2014.* Waltham, MA: Brandeis University.

Taylor, S. E. (2006). Tend and befriend biobehavioral bases of affiliation under stress. *Current Directions in Psychological Science, 15*(6), 273–277.

Thayer, J. F., & Lane, R. D. (2009). Claude Bernard and the heart–brain connection: Further elaboration of a model of neurovisceral integration. *Neuroscience and Biobehavioral Reviews, 33*(2), 81–88. doi.org/10.1016/j.neubiorev.2008.08.004

Part I
Common Sources of Parenting Stress

Chapter 2
Ethnic Variation in Poverty and Parenting Stress

Rochelle C. Cassells and Gary W. Evans

Introduction

> Poverty, misery or want is a phantom with a thousand faces that vents its fury primarily among the majority of people who live in what is referred to as the Third World and among the pockets of poor people living on the fringes of the large industrialized cities… (Santiago Barquín, 2001, p. 127)

Given poverty rates in the USA, and that 33% of the nation's poor are children (Jiang, Ekono, & Skinner, 2015), poor families are hardly on the fringes. Santiago Barquín's words speak to the indiscriminate nature of poverty—it does not differentiate between color or creed when venting its fury. Living in poverty affects not only the individual, but also every domain associated with the individual's life. An important question that has received limited research attention is how poverty affects parenting stress. We extend this question by including racial and ethnic minority groups who are disproportionately affected by poverty in the USA. Together, our chapter focuses on poverty and parenting stress in families from varied racial and ethnic backgrounds. Our discussion begins with a review of the Family Stress Model (FSM) of economic disadvantage, which is the main framework used for understanding the relationship between poverty and parenting behaviors. The bulk of the chapter is situated in the poverty and parenting literature, paying special attention to factors salient to racial and ethnic families, such as the

R.C. Cassells (✉) · G.W. Evans
Department of Human Development, Cornell University, Ithaca, NY, USA
e-mail: rcc264@cornell.edu

G.W. Evans
Department of Design and Environment Analysis, Cornell University, Ithaca, NY, USA
e-mail: gwe1@cornell.edu

K. Deater-Deckard and R. Panneton (eds.), *Parental Stress and Early Child Development*, DOI 10.1007/978-3-319-55376-4_2

neighborhood environment. We also broaden our discussion to include families that sustain livelihoods across borders, and highlight the economic pressures that traverse national lines to exert themselves upon migrant parents. In doing so, a neglected group is incorporated into the literature on parenting stress.

The Family Stress Model (FSM)

The FSM (Conger & Conger, 2008; Conger & Donnellan, 2007) guides research on the relationship between poverty and parenting. The basic tenets of the FSM are covered adeptly in several review articles (Conger & Conger, 2008; Conger & Donnellan 2007; Conger, Conger, & Martin, 2011; McLoyd, Mistry, & Hardaway, 2014) and so will only be described briefly here. The FSM suggests that economic hardship creates economic pressure, or stress, which alters parenting behaviors. Economic hardship consists of such factors as low family income, high debt to asset ratio, and adverse financial events. These economic conditions change parents' financial resources and ability to maintain their households. The result is an increase in parents' psychological distress that is positively associated with family conflict and harsh, insensitive parenting practices. Although parenting stress is not explicitly stated in the FSM, parenting stress is clearly implicated in the process. Consider for a moment the financial resources needed to manage a household. On the one hand, adequate financial resources provide parents with the ability to care for their children, whereas lack of, or limited, financial resources creates economic pressure that stresses parents.

The United States Federal Poverty Threshold guideline for a family of four in 2015 was $24,250 (Burwell, 2015). Families with annual incomes less than 100% of the poverty guideline (i.e., less than $24,250) are considered poor. Families with annual incomes between 100 and 200% of the poverty line (i.e., between $24,250 and approximately $48,258) are vulnerable to difficulties associated with economic strain and are often considered "near poor" (Huston & Bentley, 2010). The percentage of children in poverty doubles when the inclusion criterion is extended to include near-poor families. In 2013, 15.8 million (22%) children lived in poverty and 31.8 million (44%) lived in low-income households (Jiang et al., 2015). Parenting stress occurs when parenting demands are greater than the resources available to contend with them (Deater-Deckard, 2004). The imbalance between parenting demands and available resources may arouse feelings of insecurity for parents and challenge their identity as successful parents. The bidirectional relation between parenting stress and parental efficacy, and specifically the evidence linking parenting stress to lower parental self-efficacy, is explored by Crnic & Ross in Chap. 11 of this volume. However, the context of poverty produces its own parenting stress that challenges parental self-efficacy.

Poverty is a powerful driver of parenting stress because it widens the demand–resource gap by diminishing the pool of financial resources while the demands remain relatively stable, that is to say they do not diminish accordingly. Having to prioritize rent over medical insurance, or not having money for children's school trips, may build feelings of worthlessness. Mistry, Lowe, Benner, and Chien (2008) showed that parents are not only stressed by their inability to meet basic needs, but also stressed by their shortcomings in providing additional or "extra" needs (e.g., holiday presents). The authors elucidate a critical psychological difference between "making ends meet and meeting expectations," suggesting parents appraise successful parenting in ways that transcend the focus on providing basic resources.

Poverty rates vary significantly across racial and ethnic groups with some groups facing greater disadvantage than others. In the USA, 65% of Black children and 63% of Hispanic children live in low-income households, while only 31% of White and Asian children are from low-income households, (Jiang et al., 2015). Given the variation in poverty levels across racial and ethnic families, it is important to know whether poverty is expressed similarly across racial and ethnic groups, or whether there are differences among them that create distinctions in parenting outcomes.

The strength of the FSM lies in its ability to position economic strain in such a way that, conceivably, even families above the poverty line may experience economic strain. Yet, it clearly demonstrates the susceptibility of poor parents to economic pressure, or, for our purposes, parenting stress. There is also variation in parenting and child outcomes within low-income families. The FSM provides a parsimonious explanation for this heterogeneity by highlighting potential stress-buffering resources that may help some low-income families circumvent the deleterious effects of poverty.

What must also be noted is that throughout this chapter we review studies that show the effect of poverty on parenting behavior and parenting stress. Recall that parenting behaviors are part of the FSM, while parenting stress is only implicated. Economic resources impact parenting behaviors, and parenting stress is affected by parenting behavior (Abidin, 1992). Therefore, although they are separate constructs, parenting stress and parenting behaviors are indeed related; a greater number of parental stressors challenge parenting behavior (see Crnic & Ross, Chap. 11).

Extending the Family Stress Model

The FSM was developed in the context of poor, rural, White families (Conger & Donnellan, 2007). More needs to be known about the appropriateness of the model for other racial and ethnic groups. Recent scholarship has moved toward this end. Some have found success with European American, African American, and Spanish-speaking Hispanic parents, but not with Asian or English-speaking Hispanic parents (Iruka, LaForett, & Odom, 2012). Others have demonstrated the model's international applicability with a sample of Finnish parents (Solantaus, Leinonen, & Punamäki, 2004), parents from Hong Kong (Lam, 2011), and Chinese parents (Sun, Li, Zhang, Bao, & Wang, 2015). The model has been successfully replicated with African American parents from rural towns and small cities (Conger et al., 2002). The only noteworthy discrepancy relevant here is that depressive mood, which was higher in the African American population of parents, did not directly lead to low-nurturing or uninvolved parenting as was the case for European American parents.

Even though aspects of FSM were generally replicated among Mexican American parents, some important deviations were found (Parke et al., 2004). In Parke et al.'s sample, income was a weaker predictor of economic pressure for Mexican parents compared to European American parents, and Mexican American children were more greatly impacted by parental conflict than European American children. Another study was able to replicate the model in a sample of Chinese parents (Benner & Kim, 2010), but there were considerable differences between foreign-born and native parents, and between mothers and fathers. Foreign-born Chinese mothers reported greater economic pressure and higher depressive symptoms than their native counterparts. In the context of economic pressures, Chinese fathers were warmer and more nurturing, whereas mothers were more hostile and utilized coercive parenting practices.

Importantly, such findings highlight the role of culture in altering the FSM's theoretical constructs. Extending scholarship on poverty and parenting stress to racial and ethnic minority groups will be beneficial because previously overlooked factors in the relationship between poverty and family stress may be illuminated. For example, how are the mechanisms different in multi-caregiver or multi-generational households? A recent study by Landers-Potts et al. (2015) represents an effort to fulfill this gap. They examined the FSM in an African American sample with primary and secondary caregivers. Previous replications of the FSM with African American parents consisted of caregivers who were mostly romantically involved (Conger et al., 2002), which ignores the diversity in parenting arrangements that can vary greatly, especially when we begin to consider ethnic variability cross culturally, both domestically and internationally. Landers-Potts et al. (2015) showed that the impact of economic pressure on parenting behavior was stronger when caregiver conflict was high. When caregiver conflict was low, the effect was not significant. Such findings highlight the influence of family conflict and demonstrate that family conflict extends beyond typical inter-partner accounts. The authors also found that the effects of economic pressure were sustained over time. What would further advance these findings is information on whether the interaction changes across caregiver types (e.g., romantic partners versus extended kin) and also whether cultural background moderates such variability in parenting arrangements on children.

Another extension of the FSM is the repositioning of children. As it stands, children are given passive treatment within the FSM; they are acted on rather than actors themselves. However, in some families, particularly racial and ethnic minority families, children serve as secondary caregivers, and some even contribute to family income (Falicov, 2001; Orellana, 2001; Song, 1997). Pooling labor and resources are key household economic strategies for immigrant families. Moreover, considering multi-generational immigrant households, the second generation and beyond often act as bridges between first-generation immigrants and their adopted community.

Orellana (2001) showed that Hispanic immigrant children see themselves as caretakers for younger siblings and helpers around the house. When parents have to work longer hours, children take on additional responsibilities that not only affect their own outcomes, but also change their role in the family. Additionally, in her seminal study with Chinese owners of takeaway businesses in Britain, Song (1997) showed that children provide considerable help to the family business. In these families, there is an understanding that family members should help out as part of the "family work contract," which incites a desire and obligation to help among children. Another duty children perform is serving as language mediators for parents who are not proficient in English. This requires that children are heavily involved in business meetings and assist parents with day-to-day activities, which can foster dependence between parents and children. These kinds of familial arrangements position children, who may experience difficulties navigating their roles, at the center of family dynamics. Together, these studies show a need for children's role in the family to be reconceptualized.

Moving beyond a passive role for children would lead to their inclusion in family conflict and their relation to parenting stress (see also Finegood & Blair, Chap. 8). One noteworthy study incorporated adolescent evaluations of family economic circumstances into the FSM (Delgado, Killoren, & Updegraff, 2013). In a sample of Mexican American families, mother and father ratings of economic hardship significantly predicted adolescents' ratings of the same two years later. Adolescents' perceived economic hardship was negatively associated with parental warmth and positively associated with parental conflict. These findings illustrate that children are keenly aware of their family's economic situation. However, one shortcoming of this innovative study is that adolescents' perception of family's economic situation and parental warmth was related only to their own adjustment, and not to the model's other constituent parts. A worthwhile line of inquiry concerns the relation between children's knowledge of economic hardship and parenting stress.

These articles represent initial efforts to utilize more diverse samples in studies with the FSM and also embody an attempt to extend the FSM in ways that are more culturally appropriate for the diversity of family configurations. More work is needed on culturally specific factors that may alter the relationship between poverty and family stress. In the forthcoming section, we review the extant literature on poverty and parenting with specific attention given to studies with diverse samples in order to tease apart some of these factors.

Parenting in the Context of Poverty Across Racial and Ethnic Families

Race and ethnicity are predictors of income status, particularly for African American and Hispanic families (Gershoff, Aber, Raver, & Lennon, 2007). Research shows that Caucasian mothers fare better economically than other racial and ethnic groups; they have twice the income, are more likely to be homeowners and credit cardholders, and possess other financial assets (Nam, Wikoff, & Sherraden, 2013). Even though Caucasian mothers tend to achieve higher levels of education, African American mothers have the same, or higher, rates of employment. On the other hand, Hispanic mothers are least likely to be employed and achieve the least amount of education (Gershoff et al., 2007; Raver, Gershoff, & Aber, 2007). Based on these differences, how do minority groups compare to their White counterparts in regard to poverty and parenting stress?

One study found that although economic resources contribute to differences in parenting stress between White, Black, and Hispanic mothers, noneconomic factors were also a significant source of variance. For example, much of the 41% difference in parenting stress between Caucasian and African American mothers owes to high depression scores among Black mothers. If depression scores were equivalent, the difference in parenting stress would decrease by 19%. Similarly, nativity status accounted for a significant portion of the 63% difference in parenting stress between Hispanic and Caucasian mothers. If the number of native born among Hispanics were the same as Whites, then 30% of the difference in parenting stress would disappear (Nam et al., 2013).

In a diverse sample, researchers found that economic hardship, such as difficulty in paying bills and cutbacks in material spending, was significantly associated with parenting stress for mothers and fathers (Williams, Cheadle, & Goosby, 2015). Another study examined several models that linked family income and material hardship to child cognitive skills and socio-emotional competence through parent investment, stress, and behavior (Raver et al., 2007). Best-fitting models for three racial groups were compared, with high similarity found. For White, Black, and Hispanic families, higher family income corresponded to greater parental investment and less material hardship. Material hardship is characterized by food insecurity, inadequate medical care, residential instability, and financial problems. For each group, material hardship predicted elevated parent stress and lower parent investment.

Nonetheless, there were some notable differences among the three groups. First, higher material hardship was more strongly associated with higher parenting stress for Black families. Second, high parent stress was more strongly related to cold parenting for Black and Hispanic parents. Additionally, there were model-specific pathway differences. For example, family income was associated with parent stress only for White parents and was positively associated with positive parenting behaviors only for Black families. Material hardship was positively related to positive parenting behaviors for Black parents, negatively related to positive parenting behaviors for White parents, and had no impact on the parenting behaviors of Hispanic parents. Hispanic families showed some divergence from their Black and White counterparts. That neither family income nor material hardship impacted positive parenting behaviors for Hispanic parents suggests that economic factors may not always impact parenting behaviors for these families. Further research is necessary to unpack why this may be the case.

On the other hand, socioeconomic variables do impact parenting stress among Hispanic families. One recent study teased apart the structural and cultural factors contributing to parenting stress among US-born and foreign-born mothers of various ethnic origins (Nomaguchi & House, 2013; see also Nomaguchi & Milkie, Chap. 3). When controlling for structural characteristics (income, employment, and education) among foreign-born Hispanic mothers, structural factors accounted for nearly 100% of their maternal parenting stress; income and English language proficiency emerged as chief sources of maternal parenting stress. Parenting stress decreased by 32.6% for US-born Black mothers after structural factors were taken into account; single mother status and income were the most significant factors affecting maternal parenting stress for this group. Maternal parenting stress among foreign-born Asian mothers decreased by 24.1% when accounting for structural factors. Similar to foreign-born Hispanic mothers, income and English were significant determinants.

From these findings, there appears to be heterogeneity among the specific factors contributing to parenting stress for each racial and ethnic group. For example, Hispanic parents are affected more by structural economic factors than White and Black parents. For Black families, a number of noneconomic factors (like depression) affect parenting stress, and these factors are the missing mechanisms interceding between economic hardship and parenting stress. In the following section, we concentrate on specific dimensions of poverty to further assess differences in parenting stress across racial–ethnic groups.

Dimensions of Poverty and Parental Stress

When we talk about poverty, it is tempting to think only in terms of income levels. An additional value of the FSM is that it articulates the various kinds of economic hardships that influence parenting—not only income levels (Conger & Conger, 2008; Conger & Donnellan, 2007; Conger et al., 2011). In fact, low-income status is not always sufficient in creating parenting stress. In some cases, income has little to no effect on parenting stress (Gershoff et al., 2007; Gonzales et al., 2011; Nam et al., 2013; Zhang, Eamon, & Zhan, 2015). For instance, Gershoff et al. (2007) found that income captured only 3% of the variance in parenting stress, whereas 35% was accounted for by material hardship.

One reason for this difference in explanatory power is the argument that economic pressure carries a psychological dimension that absolute income level does not necessarily capture. That is, it may be the perception of economic hardship as well as feelings of relative deprivation or social comparison that drives the relationship between poverty and parenting stress. For example, in a sample of mostly African American and Hispanic mother from inner-city Milwaukee, Mistry and Lowe (2006) found that these mothers ascribed different meanings to their economic challenges according to the type of expenditure. A different psychological interpretation and emotional response was associated with balancing household accounts, spending on children, and large purchases. Keeping up with bill payments was associated with neutral feelings of satisfaction, spending on children created positive feelings, and purchasing expensive items was a source of pride.

In a recent study, Puff and Renk (2014) explored different aspects of economic disadvantage and assessed their relation to parenting stress and behaviors. Economic disadvantage included variables such as financial cutbacks, financial concerns, negative economic events, constraints on making ends meet, and constraints on satisfying material needs. With the exception of constraints on making ends meet, all factors were significantly related to parenting stress for both low- and middle-income families. This harkens back to the earlier distinction between "basic" and "extra" provisions, suggesting that making ends meet may not relate to parenting stress because it is not part of the framework for successful parenting.

Both these studies represent initial steps to capture the diversity of economic factors at play in the lives of poor parents. However, additional work would further advance our knowledge. In the first study, Mistry and Lowe (2006) did not explore whether psychological interpretations and emotional responses to household finances had racial or ethnic differences. The value of doing so would be to shed some light on how money is viewed and used across various racial and ethnic minority families. In the second study, although the sample was diverse, the majority of the participants were Caucasian, and analyses on racial or ethnic differences were not conducted (Punk & Renk, 2014). A replication that extends this work by addressing racial and ethnic differences would be useful. The potential linkages between cultural values and the salience of social comparisons, or perceived social status, may also warrant further scrutiny. The relevance of immigrant generational status can be readily imagined in this context as well. For instance, the second generation may rapidly "buy in" and acculturate to the excesses of American materialism in ways that the first generation may not, resulting in greater economic pressure among this group.

Given the results summarized thus far, it seems clear that differences in parenting stress among racial and ethnic groups will be better understood by parsing poverty-related variables. Assets, for example, are a useful way to think about economic hardship. In one study, more assets were associated with higher income, less financial demands, and less economic stressors over time (Rothwell & Han, 2010). Assets are considered more stable than income because they help to stem economic problems in times of financial crisis. Wealth can help families weather economic shocks such as job loss, rent increase, and unintended or needed expenses. Wealth may also buffer constant vigilance and worry about ongoing financial obligations and may augment feelings of control. Thus, wealth moderates, to some extent, the parenting stress uncovered when economic fortunes change. Many middle-income families have resources to mitigate economic shocks (e.g., an occasional checking account overdraft, job loss, and divorce)—an option not viable to the poor.

Homeownership and education are common types of financial assets. Research shows that low-income, African American ethnicity, and women are less likely to own their homes (Grinstein-Weiss et al., 2010; Manturuk, Riley, & Ratcliffe, 2012; Nam et al., 2013). Thus, low-income African American mothers would be expected to have increased risk for high levels of parenting stress. Manturuk et al. (2012)

compared general stress, financial stress, and financial satisfaction between homeowners and renters. They asked whether owning a home in 2008 (before the economic recession) would heighten or reduce the effect of the recession on the aforementioned dimensions. Their findings showed that although both homeowners and renters have similar financial stress, homeowners had less psychological stress and reported higher levels of financial satisfaction. Even though identifying as Black was significantly and negatively associated with homeownership, there was no such association for identifying as Hispanic.

Interesting findings were found for the impact of education on parenting stress (Cardoso, Padilla, & Sampson, 2010). White mothers with high school and some college education had significantly lower parenting stress than White mothers with less than high school education. Yet, there was no significant difference in parenting stress between White mothers with less than high school education and those with college degrees. On the other hand, Black mothers with high school and college education had lower parenting stress than Black mothers with less than high school education. No difference in parenting stress between Black mothers with some college and those with less than high school education was observed. Unlike Black and White mothers, education had no impact on parenting stress for Mexican American mothers.

Conducting more studies that discern specific economic sources of parenting stress for various ethnic groups would advance our understanding of the relationship between poverty and parenting stress and add a more nuanced portrait of this relation. In the next section, we begin that effort by highlighting three variables that seem to occupy an important place in the lives of parents from diverse, minority backgrounds.

Three Mediators in the Relationship Between Poverty and Parental Stress

Family Structure

Change in family structure is common among low-income, ethnic minority groups and is a source of parenting stress. Convention holds that resources after a family transition, like divorce, will greatly impact parenting stress. However, Cooper, McLanahan, Meadows, and Brooks-Gunn (2009) found that post-transition income had little impact on parenting stress in all racial and ethnic groups studied. Rather, mother's post-transition social resources, in particular her relationship with her child's father, reduced the effect of family structure change on parenting stress. Another study with poor and low-income black families found that father's presence reduced parenting stress for mothers (Jackson, Preston, & Thomas, 2013). Father's presence was measured by mother's satisfaction with amount of love, time, and money the father contributed to the child. Knowing which of these factors has the greatest influence on mother's parenting stress would improve our understanding of the importance of father involvement.

Nevertheless, what we see from these studies is a diminutive treatment of fathers in the literature on parenting stress. Fathers are typically included in relation to martial or relationship distress, but it is important to know how fathers respond to economic hardship and what impact it has on their parenting stress—aspects of the experience that are rarely investigated. Among the few studies to examine fathers, economic hardship was only related to lower parental warmth for Mexican fathers, whereas economic hardship was related to lower parental warmth and greater parental harshness for Mexican mothers (Gonzales et al., 2011). In another study with Mexican mothers and fathers, income was negatively associated with mother's warmth, but had no relation to father's warmth (Delgado et al., 2013). Similarly, mothers' perception of economic hardship was positively related to conflict between parents and adolescents, while no association was found between for fathers. Moreover, consistent with what we would predict from the FSM, economic hardship predicted father parenting through quality of mother–father relationship in a sample of poor, single, Black mothers (Choi & Jackson, 2012).

Mothers and fathers do not necessarily respond similarly to economic disadvantage; that is, the effect of low economic resources impacts fathers' parenting stress in ways different from mothers' parenting stress. Given the salience of family dynamics to economic hardship, more studies on mothers' and fathers' response to economic hardship would inform thinking on their unique and combined influence on parenting stress. One can also imagine that the implications of inadequate provision of economic security for families differ between men and women and likely carry considerable cultural variability. Such heterogeneity may intersect powerfully with the FSM and parenting stress.

Before concluding the discussion on family structure, a final consideration must be given to non-parental caregivers and their influence on parenting stress. Extended household structures have historically been shown to be a form of income supplementation strategy for Black and Hispanic families (Angel & Tienda, 1982). Little is known about whether these living arrangements actually buffer against parenting stress, or whether they create further burdens. One study has looked at mother and grandmother parenting in low-income households and the effect of multiple caregivers on parenting behaviors, but Barnett (2008) did not examine whether income had a direct effect on each caregiver's parenting behavior, or whether income indirectly affected each caregivers' parenting behavior though their relationship quality.

Two studies have made some strides in this regard and found that young, African American mothers have greater caregiving stress when co-parenting with grandmothers than when co-parenting with the child's biological father (Arnold, Lewis, Maximovich, Ickovics, & Kershaw, 2011; Jackson, 1998). Although other racial and ethnic groups were present in the sample in Arnold et al., the majority were African American. The authors entered socioeconomic factors and ethnicity as demographics, but did not relate to outcomes. It would be helpful to know whether the increase in parenting stress when co-parenting with grandmothers holds true for other low-income ethnic families.

Depression

Depression is a key element in the cascade of factors leading from economic pressure to negative parenting behaviors. Financial difficulties and negative life events led to higher levels of depression and the use of more negative and fewer positive parenting practices for Black, White, and Hispanic parents (Lyons, Henly, & Schuerman, 2005). For Chinese parents, depression was negatively associated with nurturing parenting and positively associated with hostile parenting for Chinese mothers. Depression also increased parental conflict, which in turn negatively impacted parenting behavior for both mothers and fathers (Benner & Kim, 2010).

In the case of African American mothers, the research on economic pressure, depressive symptoms, and parenting stress has been well documented (Jackson, 1998). In fact, in their replication of the FSM with African American parents, Conger et al. (2002) found that 19–22% of the variance in depressed mood could be attributed to economic pressure. However, the findings are mixed for Hispanic families. In another study with Latino mothers (including families of Mexican American, Puerto Rican, and South American descent), chronic poverty did predict maternal depression (Pachter, Auinger, Palmer, & Weitzman, 2006). On the other hand, Mexican mothers were least likely to be depressed when compared to Black and White mothers (Cardoso et al., 2010), and depression was only a mediator between income and child outcomes for English-speaking Hispanics, but not Spanish-speaking Hispanics (Iruka et al., 2012). These inconsistent findings among Hispanic parents may be better understood if future studies did not lump the various Hispanic cultural groups together. More clarity may also be brought to the subject if the interplay of gender, poverty, and ethnicity is further examined, especially given the traditional gender roles often found in Hispanic culture.

Neighborhoods

Although the FSM captures the effect of economic hardships on parenting, it neglects the neighborhood environment as an important context for understanding poverty and parenting. Since the 1970s, the USA has seen a steady increase in neighborhood segregation as a result of mounting income inequality (Massey, 1996; Putnam, 2015). The legacy of institutional discrimination in the housing market compounds the problem such that neighborhoods are stratified not only by wealth or poverty, but also by race. Poor neighborhoods tend to have disproportional shares of African Americans and other minority groups, while more affluent neighborhoods are primarily White (Massey, 1996).

Families in low-income neighborhoods face greater physical and psychosocial environmental risks including inadequate infrastructure, pollution, and limited resources, in addition to greater violence and crime (Evans, 2004). The psychological security of a child depends on parental availability and warmth and the emotional response of poor parents may owe to stress brought on by neighborhood conditions. In another study, African American children whose parents used nurturing parenting practices were less likely to affiliate with deviant peers (Brody et al., 2001). However Garbarino, Bradshaw, and Kostelny (2005) argue that parents in poor neighborhoods employ hypervigilant parenting techniques in an effort to protect children from neighborhood danger. Similarly, Cruz-Santiago and Ramírez García (2011) found that Mexican immigrant parents utilized strict monitoring to ensure that their adolescent children did not succumb to neighborhood pressures like gang membership. Understood in this way, the utilization of authoritarian parenting may be reinterpreted as a means for low-income parents to safeguard children from neighborhood threats.

This is yet another aspect of cross-cultural and ethnic differences to consider when thinking about poverty's impact on parent–child relationship. What may appear to be similar parenting beliefs and practices may not convey equivalent meanings in every cultural context, and there is some evidence that the degree of concordance between parental control and warmth is different across racial and ethnic groups (Bornstein, 2012; Steinberg, 2001). For instance, Asian American, African American, and Latino adolescents reported their parents as using significantly more behavioral control in parenting than adolescents with European American parents. Asian American and African American parents were also reported as significantly less warm compared to European American parents (Chao & Kanatsu, 2008). Among African American parents, highly controlling and even rigid parenting are seen as more necessary for safety, and reflecting care and a sign of child investment (Tamis-LeMonda, Briggs, McClowry, & Snow, 2008). Similarly, traditional parenting styles do not accurately represent parenting among Latino families, and Latino parents have been shown to use "protective parenting" that shows high warmth and demandingness, but low autonomy granting (Rodríguez, Donovick, & Crowley, 2009).

The neighborhood context, like economic variables, can alter parenting behavior; therefore, there is a need for its inclusion in the FSM and other theoretical models examining poverty and parenting. Indeed, some studies have begun to incorporate the neighborhood in the FSM as a key distal factor that interacts with the family environment. A recent study with families from inner-city neighborhoods in Milwaukee found that neighborhood disorder (e.g., vandalism and abandoned buildings) and housing disorder (e.g., exposed electrical wires and animal infestations) predicted psychological distress among parents (Jocson & McLoyd, 2015). Neighborhood disorder and housing disorder also predicted harsh and inconsistent parenting and less parental warmth through psychological distress. The study sample was predominantly African American single mothers who received some governmental assistance.

An earlier study with only African American families from inner-city Philadelphia found that income-to-needs ratio predicted financial strain and neighborhood stress, which then affected parent–child relations through parent psychological distress (Gutman, McLoyd, & Tokoyawa, 2005). As income declines, parents reported greater neighborhood stress and higher financial strain, inducing higher psychological stress. A higher level of psychological distress then decreased the amount of positive activities and relations between parents and adolescents and increased conflict.

A longitudinal study examined the relationship between perception of environmental stress and parenting behaviors in a sample of poor African American single mothers from inner-city New Orleans (Kotchick, Dorsey, & Heller, 2005). Perceptions of environmental stressors included gang presence, homicides, and unsanitary living conditions. Findings showed a significant indirect path of neighborhood stress to parenting behaviors through psychological distress. Neighborhood stress and maternal psychological distress were measured at time one, and parenting behaviors were measured 15 months later at time two. This suggests an enduring effect of neighborhood stress on parent's psychological well-being and subsequent parenting behaviors.

There are mixed results for the impact of low-income neighborhood environment on parenting for Mexican mothers and fathers. Gonzales et al. (2011) found that neighborhood disadvantage did not predict warm or harsh parenting, but perception of neighborhood danger decreased warm parenting. The authors also found an interesting interaction between perceptions of neighborhood danger and neighborhood disadvantage on warm parenting. Neighborhood disadvantage and mothers' warm parenting were only related when neighborhood danger was perceived to be high; the same was found for fathers. Mexican parents may attempt to stem the effects of perceived threat with positive, rather than negative, parenting. In another study with only Mexican fathers, perception of neighborhood disadvantage was not related to parental warmth or harshness (White & Roosa, 2012). Likewise, chronic poverty adversely affects parenting behaviors through neighborhood quality only for Black and White parents; no such relationship was found for Latino parents (Pachter, Auinger, Palmer, & Weitzman, 2006).

In regard to parenting stress, two important papers have explored how neighborhood factors relate to parenting stress. In the first, Guterman, Lee, Taylor, and Rathouz (2009) found that neighborhood characteristics such as presence of drug dealers or users, gang activities, and trustworthiness of neighbors predicted parenting stress for White, African American, and Hispanic parents. Although a majority of the sample was African American, this finding suggests that there may be some uniformity in the effect of low-income neighborhood context on parenting stress. In fact, the authors tested for equivalence between models with race and ethnicity constrained and another where they varied; both models were nearly identical.

Using a diverse sample, Zhang et al. (2015) recently examined the association between neighborhood disorder (e.g., gang prevalence and drug activity) and maternal stress, and the mediating role of perceived neighborhood social capital.

Again, the sample contained predominantly African American mothers (62%). Higher education was associated with less maternal stress while material hardship was related to more maternal stress. Overall, the authors found that neighborhood disorder was significantly related to maternal stress, and neighborhood disorder decreased perceived social capital. Interpretation of the potential interaction between SES, race, and ethnicity on neighborhood disorder and parenting stress was not included as these variables were controlled for in their analyses.

Given what has already been noted above about the dynamic transaction among income status, race, and neighborhood characteristics, these studies show that neighborhoods are a context in which to examine parental stress and economic processes and are deserving of more scholarship. Neighborhood conditions negatively affect parenting behaviors for Black parents, while findings with Hispanic parents do not show this trend. However, neighborhood contexts were measured in a number of different ways (e.g., neighborhood disorder, neighborhood quality, and perceived neighborhood danger). It is unclear whether Hispanics are generally less affected by neighborhood disadvantage, or whether the mixed findings relate to heterogeneity in variable measurements.

In the next section, we tackle an altogether different context—the immigration context—to illustrate how immigration contributes to the diversity among parents living in poverty. We also explore the unique stressors faced by immigrant parents, many of which go unnoticed in the literature, but have serious consequences for parent and child outcomes.

Immigration as Illustration of Diversity in Relation to Poverty and Family Stress

A chapter on parental stress among racial and ethnic families cannot ignore immigrant families who add significantly to the diversity among minority families. As of 2013, 13% of the US population consisted of immigrants. When the second generation is included, that percentage increases to 25%. This means that immigrants represent a quarter of the overall US population (Zong & Batalova, 2015). Economic factors are well-known determinants of migration. Low-income families in developing countries utilize migration as a way to stabilize incomes and diversify familial risks and resources (Stark & Bloom 1985). This strategy gives rise to the preponderance of transnational families—those separated by geographic boundaries who maintain emotional and social bonds. There are many reasons to study parenting stress in transnational families, not the least of which is its covariation with poverty.

Poor economic conditions not only induce migration, but they also shape the type of migration undertaken (see Figs. 2.1 and 2.2). Whereas middle-income families can migrate as a unit, low-income family members often have to migrate serially (i.e., one at a time) (Baptiste, Hardy, & Lewis, 1997; Crawford-Brown &

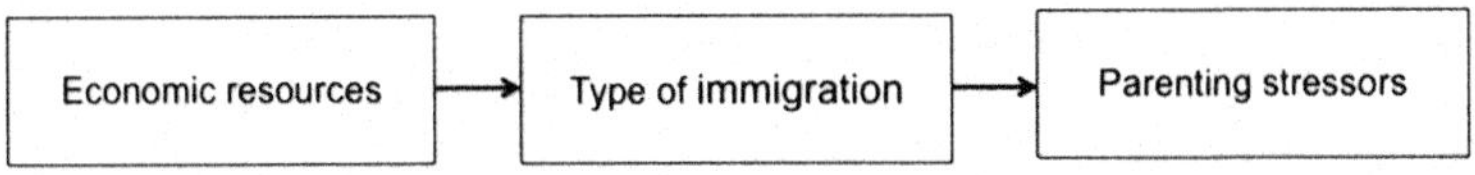

Fig. 2.1 Relations between economic resources and parenting stress

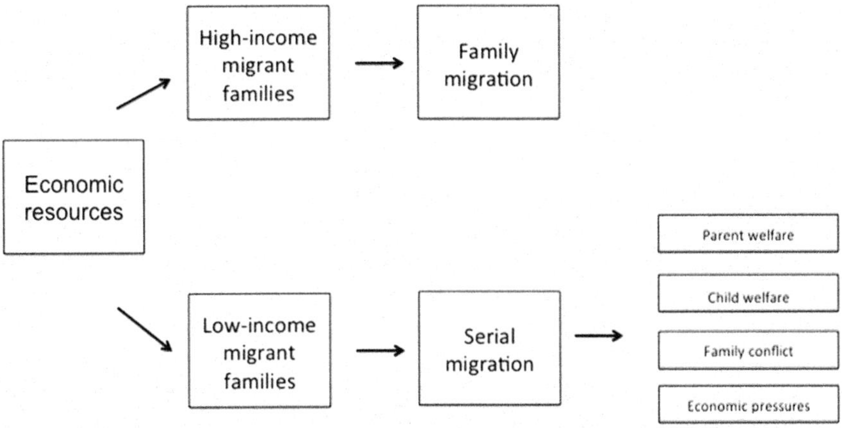

Fig. 2.2 Elaborated framework for understanding parenting stress in transnational families

Rattray, 2001). Given the global demand for female laborers, more females are initiating migration for their families (Ehrenreich & Hochschild, 2004; Benería, Berik, & Floro, 2016). When middle-class women began working outside the home, markets around the world began exporting women as nannies, domestic workers, and other kinds of care workers. This gave way to an increase in female migrants from countries such as Philippines (Arya & Roy, 2006), Jamaica (Crawford, 2003; Crawford-Brown & Rattray, 2001), and Mexico (Dreby & Stutz, 2012).

Figure 2.2 elaborates on Fig. 2.1 by specifying the types of immigration patterns and parenting stressors associated with serial migration. We draw inspiration from the FSM in order to construct a portrait of the stressors affecting immigrant parents including (1) economic pressures, (2) parent welfare (parent psychological distress in FSM), (3) child welfare, and (4) family conflict. The notable difference between our model and the model that inspires it is that children are ascribed power. They will not be fixed at an end point with unidirectional arrows pointing toward them. Likewise, though the elements in our model appear unidirectional, they are dynamic. For instance, there is a bidirectional relationship between parent and child welfare, which may lead to family conflict.

Another innovative component of our model is that we focus only on families that undertake serial migration. The reason for doing so is that, traditionally, immigrant families are discussed as one homogenous group. Differentiating between family migration and serial migration elucidates unique factors for each group and brings attention to the experiences of the latter, which often go unacknowledged. Often parents leave behind spouses and children in families that migrate serially. This means that they face tremendous economic and emotional burdens having to provide for themselves in the destination county, but also having to provide financial and emotional support to those left in the country of origin. As noted earlier, immigration also creates potentially critical inputs into the parent–child dynamic when viewed across generations. Not only are some immigrant children assisting the pioneer generation with acculturation while simultaneously navigating their own social and cultural transformations as new citizens, for some immigrant children, there are differences in how much of their childhood happened colocated with their parents both within households and across cultures and class.

To give each element there proper due would require a chapter unto itself, so we narrow the discussion to the stressors Southeast Asian, Caribbean, and Mexican transnational families. We touch only briefly on parent and child welfare. We chose to focus on mother–child relationships given the recent trend toward female migration. We then situate the majority of our discussion on economic-related stress factors, specifically the function of remittances and their relationship to family conflict. We will also briefly mention surrogate caretakers, who care for left-behind children when parents are abroad, the relationship between them and the migrant parent, and the family tensions that sometimes occur. We will also briefly allude to the role of culture within this complex ecology.

Parent and Child Welfare

Migrant mothers often contend with depression, loneliness, and grief (Best-Cummings, 2009; Kim, Agic, & McKenzie, 2014; Miranda, Siddique, Der-Martirosian, & Belin, 2005; Ornelas, Perreira, Beeber, & Maxwell, 2009). For Caribbean and Filipino mothers, their participation in the care industry often means they are responsible for other children while their own children remain in the home country. This can breed conflict in the parent–child relationship because some children feel jealous of the children in their mother's care (Parreñas, 2004), and mothers feel guilty for giving their love to these children (Hochschild, 2004).

For many Mexican and Central American families, significant parent psychological distress is brought on by the combined stress of separation from children and significant others, as well as their precarious legal status (Cervantes, Mejía, & Mena, 2010; Horton, 2009). At the same time, left-behind children in the Caribbean and Latin America face psychological distress and are vulnerable to abuse and engagement in risky behaviors (D'Emilo et al., 2007; Dillon & Walsh, 2015). Similar reports of psychological maladjustments are found with left-behind children in Southeast Asia (Graham & Jordan, 2011). Children of migrant parents feel pressure to make their parents' efforts worthwhile, sometimes to the detriment of their own well-being (Dreby & Stutz, 2012; Suârez-Orozco, Todorova, & Louie,

2002). Parents often cite their children as motivation for migration, and so many immigrant children feel a sense of obligation. They fulfill that obligation either through excelling academically or working to support the family (Fuligni, 2006). In families where separation has occurred, there may even be an extra layer of pressure because the stakes were even higher.

Together, we see that migrant mothers and their children experience psychological distress borne from life in a transitional family. Some migrant mothers also face additional psychological distress through marital conflict. When women are the ones to migrate, left-behind husbands sometimes feel threatened in their roles as providers, which can vary according to culture and whether gender roles dictate that males as breadwinners. For example, Sri Lankan custom is for women to be homemakers, while men are providers for their family (Kottegoda, 2006). When women migrate, their motives are questioned and they can sometimes be shamed and scrutinized for leaving (Gamburd, 2004). Family problems fall on the shoulders of migrant mothers as their absence receives the blame. Therefore, married migrant mothers in transnational families may be at an elevated risk for psychological distress.

Economic Pressures

Money and migration are inextricably intertwined. Economic motivations are chief reasons for migration, and financial resources are needed to pursue the journey (Massey et al., 1993). As illustrated by Fig. 2.2, low-income migrants cannot make the journey as a unit, and so remittances become "the currency of care and one of the ways in which migrants maintain their sense of belonging to the transnational family… The need for display is greater when the family is separated across borders," (Cabraal & Singh, 2013. p. 56). For the migrant parents, and specifically migrant mothers, money, gifts, and other material goods are utilized to express love and are symbolic of the promise of a better life (Crawford, 2003; Crawford-Brown & Rattray, 2001; Crawford-Brown 1999; Dreby, 2010; Gamburd, 2008; Parreñas, 2001, 2005).

Remittances are contentious for transnational families when mothers are the ones abroad. Mothers are judged more critically for their migration because their prescribed gender role is to provide emotional intimacy, not financial support (Dreby, 2006). For example, the social norm in Vietnam is for husbands to be more economically successful than their wives. Interviews with left-behind husbands in Northern Vietnam reveal that these husbands do not receive remittances from their wives, but instead work extra hours or borrow money from social networks to maintain their households (Hoang & Yeoh, 2011). The authors write that these fathers are willing to endure significant economic hardship to maintain their status as breadwinners.

While left-behind Vietnamese fathers are stressed by economic challenges due to their refusal to accept remittances from their migrant wives, the case is quite different in Sri Lanka. There, marital stress stems from the associations among migration, poverty, and male unemployment (Gamburd, 2004, 2008). In some cases, husbands use remittances on alcohol consumption instead of allocating it toward debt payment and food. This can undermine the goals of migration often by delaying economic prosperity if not exacerbating poverty (Thai, 2014). What we see then is that parent stress may operate through family conflict in transnational households that are governed by traditional gender roles. In some cases, the family economic situation does not change because husbands and wives are at odds as to who is responsible for sustaining the household.

The gender norms found in the Asian context are also seen in Mexican families as they struggle with issues of power and gender roles within the family (Dreby & Adkins, 2012; Dreby, 2006). However, in the Caribbean, many of the gender dynamics discussed do not pertain. Caribbean mothers experience support for their migration (Best-Cummings, 2009). In Jamaica, a small island nation that boasts among the highest emigration rates to OECD countries (UN Population Divison, 2013), women have long-experienced independence and economic freedom (Bauer & Thompson, 2004). Bauer and Thompson (2004) found that Jamaican women are often the main initiators of migration, and the gender divide in migration seen elsewhere is not evident in this society and likely not in other Caribbean countries either.

The "money tree syndrome" is another determinant of economic pressure and family conflict. The money tree syndrome refers to the perception held by family members in the home country that money is easily acquired abroad, even though the reality is much different (Cabraal & Singh, 2013). Family members thus place considerable economic pressure on migrant family members. When Vietnamese migrants do not meet their families' financial expectations, they are labeled as selfish or not a true "Viet Kieu" (overseas Vietnamese) (Thai, 2014).

In the Caribbean, the expectation is to provide remittances, but the sign of "making the most of the sacrifice" is when migrants are able to successfully return with substantial funds to purchase property and live out a more relaxed lifestyle (Olwig, 2012). Almost all migrants share the remittance burden in some form (Guarnizo, 2003), but migrant parents are in a worser position because their credibility as parents is contingent on their economic commitment; to not remit would be synonymous with "bad" parenting (Castaneda & Buck, 2011). When mothers do not send money home frequently, children question the extent of their love and sacrifice (Glasgow & Gouse-Sheese, 1995; Parreñas, 2001).

The problem with the money tree syndrome mentality is that it does not accurately reflect the economic conditions of many migrants. Job instability and unemployment are common among low-skilled immigrants. Many Filipino and Caribbean mothers work as nannies in New York City, a job with considerable inequities (Cheever, 2004). First, the nanny position is unstable due to children entering schools at earlier ages. Second, nannies work long hours, and many are underpaid for the services performed. For migrant parents, they endure significant economic hardship while attempting to reduce the length of separation between them and their left-behind children. Some live in overcrowded houses and work long hours in order to speed along reunification (Dreby, 2010). Caribbean mothers expressed disappointment and disillusionment when faced with the difficulty of supporting two households—their household in the destination country and their household in the home country—with low wages, and often, they had little money for themselves (Best-Cummings, 2009). Paradoxically, migrants are pressured to send money to demonstrate their love, yet family members in the home country ascribe lesser value to remittances because they are not perceived as commensurate to physical care (Singh, Robertson, & Cabraal, 2012). One can imagine that these dynamics likely vary with child age and mother's history in the origin country, as well as experience in the host country.

Family Conflict

Family separation as a result of immigration is a source of parent stress through family conflict. Conflict often occurs between separated parents and children, and between parents and caretakers. In regard to former, many left-behind children feel that the money borne from migration does not buy the emotional support needed from their parents. Research with Filipino transnational families finds that common arguments between children and their migrant mothers are about "money or family" (Parreñas, 2001). Left-behind children do not see material goods as a substitute for having the emotional support of their parents (Castaneda & Buck, 2011; Parreñas, 2004).

On the other hand, caregiving responsibilities are important considerations for parents when deciding to migrate, especially if they cannot take their children with them. When fathers migrate, the matter is relatively straightforward. However, the matter is somewhat more complicated when mothers migrate, or when both mothers and fathers migrate. In the Asian context, fathers tend to take on the child-rearing responsibilities when mothers are away (Arya & Roy, 2006). However, in Mexico and the Caribbean, both parents tend to migrate (Suárez-Orozco, Bang, & Kim, 2011). What this means is that the caregiving responsibilities are often given to other family members, most notably the maternal grandmother. In some cases, children are left with other kin. These caregiving situations are a source of stress and are more precarious in nature.

Dreby (2010) writes that grandparents offer more stable caregiving arrangements for Mexican left-behind children. When children are left with other kin, it is usually for a shorter time and parents experience greater pressure for financial contributions. In some cases, parents have to return home prematurely or take on exorbitant debt to bring their children to the USA when conflicts with these caregivers become unresolvable. Similar to the Mexican context, Caribbean mothers have to navigate relationships with caretakers of their children back at home. Although many report having good relationship with caretakers, this is likely due to their vulnerable position in the relationship and need to maintain harmony (Best-Cummings, 2009). If relations between parent and caretaker disintegrate, then reunification becomes necessary.

One may assume that reunification is always positive; however, this too is a complicated ordeal. Conflict may emerge at reunification when children's attachments to caregivers in home country put a strain on the parent–child relationship (Arnold, 2006, 2011; Santa-Maria & Cornille, 2007; Schapiro, Kools, Weiss, & Brindis, 2013). There is also the issue of new siblings or romantic partners who are unknown to the left-behind child. The change in family structure may be a source of sibling rivalry and family conflict (Best-Cummings, 2009; Dreby, 2010; Phoenix & Bauer, 2012). Studies that examine how these factors contribute to parenting stress for immigrant parents are required.

Summary

Fifty-five percent of children with immigrant parents live in low-income households (Jiang et al., 2015). In light of the discussion in the paragraphs above, we hope this figure is a call to arms for research on parenting stress and poverty among transnational families. The economic situation for many families in the developing world drives migration. This section has shown that migrant parents seek to provide a better life for their families, but encounter significant challenges due to separation from loved ones. These parents have to financially support two households, often not improving their economic condition.

The perception of a money tree in receiving countries creates much stress for the migrant person because they are pressured to send money or goods back home, often receiving little gratitude for their efforts and sacrifice. In light of the feminization of migration, questions related to gender roles within transnational families are raised, particularly regarding the ways husbands or domestic partners respond to changes in the family structure and cultural traditions concerning who is the household breadwinner. Some left-behind fathers and/or husbands struggle with expressions of masculinity when their households do not necessarily adhere to traditional patriarchal norms. Because mothers are seen as nurturer, and fathers as breadwinner, migrant women face a significant amount of pressure and stress. Nevertheless, gender roles impact transnational families with both breadwinner and nurturer roles exerting their own unique stress. In cultures where more traditional maternal care dynamics exists, the family experience may be greatly affected by these gender roles, but for cultures with high level of co-parenting, the effects may not be as great.

We touched very briefly on some of the economic-related stressors associated with parenting in the transnational context, but there is still more work to be done. A rudimentary first step would be to assess parenting stress among transnational parents and compare findings to other immigrant parents and also to the native stock. In our discussion, we showed the various ways money exerts influence in transnational families and its intersection with gendered notions of family. Another useful study would be one that compares parenting stress between migrant transnational mothers and fathers.

Conclusion

In regard to poverty and parenting, economic resources determine both the amount and kind of investments parents are able to make in order to support their children (Conger & Conger, 2008). Middle- and high-income parents are able to invest in resources that increase children's human capital, such as learning materials, educational toys, and tutoring. They are also able to afford foods high in nutrients and provide a safe home environment and medical care for children (Conger & Conger, 2008). On the other hand, low-income parents focus spending on immediate expenses related to basic needs. Much can be said about the impact of low economic resources on child outcomes, and in chapter eight of this volume, there is a rousing discussion on the impact of poverty on parent–child interactions and neurocognitive development (see Finegood & Blair, Chap. 8). Nevertheless, even though low-income parents are limited in how much they are able to provide for their children, the expectations they hold for themselves are more or less similar to their wealthier counterparts, and the desire is to provide similar experiences for their children (Hsueh, 2006; Mistry & Lowe, 2006).

We discussed family structure, depression, and the neighborhood context as factors related to poverty relevant for studies on parenting. In particular, the neighborhood context was shown to be important to the study of parenting stress, even though it is overlooked by the FSM. In light of the neighborhood findings reviewed above, one may assume that a solution would be for families to move out of low-income neighborhoods. Results from the Moving to Opportunity Program provide a more nuanced interpretation of who benefits from changing the neighbourhood environment, and provides greater clarity on some of the above mentioned findings. Chetty, Hendren, and Katz (2015) revealed that moving into a low poverty census tract did not improve economic outcomes for adults. However, children younger than age 13 whose families moved to less poor neighborhoods showed a 30.8% increase in individual earnings later in early adulthood. This suggests that after a certain point, the effects of long-term exposure to neighborhood disadvantage are difficult to moderate. Therefore, a better solution may be to improve the neighborhood conditions across America and in the meantime provide housing vouchers for families with children under the age of 13 years.

Moreover, we discussed the dimensions of poverty beyond income. One finding illustrates the power of non-income variables on parent behavior: taking a payday loan (an indicator of financial stress) reduced the odds of a parent reading to a child by 60% (Grinstein-Weiss et al., 2010). Other scholars offered novel ways of conceptualizing the relation between poverty and parenting. Mistry and Lowe (2006) suggest that poverty is not only the deprivation of needs, but also a deprivation of wants. Low-income parents express feelings of achievement when they are able to offer children more than just the necessary provisions such as food and clothing. When parents cannot afford to send their children on school trips or take them to the zoo, they become frustrated and disappointed. Therefore, subjective experience of poverty is an important topic for researchers to examine, especially in regard to parenting stress. Do parents who only provide basic needs show greater parenting stress, and are there interactions based on race and ethnicity? Further, how do conceptualizations of poverty affect this relationship? For example, do absolute or relative views of poverty dictate feelings of what should be provided? Do parents with more relative views of poverty experience greater parenting stress than those with absolute views, or vice versa? This is one direction research on poverty and parenting stress may seek to orient itself, especially given the sociocultural inputs that create and influence the subjective experience of poverty.

Furthermore, our review shows that there is important research yet to be done regarding poverty and parenting stress. Many of the published studies treat ethnicity and income as a covariates rather than examining their possible interactions. Future studies need to see this interaction as an important source of information regarding differences in the kinds of economic stressors faced by parents from racial and ethnic families. Furthermore, a major criticism of the current literature on poverty and parenting stress is the overall lack of studies with Asian families. The "model minority" myth may obscure research with poor Asian families because Asians are presumed to possess high levels of income and education. There is a tendency to treat Asians, and also Hispanics, as monolithic when there are considerable cultural and economic differences among such subgroups.

Takei and Sakamoto (2011) demonstrated that there is considerable heterogeneity in Asians in regard to their poverty levels. For example, some Asian subgroups such as Asian Indians, Japanese, and Filipinos are less likely to be poor than Whites. Others (Indonesians, Malaysians, and Thai) show no difference to Whites, while some (Bangladeshi, Cambodians, Chinese, Laotian, Korean, Vietnamese, Sri Lankan, Pakistani, Hmong, and Other Asian) are likely to be poorer. The highest poverty rates are found among Bangladeshi, Cambodians, and Hmong. Foreign-born Asian Americans have higher poverty rates than native-born Asian Americans. In fact, poverty rates are highest among the most recent arrivals, illustrating diversity among Asian families and dispelling illusions of widespread wealth.

Moreover, another form of lumping occurs when immigration, and more specifically the type of migration, is ignored. There are profound impacts on parenting depending on whether the family came as a unit or were separated during immigration. Power emerges as a critical source of conflict as family members negotiate their roles when the family structure changes, yet the social structures remain. For example, even as social changes lead to greater agency for women, in traditional cultures parenting roles remain constrained by gender roles. Additionally, left-behind children exert their influence on parents during separation, and parents and surrogate caregivers strive to maintain amicable relations in order to ensure the welfare of children left behind.

Although the FSM informs much of our thinking about the impact of poverty and economic pressure on parenting, there are some important criticisms to be noted. The first line of criticism is a methodological one. In many of the studies, greater explanatory power is found when using an index of financial strain. Given that the parent is the source of information for material hardship, family conflict, and psychological distress, issues of mono-method bias demand further exploration. For example, the parent may feel inadequate and report greater economic pressure. Or a parent may have high levels of neuroticism and therefore report more money worries. Future studies may want to include measures that rule out these possibilities and strengthen the internal validity.

A second line of criticism concerns the treatment of children as passive actors in the FSM. The model situates the child at the outcome. Economic stressors affect parents, and children are affected by their parents. Children are not considered active in the model. Our discussion of transnational families shows the influence children have on their parents. In our model, we allow children to be fluid; they are as much affected by their parents as they affect them. Sometimes, migrant parents with children left behind make decisions about returning home or bringing a child abroad based on the influence of the child (Dreby, 2010). This is not done without conflict or stress, but it speaks to the power of children in family dynamics.

In the FSM, children are done to rather than doers. The chapter encourages us to abandon such unidirectional conceptions. For many immigrant families, it is cost-effective to hire children as labor. This keeps money in the family and helps to stem some of the effects of financial hardship. However, family tensions are borne from such practices (Falicov, 2001). When we consider that the conflict may be between parents and children, and not only between adults, the FSM falls short in addressing bidirectional, dynamic effects between parental stress and child stress. We see that poverty affects all family members, and household strategies to combat poverty may contribute to different kinds of family conflict that are likely to impact parenting behavior.

A final criticism of the FSM relates to a point made by Parke et al. (2004) who hypothesized that the reason for the weaker association between income and economic pressure in a replication of the FSM with Mexican parents was due to their frame of reference. Research shows that immigrants do compare their economic situation to others, but to their compatriots back home and not to the native stock (Rogers, 2006). A dollar in the USA is worth more than a dollar back home. Therefore, even if immigrants have lower incomes compared to Americans, they may perceive themselves as doing quite well because their income levels are higher than those in their origin country. Therefore, for immigrant families in particular, income may not be the driver of parenting stress. Uncovering exactly what economic factors contribute most to the parenting stress for immigrant parents is needed. This is one direction research on poverty and parenting stress may seek to orient itself.

Before concluding our chapter, we want to bring attention to two overlooked factors in the literature that require future investigation for their relationship to parenting stress—suburban poverty and shift work. Regarding suburban poverty,

Kneebone and Berube (2013) address the fallacy of suburban wealth in their recent book "Confronting Suburban Poverty in America." They explain that the imagery conjured when poverty is discussed in the USA is one of inner-city slums. More still, discussions on the "intersection of poverty and place" mostly center on the rural–urban contrast, even though there has been a decline in the poor population in rural areas from 1970 to 2000 where suburban areas have been on a steady increase in the last few decades. Despite the fact that low-income residents have always been part of suburban development, the discussion fails to include this neighborhood type.

One reason for the neglect owes to the perception that poverty is not a feature of suburban areas. Suburbia invokes quintessential trappings of the American Dream. However, their findings show that, in fact, suburban areas are subject to significant poverty. Since the 1980s, the rate of growth in the amount of poor people living in suburban areas has been faster than in cities. For example, between 2000 and 2010, the percent change in the growth rate for suburban areas was approximately 53% compared to roughly 24% in cities (Kneebone & Berube, 2013). In 2010, 15 million people were poor and 22 million people were "near poor" in suburban areas. In other words, by 2010, one in four persons in a suburban area was poor.

Forty-seven percent of poor minorities live in the suburbs, and their rate of change is much greater than for poor Whites. In general, Blacks are least likely to live in suburbs (39%), yet 51% of all immigrants live in suburban areas, whereas only 33% live in cities (Kneebone & Berube, 2013). For Blacks and Hispanics, access to affordable housing induces a move to the suburbs, whereas high employment attracts Whites and Asians to suburban neighborhoods (Howell & Timberlake, 2014). A significant problem with living in a suburban area is transportation. Transportation system investments are low in these areas, and cars are a necessity. Poor families without cars are at a severe disadvantage. The perception that there is no poverty leads to lack of service provision, political response, and donations for poor suburban people (Kneebone & Berube, 2013).

There are many unknown questions regarding parenting stress for families from suburban areas since little work has been done in this regard. One question we would like to see answered is whether the perception of the suburbs as wealthy leads poor parents living in these areas to spend more and accumulate more debt in an effort to match the lifestyle of the suburban ideal, and whether this increase in economic pressure also increases parenting stress.

The second area for future research is on shift work. In the literature on poverty and parenting stress, there tends to be a focus on the employed versus unemployed. Employment among poor parents tends to be differentiated between shift work and nonstandard hours (Hsueh, 2006). In her ethnographic work with a subset of mothers from the Child Family Study, mostly African American and Hispanic single mothers receiving some form of government assistance, Hsueh (2006) found that 45% of the sample worked fixed standard hours, 26% worked nonstandard, 15% worked variable standard, and 14% worked variable nonstandard.

Standard hours are those that occur between 8 AM and 4 PM. Nonstandard hours fall outside this range, and also anytime on weekends. Mothers who worked fixed nonstandard schedules reported less maternal stress than mothers with fixed standard work schedules; however, this effect depended on choice. That is, if mothers did not chose to work nonstandard hours, then maternal stress was higher (Hsueh, 2006). According to the qualitative data, many mothers who worked nonstandard hours were those working multiple jobs and overtime to supplement their regular hours. Many were doing so in order for their children not to feel "poor" or "deprived." There are serious costs to nonstandard hours. These include fatigue and stress, time away from children, and difficulties arranging childcare (see Crnic & Ross, Chap. 11 of this volume). Given the paucity of research on shift work and parenting stress in ethnic minority groups, this is a fruitful research area.

As we have shown, poverty is an important factor contributing to parental stress. Many of the individual factors considered in this volume such as material hardship, family structure, and neighborhood environment covary with poverty. A less understood but critical contributor to poverty and parenting stress is culture. Both different cultural traditions themselves as well as their intersections with caregiver roles as nurturer, breadwinner, and marital partners all overlap in potentially powerful ways with poverty to affect parenting (see Nomaguchi & Milkie, Chap. 3, for a robust discussion on the social intuitions and ideologies that bring to bear on parents, particularly in the context of social and economic change). We have also introduced to the discussion an important but neglected role of immigration in family dynamics and parenting. Many families from low-income countries move to high-income countries in search of a better life. There are profound implications for child rearing, especially when families cannot move together due to economic constraints. Lastly, children are not simply the passive recipients of parenting. They themselves play an active, dynamic role in family systems. Income, culture, age, and immigrant status converge to create an experience of disadvantage for families.

Acknowledgements This research is supported by the National Science Foundation Graduate Research Fellowship Grant No. DGE-1144153 awarded to the first author. This research was also supported by the W.T. Grant Foundation, the John D. and Catherine T. MacArthur Foundation Network on Socioeconomic Status and Health, and National Institute for Minority Health and Health Disparities Grant No. 5RC2MD00467 granted to the second author.

References

Abidin, R. R. (1992). The determinants of parenting behavior. *Journal of Clinical Child Psychology, 21*(4), 407–412.

Angel, R., & Tienda, M. (1982). Determinants of extended household structure: Cultural pattern or economic need? *American Journal of Sociology, 87*(6), 1360–1383. doi:10.1086/227597.

Arnold, E. (2006). Separation and loss through immigration of African Caribbean women to the UK. *Attachment & Human Development, 8*(2), 159–174. doi:10.1080/14616730600789472.

Arnold, E. (2011). Clinical implications of attachment in immigrant communities. In P. Holmes & S. Farnfield (Eds.), *The routledge handbook of attachment: Implications and interventions* (pp. 117–131). London: Routledge.

Arnold, A., Lewis, J., Maximovich, A., Ickovics, J., & Kershaw, T. (2011). Antecedents and consequences of caregiving structure on young mothers and their infants. *Maternal and Child Health Journal, 15*(7), 1037–1045. doi:10.1007/s10995-010-0650-3.

Arya, S., & Roy, A. (Eds.). (2006). *Poverty, gender and migration* (2nd ed.). New Delhi, IN: SAGE Publications.

Baptiste, D. A. J., Hardy, K. V., & Lewis, L. (1997). Clinical practice with Caribbean immigrant families in the United States: The intersection of emigration, immigration, culture, and race. In J. L. Roopnarine & J. Brown (Eds.), *Caribbean families: Diversity among ethnic groups* (pp. 275–303). Greenwich: Ablex Publishing Corporation.

Barnett, M. A. (2008). Economic disadvantage in complex family systems: Expansion of family stress models. *Clinical Child and Family Psychology Review, 11*(3), 145–161.

Bauer, E., & Thompson, P. (2004). "She's always the person with a very global vision": The gender dynamics of migration, narrative interpretation and the case of Jamaican transnational families. *Gender & History, 16*(2), 334–375. doi:10.1111/j.0953-5233.2004.00344.x.

Benería, L., Berik, G., & Floro, M. S. (Eds.). (2016). *Gender, development, and globalisation: Economics as if all people mattered* (2nd ed.) New York, NY: Routledge. 10.1080/02255189.2016.1146130

Benner, A. D., & Kim, S. Y. (2010). Understanding Chinese American adolescents' developmental outcomes: Insights from the family stress model. *Journal of Research on Adolescence, 20*(1), 1–12. doi:10.1111/j.1532-7795.2009.00629.x.

Best-Cummings, C. (2009). *The long goodbye: Challenges of transnational parenting*. Saarbrucken, DE: VDM Publishing.

Bornstein, M. H. (2012). Cultural approaches to parenting. *Parenting, Science and Practice, 12*(2–3), 212–221. doi:10.1080/15295192.2012.683359.

Brody, G. H., Ge, X., Conger, R., Gibbons, F. X., Murry, V. M., Gerrard, M., et al. (2001). The influence of neighborhood disadvantage, collective socialization, and parenting on African American children's affiliation with deviant peers. *Child Development, 72*(4), 1231–1246. doi:10.1111/1467-8624.00344.

Burwell, S. M. (2015). Annual update of the HHS poverty guidelines, 80 Federal Register: The Daily Journal of the United States Government 3236–3237. Retrieved from https://www.federalregister.gov/articles/2015/01/22/2015-01120/annual-update-of-the-hhs-poverty-guidelines

Cabraal, A., & Singh, S. (2013). Contested representations of remittances and the transnational family. *South Asia, 36*(1), 50–64. 10.1080/00856401.2012.710304

Cardoso, J. B., Padilla, Y. C., & Sampson, M. (2010). Racial and ethnic variation in the predictors of maternal parenting stress. *Journal of Social Service Research, 36,* 429–444. doi:10.1080/01488376.2010.510948.

Castaneda, E., & Buck, L. (2011). Remittances, transnational parenting, and the children left behind: Economic and psychological implications. *The Latin Americanist, 55*(4), 85–110. doi:10.1111/j.1557-203X.2011.01136.x.

Cervantes, J. M., Mejía, O. L., & Mena, A. G. (2010). Serial migration and the assessment of extreme and unusual psychological hardship with undocumented Latina/o families. *Hispanic Journal of Behavioral Sciences, 32*(2), 275–291. doi:10.1177/0739986310366286.

Chao, R., & Kanatsu, A. (2008). Beyond socioeconomics: Explaining ethnic group differences in parenting through cultural and immigration processes. *Applied Developmental Science, 12*(4), 181–187. doi:10.1080/10888690802388102.

Cheever, S. (2004). The nanny dilemma. In B. Ehrenreich & A. R. Hochschild (Eds.), *Global woman: Nannies, maids, and sex workers in the new economy* (pp. 31–38). New York: Metropolitan/Owl Books.

Chetty, R., Hendren, N., & Katz, L. F. (2015). The effects of exposure to better neighborhoods on children: New evidence from the moving to opportunity experiment. *American Economic Review*. doi:10.3386/w21156.

Choi, J. K., & Jackson, A. P. (2012). Nonresident fathers' parenting, maternal mastery and child development in poor African American single-mother families. *Race and Social Problems, 4*(2), 102–111. doi:10.1007/s12552-012-9070-x.

Conger, R. D., & Conger, K. J. (2008). Understanding the process through which economic hardship influences families and children. In T. B. Heaton (Ed.), *Handbook of families and poverty* (pp. 64–81). Thousand Oaks, CA: Sage Publications.

Conger, R. D., & Donnellan, M. B. (2007). An interactionist perspective on the socioeconomic context of human development. *Annual Review of Psychology, 58,* 175–199. doi:10.1146/annurev.psych.58.110405.085551.

Conger, R. D., Conger, K. J., & Martin, M. J. (2011). Socioeconomic status, family processes, and individual development. *Journal of Marriage and Family, 72*(3), 685–704. doi:10.1111/j.1741-3737.2010.00725.x.Socioeconomic.

Conger, R. D., Wallace, L. E., Sun, Y., Simons, R. L., McLoyd, V. C., & Brody, G. H. (2002). Economic pressure in African American families: A replication and extension of the family stress model. *Developmental Psychology, 38*(2), 179–193. doi:10.1037/0012-1649.38.2.179.

Cooper, C., McLanahan, S. S., Meadows, S. O., & Brooks-Gunn, J. (2009). Family structure transitions and maternal parenting stress. *Journal of Marriage and Family, 71*(3), 558–574. doi:10.1111/j.1741-3737.2009.00619.x.

Crawford, C. (2003). Sending love in a barrel: The making of transnational Caribbean families in Canada. *Canadian Woman Studies, 22*(3), 104–109.

Crawford-Brown, C. P. J. (1999). *Who will save our children? The plight of the Jamaican child in the nineties.* Kingston, JM: University of the West Indies Press.

Crawford-Brown, C. P. J., & Rattray, J. M. (2001). Parent-child relationships in Caribbean families. In N. B. Webb & D. Lum (Eds.), *Culturally diverse parent-child and family relationships: A guide for social workers and other practitioners* (pp. 107–130). New York: Columbia University Press.

Cruz-Santiago, M. A., & Ramírez García, J. I. (2011). Adaptive parenting of adolescent children among Mexican-American parents residing in a dangerous neighborhood. *Family Process, 50*(1), 92–115.

D'Emilo, A. L., Cordero, B., Bainvel, B., Skoog, C., Comini, D., Gough, J., … Kilbane, T. (2007). *The impact of international migration: children left behind in selected countries of Latin America and the Caribbean.* Working Paper, Division of Policy and Planning. New York, NY. Retrieved from http://www2.unicef.org:60090/socialpolicy/index_46050.html

Deater-Deckard, K. D. (2004). *Parenting stress.* New Haven, CT: Yale University Press.

Delgado, M. Y., Killoren, S. E., & Updegraff, K. A. (2013). Economic hardship and Mexican-origin adolescents' adjustment: Examining adolescents' perceptions of hardship and parent-adolescent relationship quality. *Journal of Family Psychology, 27*(5), 827–837. doi:10.1037/a0033737.

Dillon, M., & Walsh, C. A. (2015). Left behind: The experiences of children of the Caribbean whose parents have migrated. *Journal of Comparative Family Studies, 43*(6), 871–902.

Dreby, J. (2006). Honor and virtue: Mexican parenting in the transnational context. *Gender & Society, 20*(1), 32–59. doi:10.1177/0891243205282660.

Dreby, J. (2010). *Divided by borders: Mexican migrants and their children.* Berkeley, CA: University of California Press.

Dreby, J., & Adkins, T. (2012). The strength of family ties: How US migration shapes children's ideas of family. *Childhood, 19*(2), 169–187. doi:10.1177/0907568211411206.

Dreby, J., & Stutz, L. (2012). Making something of the sacrifice: Gender, migration and Mexican children's educational aspirations. *Global Networks, 12*(1), 71–90. doi:10.1111/j.1471-0374.2011.00337.x.

Ehrenreich, B., & Hochschild, A. R. (Eds.). (2004). *Global woman: Nannies, maids, and sex workers in the new economy.* New York, NY: Metropolitan/Owl Books. doi:10.1177/026327640402100612.

Evans, G. W. (2004). The environment of childhood poverty. *American Psychologist, 59*(2), 77–92. doi:10.1037/0003-066X.59.2.77.

Falicov, C. J. (2001). The cultural meanings of money: The case of Latinos and Anglo-Americans. *American Behavioral Scientist, 45*(2), 313–328. doi:10.1177/00027640121957088.

Fuligni, A. J. (2006). Family obligation among children in immigrant families. Retrieved from http://www.migrationpolicy.org/article/family-obligation-among-children-immigrant-families
Gamburd, M. R. (2004). Breadwinner no more. In B. Ehrenreich & A. R. Hochschild (Eds.), *Global woman: Nannies, maids, and sex workers in the new economy* (pp. 190–206). New York, NY: Metropolitan/Owl Books.
Gamburd, M. R. (2008). Milk teeth and jet planes: Kin relations in families of Sri Lanka's transnational domestic servants. *City & Society, 20*(1), 5–31. doi:10.1111/j.1548-744X.2008.00003.x.
Garbarino, J., Bradshaw, C. P., & Kostelny, K. (2005). Neighborhood and community influences on parenting. In T. Luster & L. Okagaki (Eds.), *Parenting: An ecological perspective* (2nd ed., pp. 297–318). Mahwah, NJ: Lawrence Erlbaum Associates.
Gershoff, E. T., Aber, J. L., Raver, C. C., & Lennon, M. C. (2007). Income is not enough: Incorporating material hardship into models of income associations with parenting and child development. *Child Development, 78*(1), 70–95. doi:10.1111/j.1467-8624.2007.00986.x.
Glasgow, G. F., & Gouse-Sheese, J. (1995). Themes of rejection and abandonment in group work with Caribbean adolescents. *Social Work with Groups, 17*(4), 3–27.
Gonzales, N. A., Coxe, S., Roosa, M. W., White, R. M. B., Knight, G. P., Zeiders, K. H., et al. (2011). Economic hardship, neighborhood context, and parenting: Prospective effects on Mexican-American adolescent's mental health. *American Journal of Community Psychology, 47*(1), 98–113. doi:10.1007/s10464-010-9366-1.
Graham, E., & Jordan, L. P. (2011). Migrant parents and the psychological well-being of left-behind children in Southeast Asia. *Journal of Marriage and Family, 73*(4), 763–787. doi:10.1111/j.1741-3737.2011.00844.x.
Grinstein-Weiss, M., Williams Shanks, T. R., Manturuk, K. R., Key, C. C., Paik, J. G., & Greeson, J. K. P. (2010). Homeownership and parenting practices: Evidence from the community advantage panel. *Children and Youth Services Review, 32*(5), 774–782. doi:10.1016/j.childyouth.2010.01.016.
Guarnizo, L. E. (2003). The economics of transnational living. *International Migration Review, 37* (3), 666–699. doi:10.2307/30037753.
Guterman, N. B., Lee, S. J., Taylor, C. A., & Rathouz, P. J. (2009). Parental perceptions of neighborhood processes, stress, personal control, and risk for physical child abuse and neglect. *Child Abuse and Neglect, 33*(12), 897–906. doi:10.1016/j.chiabu.2009.09.008.
Gutman, L. M., McLoyd, V. C., & Tokoyawa, T. (2005). Financial strain, neighborhood stress, parenting behaviors, and adolescent adjustment in urban African American families. *Journal of Research on Adolescence, 15*(4), 425–449. doi:10.1111/j.1532-7795.2005.00106.x.
Hoang, L. A., & Yeoh, B. S. A. (2011). Breadwinning wives and "left-behind" husbands: Men and masculinities in the Vietnamese transnational family. *Gender & Society, 25*(6), 717–739. Retrieved from http://www.jstor.org/stable/23212197
Hochschild, A. R. (2004). Love and gold. In B. Ehrenreich & A. R. Hochschild (Eds.), *Global woman: Nannies, maids, and sex workers in the new economy* (pp. 15–30). New York, NY: Metropolitan/Owl Books.
Horton, S. (2009). A mother's heart is weighed down with stones: A phenomenological approach to the experience of transnational motherhood. *Culture, Medicine and Psychiatry, 33*(1), 21–40. doi:10.1007/s11013-008-9117-z.
Howell, A. J., & Timberlake, J. M. (2014). Racial and ethnic trends in the suburbanization of poverty in U.S. metropolitan areas, 1980–2010. *Journal of Urban Affairs, 36*(1), 79–98. doi:10.1111/juaf.12030.
Hsueh, J. (2006). Mothers at work in a 24/7 economy: Exploring implications for family and child well-being. In H. Yoshikawa, T. S. Weisner, & E. D. Lowe (Eds.), *Making it work: Low-wage employment, family life, and child development* (pp. 97–123). New York, NY: Russell Sage Foundation.
Huston, A. C., & Bentley, A. C. (2010). Human development in societal context. *Annual Review of Psychology, 61*(1), 411–437. doi:10.1146/annurev.psych.093008.100442.

Iruka, I. U., LaForett, D. R., & Odom, E. C. (2012). Examining the validity of the family investment and stress models and relationship to children's school readiness across five cultural groups. *Journal of Family Psychology, 26*(3), 359–370. doi:10.1037/a0028290.

Jackson, A. P. (1998). The role of social support in parenting for low-income, single. *Black mothers. Social Service Review, 72*(3), 365–378. doi:10.1086/515763.

Jackson, A. P., Preston, K. S. J., & Thomas, C. A. (2013). Single mothers, nonresident fathers, and preschoolers' socioemotional development: Social support, psychological well-being, and parenting quality. *Journal of Social Service Research, 39*(1), 129–140. doi:10.1080/01488376.2012.723241.

Jiang, Y., Ekono, M., & Skinner, C. (2015). *Basic facts about low-income children: Children under 18 Years, 2013. National Center for Children in Poverty*. New York, NY. Retrieved from http://www.nccp.org/publications/pub_1099.html

Jocson, R. M., & McLoyd, V. C. (2015). Neighborhood and housing disorder, parenting, and youth adjustment in low-income urban families. *American Journal of Community Psychology, 55,* 304–313. doi:10.1007/s10464-015-9710-6.

Kim, J., Agic, B., & McKenzie, K. (2014). The mental health of Korean transnational mothers: A scoping review. *The International Journal of Social Psychiatry, 60*(8), 783–794. doi:10.1177/0020764014522775.

Kneebone, E., & Berube, A. (2013). *Confronting suburban poverty in America*. Washington, DC: Brookings Institution Press.

Kotchick, B. A., Dorsey, S., & Heller, L. (2005). Predictors of parenting among African American single mothers: Personal and contextual factors. *Journal of Marriage and Family, 67,* 448–460. doi:10.1111/j.0022-2445.2005.00127.x.

Kottegoda, S. (2006). Bringing home the money: Migration and poverty in gender politics in Sri Lanka. In *Poverty, gender and migration* (2nd ed., pp. 49–71). New Delhi, IN: SAGE Publications.

Lam, C. M. (2011). Psychological stress and parenting behavior among Chinese families: Findings from a study on parent education for economically disadvantaged families. *Social Indicators Research, 100*(3), 451–462.

Landers-Potts, M. A., Wickrama, K. A. S., Simons, L. G., Cutrona, C., Gibbons, F. X., Simons, R. L., et al. (2015). An extension and moderational analysis of the family stress model focusing on African American adolescents. *Family Relations, 64*(2), 233–248. doi:10.1111/fare.12117.

Lyons, S. J., Henly, J. R., & Schuerman, J. R. (2005). Informal support in maltreating families: Its effect on parenting practices. *Children and Youth Services Review, 27,* 21–38. doi:10.1016/j.childyouth.2004.08.010.

Manturuk, K., Riley, S., & Ratcliffe, J. (2012). Perception vs. reality: The relationship between low-income homeownership, perceived financial stress, and financial hardship. *Social Science Research, 41*(2), 276–286. doi:10.1016/j.ssresearch.2011.11.006.

Massey, D. S. (1996). The age of extremes: Concentrated affluence and poverty in the twenty-first century. *Demography, 33*(4), 395–412. doi:10.2307/2061774.

Massey, D. S., Arango, J., Hugo, G., Kouaouci, A., Pellegrino, A., & Taylor, J. E. (1993). Theories of international migration: A review and appraisal. *Population English Edition, 19*(3), 431–466. doi:10.2307/2938462.

McLoyd, V. C., Mistry, R. S., & Hardaway, C. R. (2014). Poverty and children's development: Familial processes as mediating influences. In E. T. Gershoff, R. S. Mistry, & D. A. Crosby (Eds.), *Societal contexts of child development: Pathways of influence and implications for practice and policy* (pp. 109–138). Oxford: Oxford University Press.

Miranda, J., Siddique, J., Der-Martirosian, C., & Belin, T. R. (2005). Depression among Latina immigrant mothers separated from their children. *Psychiatric Services (Washington, D.C.), 56* (6), 717–720. http://doi.org/10.1176/appi.ps.56.6.717

Mistry, R. S., & Lowe, E. D. (2006). What earnings and income buy—the "basics" plus "a little extra": Implications for family and child well-being. In H. Yoshikawa, T. S. Weisner, & E. D. Lowe (Eds.), *Making it work: Low-wage employment, family life, and child development* (pp. 173–205). New York, NY: Russell Sage Foundation.

Mistry, R. S., Lowe, E. D., Benner, A. D., & Chien, N. (2008). Expanding the family economic stress model: Insights from a mixed-methods approach. *Journal of Marriage and Family, 70* (1), 196–209. doi:10.1111/j.1741-3737.2007.00471.x.

Nam, Y., Wikoff, N., & Sherraden, M. (2013). Racial and ethnic differences in parenting stress: Evidence from a statewide sample of new mothers. *Journal of Child and Family Studies, 24* (12), 278–288. doi:10.1007/s10826-013-9833-z.

Nomaguchi, K. M., & House, A. N. (2013). Racial-ethnic disparities in maternal parenting stress: The role of structural disadvantages and parenting values. *Journal of Health and Social Behavior, 54*(3), 386–404. doi:10.1177/0022146513498511.

Olwig, K. F. (2012). The "successful" return: Caribbean narratives of migration, family, and gender. *Journal of the Royal Anthropological Institute, 18*(4), 828–845. doi:10.1111/j.1467-9655.2012.01794.x.

Orellana, M. F. (2001). The work kids do: Mexican and Central American immigrant children's contributions to households and schools in California. *Harvard Educational Review, 71*(3), 366–389.

Ornelas, I. J., Perreira, K. M., Beeber, L., & Maxwell, L. (2009). Challenges and strategies to maintaining emotion health: Qualitative perspectives of Mexican immigrant mothers. *Journal of Family Issues, 30*(11), 1556–1575. doi:10.1177/0192513X09336651.

Pachter, L. M., Auinger, P., Palmer, R., & Weitzman, M. (2006). Do parenting and the home environment, maternal depression, neighborhood, and chronic poverty affect child behavioral problems differently in different racial-ethnic groups? *Pediatrics, 117*(4), 1329–1338. doi:10.1542/peds.2005-1784.

Parke, R. D., Coltrane, S., Duffy, S., Buriel, R., Dennis, J., Powers, J., … Widaman, K. F. (2004). Economic stress, parenting, and child adjustment in Mexican American and European American families. *Child Development, 75*(6), 1632–1656.

Parreñas, R. (2001). Mothering from a distance: Emotion, gender and inter-generational relationships in Filipino transnational families. *Feminist Studies, 27*(2), 361–390. doi:10.1017/CBO9781107415324.004.

Parreñas, R. S. (2004). The care crisis in the Philippines: Children and transnational families in the new global economy. In B. Ehrenreich & A. R. Hochschild (Eds.), *Global woman: Nannies, maids, and sex workers in the new economy* (pp. 39–54). New York, NY: Metropolitan/Owl Books.

Parreñas, R. (2005). *Children of global migration: Transnational families and gendered woes.* Stanford, CA: Stanford University Press.

Phoenix, A., & Bauer, E. (2012). Challenging gender practices: Intersectional narratives of sibling relations and parent-child engagements in transnational serial migration. *European Journal of Women's Studies, 19*(4), 490–504. doi:10.1177/1350506812455994.

Puff, J., & Renk, K. (2014). Relationships among parents' economic stress, parenting, and young children's behavior problems. *Child Psychiatry and Human Development, 45,* 712–727. doi:10.1007/s10578-014-0440-z.

Putnam, R. D. (2015). *Our kids: The American Dream in crisis.* New York, NY: Simon & Schuster.

Raver, C. C., Gershoff, E. T., & Aber, J. L. (2007). Testing equivalence of mediating models of income, parenting, and school readiness for white, black, and Hispanic children in a national sample. *Child Development, 78*(1), 96–115. doi:10.1111/j.1467-8624.2007.00987.x.

Rodríguez, M. M. D., Donovick, M. R., & Crowley, S. L. (2009). Parenting styles in a cultural context: Obersevations of "protective pareting" in first-generation Latinos. *Family Process, 48* (2), 195–211.

Rogers, R. R. (2006). Black like who? Afro-Caribbean immigrants, African Americans, and the politics of group identity. In *Afro-Caribbean immigrants and the politics of incorporation* (pp. 170–202). Cambridge, MA: Cambridge University Press. http://dx.doi.org/10.1017/CBO9780511606694.007

Rothwell, D. W., & Han, C.-K. (2010). Exploring the relationship between assets and family stress among low-income families. *Family Relations, 59*(4), 396–407. doi:10.1111/j.1741-3729.2010.00611.x.

Santa-Maria, M. L., & Cornille, T. (2007). Traumatic stress, family separations, and attachment among Latin American immigrants. *Traumatology, 13*(2), 26–31.

Santiago Barquín, C. (2001). The poor: The theological perspective of the Vincentian charism. Retrieved from http://famvin.org/wiki/The_Poor:_the_theological_perspective_of_the_Vincentian_charism

Schapiro, N. A., Kools, S. M., Weiss, S. J., & Brindis, C. D. (2013). Separation and reunification: The experiences of adolescents living in transnational families. *Current Problems in Pediatric and Adolescent Health Care, 43*(3), 48–68. doi:10.1016/j.cppeds.2012.12.001.

Singh, S., Robertson, S., & Cabraal, A. (2012). Transnational family money: Remittances, gifts and inheritance. *Journal of Intercultural Studies, 33*(5), 475–492. doi:10.1080/07256868.2012.701606.

Solantaus, T., Leinonen, J. A., & Punamaki, R.-L. (2004). Children's mental health in times of economic recession: Replication and extension of the family economic stress model in Finland. *Developmental Psychology, 40*(3), 412–429. doi:10.1037/0012-1649.40.3.412.

Song, M. (1997). Children's labour in ethnic family businesses: the case of Chinese take-away businesses in Britain. *Ethnic and Racial Studies, 20*(4), 690–716.

Stark, O., & Bloom, D. E. (1985). The new economics of labor migration. *The American Economic Review, 75*(2), 173–178.

Steinberg, L. (2001). We know some things: Parent–adolescent relationships in retrospect and prospect. *Journal of Research on Adolescence, 11*(1), 1–19. doi:10.1111/1532-7795.00001.

Suárez-Orozco, C., Bang, H. J., & Kim, H. Y. (2011). I felt like my heart was staying behind: Psychological implications of family separations & reunifications for immigrant youth. *Journal of Adolescent Research, 26*(2), 222–257. doi:10.1177/0743558410376830.

Suârez-Orozco, C., Todorova, I. L. G., & Louie, J. (2002). Making up for lost time: The experience of separation and reunification among immigrant families. *Family Process, 41*(4), 625–643. doi:10.1111/j.1545-5300.2002.00625.x.

Sun, W., Li, D., Zhang, W., Bao, Z., & Wang, Y. (2015). Family material hardship and Chinese adolescents' problem behaviors: A moderated mediation analysis. *PLoS ONE, 10*(5), 1–22. doi:10.1371/journal.pone.0128024.

Takei, I., & Sakamoto, A. (2011). Poverty among Asian Americans in the 21st century. *Sociological Perspectives, 54*(2), 251–276. doi:10.1525/sop.2011.54.2.251.

Tamis-LeMonda, C. S., Briggs, R. D., McClowry, S. G., & Snow, D. L. (2008). Challenges to the study of African American parenting: Conceptualization, sampling, Research approaches, measurement, and design. *Parenting, 8,* 319–358. doi:10.1080/15295190802612599.

Thai, H. C. (2014). *Insufficient funds: The culture of money in low-wage transnational families*. Stanford, CA: Stanford University Press.

UN Population Divison. (2013). *World Migration in Figures*.

White, R. M. B., & Roosa, M. W. (2012). Neighborhood contexts, fathers, and Mexican American young adolescents' internalizing symptoms. *Journal of Marriage and Family, 74*(1), 152–166. doi:10.1111/j.1741-3737.2011.00878.x.

Williams, D. T., Cheadle, J. E., & Goosby, B. J. (2015). Hard times and heart break: Linking economic hardship and relationship distress. *Journal of Family Issues, 36*(7), 924–950. doi:10.1177/0192513X13501666.

Zhang, S., Eamon, M. K., & Zhan, M. (2015). Neighborhood disorder, perceptions of neighborhood social capital, and maternal stress: Exploration of a mediating mechanism. *Journal of Community Pscyhology, 43*(3), 278–295. doi:10.1002/jcop.

Zong, J., & Batalova, J. (2015). Frequently requested statistics on immigrants and immigration in the United States. *Migration Policy Institute*. Retrieved from http://www.migrationpolicy.org/article/frequently-requested-statistics-immigrants-and-immigration-united-states

Chapter 3
Sociological Perspectives on Parenting Stress: How Social Structure and Culture Shape Parental Strain and the Well-Being of Parents and Children

Kei Nomaguchi and Melissa A. Milkie

Introduction

The parent-child relationship is perhaps the most central and enduring tie for most adults and as such, parenting carries with it enormous emotional weight (Pearlin, 1983). Raising children involves both challenges and joys over many years (Nomaguchi & Milkie, 2003). When burdens overweigh rewards of parenting, mothers and fathers may feel it difficult to carry on within this key social role and they may experience what researchers commonly call parenting stress (Deater-Deckard, 2004). Describing and explaining social patterns of exposure to stressors (or strains) and their consequences for mental health among parents are primary goals in sociological studies of parenting stress (Pearlin, 1989). Research within this discipline centers on understanding the social origins of parenting stress, more specifically, how stressors experienced by individual parents—parental strains—are shaped by parents' locations in the structured arrangements of statuses and roles in society (Pearlin, 1989) and the cultural ideologies or larger belief systems about parenting (Milkie & Denny, 2014). Sociologists thus investigate gradations in levels and types of parental strains, the moderating resources parents may have in order to help buffer those strains, and ultimately the mental health of parents, each of which are influenced by social loca-

Research for this chapter was supported in part by a funding by the Eunice Kennedy Shriver National Institute of Child Health and Human Development (1R15HD083891-1 PI: Kei Nomaguchi)

K. Nomaguchi (✉)
Department of Sociology, Bowling Green State University,
Bowling Green, OH 43402, USA
e-mail: knomagu@bgsu.edu

M.A. Milkie
Department of Sociology, University of Toronto, Toronto, ON M5S 2J4, Canada
e-mail: melissa.milkie@utoronto.ca

K. Deater-Deckard and R. Panneton (eds.), *Parental Stress and Early Child Development*, DOI 10.1007/978-3-319-55376-4_3

tions or social groups to which parents belong (Mirowsky & Ross, 2003; Pearlin, 1989). Social groups that are important to examine among parents include, but are not limited to, social class, race-ethnicity, gender, and sexual orientation. Findings of sociological studies inform policy-makers about the current reality of parents' needs that are specific to different social groups, and social policies are able to shape the context of parenting in important ways. For example, studies show that the negative association between parenthood and life satisfaction or depression is weaker in countries with better state supports for parents to raise children (e.g., Sweden and Denmark) than in countries with less support (e.g., the USA) (Glass, Simon, & Andersson, 2016; Margolis & Myrskylä, 2011).

In this chapter, we highlight key features of *sociological* approaches to understanding sources, mechanisms, and manifestation of stress among parents, the advantages of these approaches, and future research directions. Other chapters in this volume expand this discussion by addressing research on the link between parenting stress and child development more directly. In the service of our own goals, we first discuss major theoretical frameworks and research methods used by sociologists, including unique ways in which those in the field investigate, conceptualize, and measure stressors that parents experience in a rapidly changing society. Then, we discuss theoretical perspectives and empirical work that help to explain the variation in levels and types of parenting stress across major social groups and institutions. We also discuss how disparities in availability of moderating resources lead to differential vulnerability to parenting stress across social groups. We touch on two other ways through which sociologists examine how the parenting role influences adults' well-being: comparisons between parents and non-parents and cross-national comparisons. We end this chapter by discussing future directions in parenting stress research.

How Sociologists Study Parenting Stress

Theoretical Frameworks and Research Methods

A major sociological perspective on parenting stress is the *stress process model*. This model is a conceptual and analytical framework that helps to explain socially patterned distributions of strains and mental health (Pearlin, 1989, 1999; Pearlin & Bierman, 2013; Pearlin, Menaghan, Lieberman, & Mullan, 1981). The stress process model draws on the theories of human stress and coping in psychology (Lazarus & Folkman, 1984) as well as the social structure and personality perspective in sociological social psychology (House, 1981). Pearlin (1989, 1999) argues that stress is an overall process with three central components: sources of stress (i.e., stressors or strains), moderating resources (e.g., supports and coping mechanisms), and manifestation or outcomes of stress (i.e., mental health). As Fig. 1.1 shows, the stress process model shows how stressors link to negative mental health outcomes. Notably, the word "stress" is often ambiguous in the

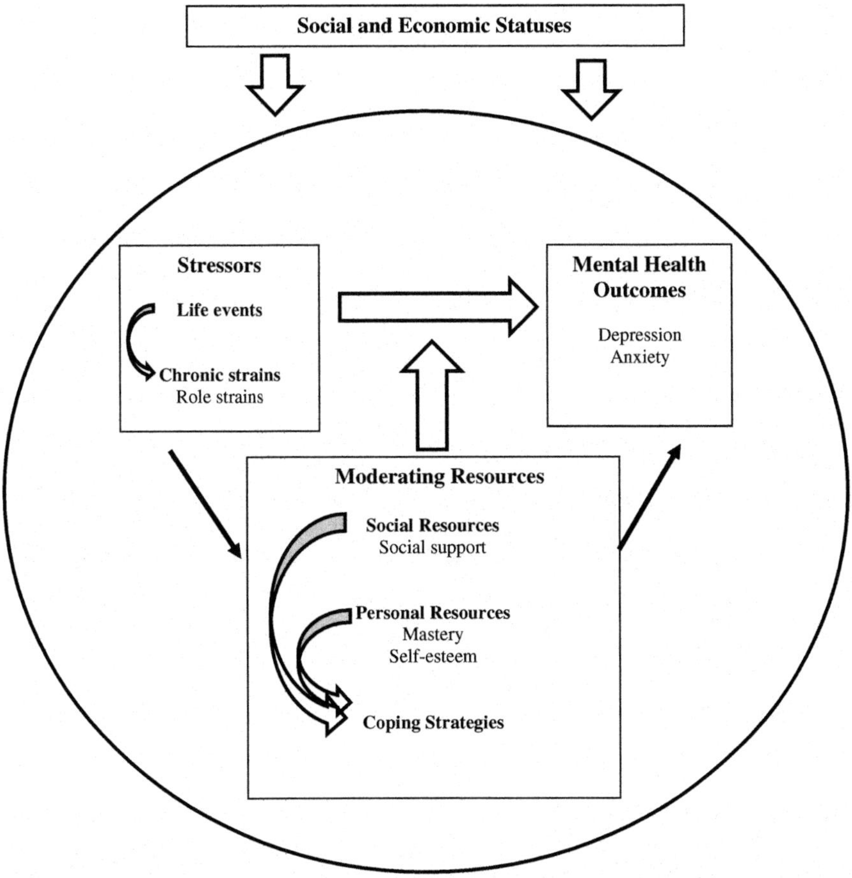

Based on Pearlin et al. (1981), Pearlin (1989)

Fig. 3.1 Stress process model

literature and can impede conceptual advancement. Its use sometimes conflates independent variables (i.e., stressors) with dependent variables or outcomes of stressors (i.e., mental health), such as depression, anxiety, anger, or substance use. Thus, sociologists tend to use phrases such as "stressors parents experience" or "parental strains" to refer to what is typically called parenting stress elsewhere.

Of particular interest to sociologists is the nature and the origins of stressors (Pearlin, 1989). Stressors appear in the form of life events, daily hassles, and role strains (Deater-Deckard 2004; Wheaton, Young, Montazer, & Stuart-Lahman, 2013). Sociologists are especially interested in role strains given that social roles tie people to major social institutions. Parental role strain refers to the enduring hardships, challenges, and conflicts or other problems that parents come to experience in their daily lives (Pearlin, 1983). The central idea is that normal aspects of individuals' experiences in the parenting role can have consequences for parents' mental health—which has important implications for child's well-being (see also Chap. 12 by Havighurst & Kehoe in this volume). Parental role strain involves multiple dimensions, including feeling overwhelmed or trapped by one's level of responsibilities, feeling frustrated by children's behaviors in comparison with parent's expectations, and feeling strained by the parent–child relationship (Pearlin, 1983, 1989). Pearlin (1989) identifies several general aspects of role strain, including role overload, role captivity, and interpersonal conflict. *Role overload* involves the extent to which the amount of demand exceeds the individual's capacity. To measure role overload, sociologists ask people about their subjective feelings of being overwhelmed (e.g., "Being a parent is harder than I thought it would be."). Sociologists also use objective measures of high demands of parenting, such as the number of children in the household, child illness, or single parenthood (e.g., Simon, 1992) as a way of approaching role overload. *Role captivity* refers to the extent to which individuals feel unwilling to fulfill their parenting role(s). Sociologists ask people about their feelings of being trapped by responsibilities as a parent, or having no time for themselves because of children, not being able to spend their time the way they want to (e.g., Nomaguchi & Brown, 2011). This concept may be similar to "parenting distress" in Abidin's (2012) parenting stress index. *Parent–child relationship quality*—or interpersonal conflict—(Pearlin, 1983) may be equivalent to the "parent-child dysfunction interaction scale" in Abidin's (2012) classification. The quality of the parent–child relationship plays a strong role in influencing parents' mental health (Milkie et al. 2008; Nomaguchi, 2012a; Umberson, 1992; Umberson & Gove, 1989; Ward, 2008). *Inter-role conflict*, especially difficulties in balancing paid work and parenting responsibilities, is a key challenge for today's parents in North America (Bianchi & Milkie 2010; Milkie, Kendig, Nomaguchi, & Denny, 2010; Nomaguchi, 2009). Besides direct parenting strain in the form of overload, captivity, and conflict within and across roles, being a parent (versus not) creates additional strains, such as greater workload in the home, significant financial obligations, conflicts with partners, and time strains, that may result in poorer mental health.

A major research method in sociological studies is the use of population-based surveys, which is quite different from many psychological studies of parents that may include clinical samples. Sociologists typically use a representative sample of a large-scale population, largely because the purpose of sociological studies is, as discussed earlier, to look for social patterns in the levels of strains and mental health experienced by parents. In past decades, a series of longitudinal national surveys have collected information regarding parenting stress, such as the NICHD Study of Early Child Care and Youth Development (SECCYD), the Fragile Families and Child Well-being Study (FFCWS), the Early Childhood Longitudinal Study, Kindergarten Cohort (ECLS-K), Birth Cohort (ECLS-B), and the Child Development Supplement to the Panel Study of Income Dynamics (PSID-CDS). These data sets typically include three to five question items that are derived from the well-known Abidin's (2012) parenting stress index.

Other major methods of sociological research are observing the natural settings of parents' lives (ethnographies) and conducting in-depth interviews (e.g., Coles, 2009; Dow, 2016; Hays, 1996; Nelson, 2010). Studies using these qualitative methods can reveal nuanced sources and processes of parenting stress. Moreover, qualitative studies are useful in finding emerging issues that serve as new sources of strain experienced by parents. This is especially important given the rapid pace of changing economic, family, or cultural circumstances of parenting in contemporary USA and other societies, as we discuss below. Measuring cultural changes in surveys is challenging. Content analysis of books (Hays, 1996), magazines (Denny, Brewton-Tiayon, Lykke, & Milkie, 2014; Milkie & Denny, 2014; Rutherford, 2011), and other documents over time, coupled with ethnographic studies and in-depth interviews with parents today, has been used to analyze changes in socially expected parenting practices.

Social Change and the Changing Nature and Sources of Parental Strain

In addition to using conventional concepts and measures of parental strain (briefly discussed above), sociologists strive to identify new types of challenges (i.e., stressors) that parents in contemporary society face. A life course perspective (Elder, 1999) argues that the levels and the types of challenges and rewards of parenting change across different historical times. This is in part because of economic changes that lead to increases or decreases in available material or social resources that parents can invest in parenting (Beck & Beck-Gernsheim, 1995). Types of demands and rewards of parenting also vary by historical time because of changes in parenting values (Alwin, 1989; Nomaguchi & Milkie, 2016). As Goode (1960) notes, parental role strain involves individuals' subjective perception that they are unable to meet *socially expected* demands of the parenting role. What parents are expected to do for children and children's place in the world changes over time as economic circumstances and parenting values shift (Beck & Beck-Gernsheim, 1995; Hays, 1996). In this section, we discuss examples of major social changes that have led to changes in stressors that parents may experience.

First, the increase in mothers' labor force participation has led many parents, particularly mothers, to experience an additional source of strain: arranging quality childcare. Research shows that difficulty in arranging childcare is a major stressor that has consequences for parents' mental health (Bird, 1997; Ross & Mirowsky, 1988). These research findings have important policy implications in the USA, which suggest that it is critical to increase the availability of affordable, quality childcare as well as employees' ability to take family leaves and to have control over their work schedules. Although research and policy discussions tend to focus on childcare problems during early childhood, Kurz's (2000, 2006) qualitative studies find that how to supervise children after school is in fact a central concern among employed parents with older children. Childcare arrangements are complex, change frequently over the seasons of the year and as children grow, and are often different for siblings in the same family (Kurz, 2000). In general, control over their work schedules—control over the timing of their work, the number of hours they work, and the location of their work—allows parents to reduce work–family conflict (Kelly et al., 2014), although as discussed in the next section, the effects of flexible work schedules on work–family conflict and mental health depend on occupational status.

Second, since the late 1980s, US parenting culture has increasingly emphasized parents' close involvement in children's day-to-day lives, which has created the norms of "intensive mothering" and "involved fathering" (Hays, 1996; Milkie & Denny, 2014). Spending time with children has become a central perceived requirement of a being a "good" parent. Intensive mothering and involved fathering ideology has created high standards regarding the adequate amount of time parents "ought to" spend with their children, which may clash with the ideal of breadwinning for fathers and may be considered "never enough" for mothers. Using data from the National Survey of Parents (NSP), the 2010 General Social Survey (GSS), and the National Study of Changing Workforce (NSCW), we have found that a majority of mothers and fathers report feeling that they spend too little time with their children (Milkie, Mattingly, Nomaguchi, Bianchi, & Robinson, 2004; Nomaguchi, Milkie, & Bianchi, 2005). Time strains with children appear to be a stressor in the parenting role (Milkie, Nomaguchi, & Schieman, 2016). Full-time employed mothers with young children report always feeling rushed (Milkie, Raley, & Bianchi, 2009).

Intensive mothering ideology is linked to a world that feels increasingly unsafe and less predictable due to economic, job and relationship insecurities and few social safety nets (Milkie & Warner, 2014; Villalobos, 2014). Milkie and Warner (2014) argue that mothers increasingly feel pressure to work to "safeguard" children's futures in a world where social programs are weak. Middle-class parents push children more to work hard toward academic achievement in school and at developing their unique talents through extra-curricular activities (Lareau, 2003; Putnam, 2015). The idealization of mothers as sole champion of children perpetuates an individualistic approach to parenting and places enormous pressures on mothers to protect children from harms and create "successful" children (Elliott, Powell, & Brenton, 2015; Nelson, 2010; Villalobos, 2014). When children are not succeeding, parents' own well-being suffers. For example, adult children having problems at their workplaces, in marriage and romantic partnerships, or with the law is a powerful source of parental strain among older adults (Greenfield & Marks, 2006; Milkie et al., 2008; Pillemer, & Suitor, 1991; Spitze, Logan, Deane, & Zerger, 1994). For mothers with minor children, Milkie and colleagues (2010) found that when employed parents perceive that their children are not doing well, they feel imbalanced. More research is needed to investigate how parents' perceptions as to how their children who are minors are succeeding (e.g., with peers, with teachers, and with school work) may influence parental strain.

Third, another trend in the USA that has implications for parental strain and the well-being of parents and children is the increase in incarceration rates in the past several decades, in part as a policy response to the "war on drugs" (Carson & Golinelli, 2013). The majority of inmates have children (Glaze & Maruschak,

2008). Researchers have begun investigating the consequences of incarceration for parental strains and mental health. Parents who have been incarcerated face great challenges in providing their children with financial or emotional support (Swisher & Waller, 2008). Incarceration of a partner also leads to increases in financial, instrumental, and emotional burdens in parenting (Wildeman, Schnittker, & Turney, 2012). In addition, incarceration often leads to relationship dissolution and new partnerships (Turney & Wildeman, 2013), which creates family complexity that has a range of challenges in parenting as we discuss below. Fewer studies have examined the question as to how (adult) children's arrest, detention, or incarceration relates to parents' stress. Children's incarceration brings a lot of challenges to parents, including financial difficulty to pay legal fees, travel to a prison to visit their children, keeping close contact with their children, and taking care of grandchildren (Green, Ensminger, Robertson, & Juon, 2006). Because incarceration has become part of the life course of many people in low-income families, research should not ignore the role of incarceration in influencing parental strain and child's well-being.

In sum, from a sociological point of view, stressful experiences in parenting may derive from structural arrangements and its changes, cultural ideology and its shifts, and social policies (or lack thereof). These structural, cultural and policy factors are embedded in key social institutions such as the economy, the criminal justice system, and the workplace. Sociologists strive to address new sources of parental strain that are often a product of larger social changes.

Parental Strain: Variation Across Social Groups

Strain arises from certain experiences that individuals encounter repeatedly, which are often deeply rooted in social structural contexts and individuals' locations within such contexts (Pearlin, 1989). Sociological research is concerned with how parental strain is unevenly distributed across major indicators of stratification within society (Pearlin, 1989; Umberson, Pudrovska, & Reczek, 2010). In this section, we discuss variations in parental strain by some of such major indicators, including social class, race-ethnicity, gender, sexual orientation, marital status, and child's life stage.

Social Class—Education, Employment, and Occupation

Financial strain is a key factor that explains why parents raising children report poorer mental health and unhappiness compared with non-parents (Bird, 1997; Pollmann-Schult, 2014). Parents who do not earn a sufficient income, who are unable to secure a home, food, and health insurance, tend to suffer from high parental strain and poorer mental health. In this chapter, however, we do not focus on poverty as other chapters have extensive discussions on it (Cassells & Evans; Finegood & Blair in this volume). We discuss other indicators of social class: education, employment, and occupation.

In general, lower socio-economic status (SES) is related to more stressors (Pearlin, 1999). Yet how education is related to parental strain level depends on the arena of parenting strains examined (Nomaguchi & Brown, 2011). More education may reflect higher levels of material, social, and psychological resources that mothers can use to deal with or buffer stressors (Ross & Van Willigen, 1997). Adults with a higher level of education are more likely to be able to postpone their childbearing until they are settled with financial goals and careers (Cherlin, 2010). Education is related to intended childbearing (Musick, England, Edgington, & Kangas, 2009), and intended births are associated with less depression among fathers and more happiness among mothers (Su, 2012). However, more education is often associated with more demands or expectations for parents to invest in childrearing (Lareau, 2003; Nelson, 2010; Putnam, 2015). Nelson (2010) called today's parenting among the professional middle class "out of control" in that mothers with teenagers are supposed to observe, discuss, and negotiate a range of activities in their children's daily lives. Based on her in-depth interviews, Nelson found that the professional-middle-class mothers are more likely than working-class mothers to doubt themselves and worry a lot about consequences of their parenting for their children's future. In addition, mothers with a higher level of education are more likely to have greater career demands, which increase work–family conflict (Schieman & Glavin, 2011). Using data from SECCYD, Nomaguchi and Brown (2011) found that mothers with college degrees reported more role captivity (e.g., feeling trapped), whereas mothers who did not have college education reported more parenting anxiety (e.g., worried about their children's safety and their parenting). These findings suggest that it is important to investigate how differential SES is linked to different types of parental strain.

Typically, having a paid job is negatively related to parental strain for both fathers and mothers (Nomaguchi & Brown, 2011; Nomaguchi & Johnson, 2016), perhaps because it increases material, social, and psychological resources for parents. Job loss and unemployment, especially fathers' unemployment, are related to more parental strains for both mothers and fathers (Conger, Ge, Elder, Lorenz, & Simons, 1994). Yet, employment could become a source of parental strain depending on its characteristics. For example, long work hours is a strong predictor of parents' senses of time deficits with children (Milkie et al., 2004). An inflexible schedule is also positively related to parental strain for both fathers and mothers (Nomaguchi & Johnson, 2016). This makes sense, given that many parents, mostly mothers, change their work hours to meet their children's needs (Bianchi, 2011; Gerstel & Clawson, 2015; Nomaguchi & Fettro, 2016). Non-standard work schedules—e.g., working in the evening, at night, or rotating shifts—bring depression and strain to the mother–father relationship (Presser, 2000; Strazdins, Clements, Korda, Broom, & D'Souza, 2006), and, as we will see below, partner problems are related to parental strain (Deater-Deckard, 2004; Nomaguchi, Johnson, Minter, & Aldrich, 2017).

Types of issues parents face in balancing work and family life vary markedly across occupations. In non-professional positions, for example, in the service industry, work schedules are increasingly unpredictable (Gerstel & Clawson, 2015). With short notice, employees are told to stay at work late or come to work early; they are sent home between shifts or their shifts are cancelled because there are not enough customers. Unpredictability in work schedules disrupt parents' and children's daily routine and create challenges with arrangements of childcare. In professional positions, control over one's schedule along with the responsibility for overseeing others may create more interference with family, as today's jobs and technologies may be more likely to spill over into home life (Schieman, Milkie & Glavin, 2009). Future research should investigate how specific occupations and workplace dynamics influence differences in levels of parental strain.

Race-Ethnicity and Nativity

Sociologists have long been interested in Black-White disparities in adult and child's well-being (Brown, Donato, Laske, & Duncan, 2013). More recently, the increase in immigration from Asia and Latin America has expanded the racial–ethnic diversity of US families (Grieco, 2010). Although sociological stress research suggests that in general racial–ethnic minorities are more likely to be exposed to various kinds of stressors than whites, little research has examined variation in parental strain by racial–ethnic group.

One explanation for variations in parenting experiences by race-ethnicity is disparities in structural resources (Nomaguchi & House, 2013). There are marked differences in structural factors across racial–ethnic groups in the USA. Black and Latino mothers are more likely than White and Asian mothers to be young, be single, have more children, and have lower family income (Aud, Fox, & KewalRamani, 2010), all of which reflect more burdens of parenting and lower levels of resources that mothers can use to deal with burdens, and thus are positively related to parental strain (Nomaguchi & Brown, 2011). Another explanation is racial–ethnic differences in parenting values (Nomaguchi & House, 2013). Prior research on parental strain has shown that mothers with an authoritarian parenting style are more likely than mothers with an authoritative parenting style to report frustration and conflict with their children (Nomaguchi & Brown, 2011). Blacks, Latinos, and Asians are more likely than Whites to use an authoritarian style of parenting, which is less tolerant of children's disrespectful behaviors and more likely to expect obedience and loyalty to parents and elders (Chao & Kanatsu, 2008; Dixon, Brooks-Gunn, & Graber, 2008). Thus, observed racial–ethnic differences in parental strain may be explained (in part) by differences in structural factors and parenting values.

One overlooked but critical note is that racial–ethnic variations are often compounded by differences in nativity. Using longitudinal data from the 1998–99 ECLS-K, Nomaguchi and House (2013) found that US-born Hispanics and

US-born Asians differed little from US-born Whites in structural factors, parenting values, and parental strain. This is not surprising given that Hispanic and Asian immigrants are likely to assimilate into the mainstream White culture, as seen in their high rates of intermarriage with Whites (Qian & Lichter, 2011). In their children's kindergarten year, foreign-born Hispanic mothers reported more parental strain than US-born White mothers because of structural factors, such as single parenthood and lower family income. Foreign-born Asian-American mothers reported more parental strain than US-born White mothers because of more authoritarian parenting values. US-born Black mothers, but not foreign-born Black mothers, reported more parental strain than US-born White mothers. From kindergarten to third grade years, only Black mothers experienced an increase in parental strain and their higher level of parental strain than other mothers was not explained by structural factors or parenting values (Nomaguchi & House, 2013).

In order to better understand these patterns, we need more research to investigate variations across racial–ethnic groups *and* nativity status in terms of specific concerns regarding raising children. Qualitative studies have illustrated that, for African-American parents, as children move from early childhood into school age, how to protect their children—especially boys—from discrimination may be a constant burden (Blum, 2015; Lareau, 2003; Putnam, 2015). Warner (2010) found that African-American parents report complex layers of safeguarding necessary to ensure the emotional health of their children in a racist world. Dow (2016) also reported that raising African-American boys, even in middle-class contexts, involves a constant pressure for mothers to protect their children from the reality that their sons are seen as dangerous and thus are likely to be subjected to harsher discipline in school and on the street. In contrast, for Asian immigrant parents, given the strong emphasis on academic achievement in the community, a primary concern may center on their children's academic success (Lee & Zhou, 2013). Further, Nomaguchi and House (2013) found that American Indian mothers report less parental strain than other mothers despite having structural disadvantages and authoritarian parenting values. Cultural differences, such as a closer kinship network and a more communal approach to childrearing (MacPhee, Fritz, & Miller-Heyl, 1996), may explain the lower level of parental strain among American Indian mothers. These studies suggest that besides common stressors, such as lack of material resources, there may be stressors that are specific to certain racial–ethnic groups due to their unique locations in a given society.

Gender and Sexual Orientation

In sociological research, gender is defined as a basic aspect of structure and culture in which "the patterning of difference and domination [is]… integral to many social processes" (Acker, 1992, p. 565). Despite expansion in women's economic roles and changes in American's attitudes about gender toward more egalitarianism, parenting remains gendered (Bianchi, Robinson, & Milkie, 2006; Milkie, Bianchi,

Mattingly, & Robinson, 2002) in terms of behaviors and cultural beliefs. Mothers are much more likely than fathers to take the primary responsibility for caring for their children (Bianchi, Robinson & Milkie, 2006). Additionally, the belief that mothers are better suited to the caregiving role than fathers appears to be persistent in the USA and other nations (Doucet, 2006), although some countries such as Sweden have striven to change this gendered belief (Johansson & Klinth, 2007). At the same time, ideal fatherhood increasingly emphasizes nurturing and involved fathers (Lamb, 2000) and fathers have increased their time in the care of children in many countries (Bianchi et al., 2006).

Despite the primary role that gender plays in influencing the levels and types of parental strain that parents experience, empirical studies that focus on gender differences in strains are scarce. National surveys often ask only one "primary" parent, which in the majority of cases are mothers, and thus many studies do not examine fathers. Very little research examines parenting stress for single fathers compared to that for single mothers. Using data from the FFCWS, which collected information regarding parental strains from both mothers and fathers, Nomaguchi and Johnson (2016) found more gender similarities than differences in the role of employment characteristics in influencing parental strain among parents with preschool children—with unemployment and inflexible work schedules being major characteristics that are related to higher levels of parental strain. In contrast, using data from the National Survey of Parents, Milkie and colleagues (2010) found gender differences in the associations between types of time spent with children and employed parents' sense of work–family balance. This is interesting, given that work–family balance is a good indicator of lower stressors for employed parents, in that interactive "quality" time is associated with mothers' feelings of balance more than fathers'. We strongly urge researchers to collect information regarding parenting stressors and mental health outcomes from both mothers and fathers.

Parents' sexual orientation is another key status that is of emerging research interest. Gays or lesbians raising children may experience stressors related to being a discriminated against sexual minority—this "minority" stress may link to their parenting experiences and their mental health (LeBlanc, Frost & Wight, 2015). Some of the challenges for gay or lesbian parents are related to different ways through which they become parents, such as through artificial insemination, surrogacy, adoption, and/or past heterosexual relationships (Manning, Fettro, & Lamid, 2014; Meezan & Rauch, 2005). In multiple ways, gay and lesbian parents may have to overcome various difficulties like discrimination or stigma in raising children that heterosexual parents may not experience. In addition, prior research on gay and lesbian parents, which mostly focused on the well-being of children, identifies various methodological challenges in studying same-sex parents, including the difficulty in obtaining a representative sample with a large enough sample size, measuring sexual orientation, and using an adequate comparison group (Carpenter & Gates, 2008; Manning et al., 2014; Meezan & Rauch, 2005; Patterson, 2006). Future studies need careful research designs to understand how the links among parenting strains, supports and mental health may depend upon sexual orientation.

Marriage and Romantic Partnerships

Marriage and romantic partnerships play an important role in influencing parental strain and mental health (Umberson, Pudovska, & Reczek, 2010). There have been notable changes in romantic partnerships in the past several decades in the USA and other Western countries (Cherlin, 2010). A relatively larger share of couples cohabitate rather than marry compared to the past. In the 2011 National Study of Family Growth (NSFG), 65% of US women aged 19–44 reported that they had ever cohabited (Manning & Stykes, 2015). And having children within a cohabiting union is increasingly common. The share of births to cohabiting women in the USA increased from 6% in the early 1980s to 25% in 2009–2013 (Manning, Brown, & Stykes, 2015). Many of these cohabiting unions do not last long. Data from the 2006–2010 NSFG showed that 40% of women's first cohabitations ended in marriage and 27% ended in dissolution, whereas 32% remained cohabiting within the three years after union formation (Copen, Daniels, & Mosher, 2013). Adults who dissolved their cohabiting unions as well as those who divorced typically recouple or remarry. In 2013, 40% of all marriages were remarriages (Lewis, Jamie, Rose, & Kreider, 2015) and close to half (46%) of adults who remarry have children from a previous marriage or relationship. Previously married adults are likely to choose to cohabitate before they remarry. In 2013, 47% of cohabiting adults were previously married (Manning, 2015). These changes in romantic partnerships may make parenting more complex. Many studies investigate how these diverse and increasingly complex mother–father relationship contexts influence child's well-being, but fewer investigate how these changes influence parental strain.

The increase in cohabitation has led to a question as to differences in parental strain between married and cohabiting parents. Using the 1999 National Survey of American Families, Brown (2004) showed that cohabitating parents were more likely to report a higher level of parental strain than married parents at the descriptive level. Using the FFCWS, Gibson-Davis (2008) found that at the bivariate level, mothers without a partner and mothers cohabiting with a new partner (i.e., their children's stepfather) reported more parental strain than mothers who live with their children's fathers. Cohabiting stepfathers reported more parental strain than fathers who are married to the mother of their children and lived with them. One question is to what extent these associations are due to what sociologists call a "selection effect." That is, men who become cohabiting stepparents are less advantaged in many ways compared to those who remain married to their children's mother or those who remarry their stepchildren's mother, including having less education and lower income (Hofferth, 2006). These antecedent differences may shape the differences in parenting stress between cohabiting stepfathers and residential biological fathers or married stepparents. Gibson-Davis (2008) used fixed-effects models, which control for unobserved antecedent characteristics that might be related to step-parenthood, cohabitation, and parental strain, and found that there was little difference in parental strain levels by family structure except that cohabiting stepfathers reported less parental strain than biological married fathers. This may be because cohabiting stepfathers assume fewer parenting responsibilities—they may be less worried about financial or emotional aspects of raising stepchildren, particularly if there is a biological father who remains connected to those children. As cohabitation becomes more common in the USA and a "legitimate" form of parental union, such differences in parenting stress between cohabiting and married (step)parents may diminish (Stavrova & Fetchenhauer, 2015).

The increase in cohabitation, which is a less stable form of union, has led to an increase in the percentage of mothers and fathers who experience more than one partnership dissolution and have children from multiple partners (Guzzo, 2014). This "multiple partner fertility" (MPF) often leads to complex co-parenting arrangements across multiple biological and social parents, which presumably leads to more strains and poorer mental health. Again, because MPF is far more likely to be experienced by economically and socially disadvantaged adults than those who are more advantaged (Guzzo, 2014), both MPF, including family complexity that MPF creates, and poorer mental health are results of such disadvantages (Turney & Carlson, 2011).

At the descriptive level, single mothers report higher parental strain than partnered mothers (Avison, Ali, & Walters, 2007). Explanations for this discrepancy focus on two different perspectives—resource versus crisis models (Amato, 2010; Williams, 2003). The resource model contends that single mothers are more likely than partnered mothers to have fewer economic resources and weaker social support, which leads to greater financial strain, overload, and work–family conflict (Nomaguchi, 2012b). Some studies support this perspective, showing that differences in parental strain by partnership status were no longer significant once SES was controlled for (Nomaguchi & Brown, 2011; Nomaguchi & Johnson, 2016). Other studies, however, show that single motherhood is related to more parental strain even after controlling for SES (Nomaguchi & House, 2013). The crisis model posits that divorce or the termination of a relationship is a stressful event, but most people are able to adjust after a while. Using longitudinal data from the FFCWS, a couple of studies (Cooper et al., 2009; Halpern-Meekin & Turney, 2016) found support for the crisis model, suggesting that longitudinal examination is critical in understanding the link between single parenthood and parental strain.

Residency status with children is important for understanding parental strain. Non-resident parents tend to feel more, not less, parental strain and poorer mental health than resident parents, perhaps because they face many constraints to support or spend time with their children and thus they feel they are not adequate as a parent (Evenson & Simon, 2005; Gibson-Davis, 2008; Nomaguchi & Milkie, 2003). Increasingly, post-divorce arrangements involve joint custody and co-parenting, which has led to an increasing diversity in living arrangements among separated parents and their children (Bakker & Karsten, 2013). Yet, we do not know much about how joint custody arrangements, which may involve coordination of childcare responsibilities and children's residential transitions between two households, influence parental strain. Based on in-depth interviews with formerly married or cohabiting parents in the Netherlands, Bakker and Karsten (2013) found that mothers with a joint custody arrangement, in which their children alternate living between parents, experience fewer constraints in combining work, childcare, and leisure. Also using Dutch data, van der Heijden, Poortman, and Van der Lippe (2016) report that for mothers, a joint custody arrangement is related to less time pressure than a sole custody (i.e., their children live mostly with them) arrangement.

The quality of the mother–father relationship plays a primary role in influencing parental strain (Umberson et al., 2010). The concepts and measures that capture relationship quality vary, including emotional support, conflict, intimate partner violence, and cooperative co-parenting (Crnic & Ross in this volume; Nomaguchi, Brown, & Leyman, 2015; Nomaguchi, Johnson, Minter, & Aldrich, 2017). To better understand how partners affect each other's stress and mental health, it is important to examine how fathers' contributions to childcare influence mothers' parental strain. Using data from the FFCWS, Nomaguchi, Brown, and Leyman (2015) found that two aspects of fathers' participation in parenting—engagement with children and participation in child-related chores—were negatively related to maternal parental strain regardless of mother–father relationship statuses (i.e., married, cohabiting, dating, separated, and repartnered). Van der Heijden, Poortman, and Van der Lippe (2016), in the Dutch study mentioned earlier, reported that sole-resident mothers experienced less time pressure when their former partner saw their child more often. Thus, given that engagement with children is related to less parental strain levels for fathers (Nomaguchi & Johnson, 2016), there is a gain for both mothers and fathers when fathers participate more. As briefly discussed earlier, however, fathers often face challenges in spending time engaged with children in daily lives due to long work hours and inflexible work schedules (Fox, 2009; Gerstel & Clawson, 2015).

There are other changes in mother–father relationship contexts that may have important implications for parental strain. One trend toward diversity in romantic relationships is the increase in interracial marriage and romantic partnership (Qian & Lichter, 2011). Research that examines parental strain among interracial or interethnic couples is rare. Interracial or interethnic couples are more likely than same-race or same-ethnic couples to have different values in childbearing and other issues (Hohmann-Marriott, & Amato, 2008), which may add another layer of challenge to parenting. Finally, it is possible that factors that are salient to parental strain may vary across family structure, family type, and residential status. For partnered parents, fairness in the division of labor and the quality of partnership may be salient sources of parental strain, whereas for single parents, lower levels of social support both in the workplace and in the household may be more relevant (e.g., Nomaguchi, 2012b). Identifying specific stressors or needs of parents that differ across different family structures is critical in informing policy-makers about effective social policies that help parents raise their children.

Life Stage

Although researchers and the public tend to focus on early childhood as the period when parenting is most stressful, sociologists using a life course perspective argue that parental strain does not stop when children reach a certain age (Pearlin, 1983). Parenthood continues throughout the entire life course, and the emotional stakes of relationships with children are high even after children are far into adulthood (Milkie et al., 2008; Umberson, 1992). However, parents' specific concerns about children change as children get older. For parents of newborns, for example, sources of strain may have more to do with physical exhaustion, and the fears of making sure the baby is properly cared for (Fox 2009; LaRossa & LaRossa, 1981). Parents of school-aged children may be more concerned about misbehavior at school, failure to achieve acceptable grades, and relationships with friends. Moreover, parent–child relationship quality begins to decline as children move from preschool to school-age as well as from school-age to adolescence (Nomaguchi, 2012a). For parents with adolescents, there are many new forms of strain potentially introduced. For example, monitoring teenagers' behavior can be quite difficult, and the kinds of trouble that adolescents may encounter (e.g., experimenting with drugs and alcohol, sex, skipping school, law breaking) can have serious consequences (Lanctôt, Cernkovich, & Giordano, 2007). Negative events in youths' lives can have a long reach—even elderly parents whose adult children had trouble years back when those offspring were adolescents are more depressed than the elderly whose adult children had fewer problems as teens (Milkie, Norris, & Bierman, 2011). Recent studies have suggested that parents of young adults continue to be heavily involved ("helicopter parents") or are relied upon as a safety net when misfortunes such as job loss or relationship dissolution happen in their children's lives (Kirkpatrick Johnson, 2013; LeMoyne & Buchanan, 2011). For aging parents, major sources of potential stressors include whether their adult children are economically independent, staying clear of legal issues, and have strong social support (e.g., Greenfield & Marks, 2006). Poorer relationship quality with adult children—conflict, unpleasant treatments, or ambivalence—is another key stressor for aging parents (Fingerman et al., 2008; Milkie et al., 2008; Umberson 1992). These studies indicate that children in each life stage may create unique stressors for parents.

Moderators in the Stress Process

As Pearlin (1989) noted, not all parents who are exposed to the same level of stressors show manifestations of stress, such as increased depression, anxiety, or anger. One reason for such differential vulnerability to stressors is differential distributions of coping resources. Although research typically focuses on social support, mastery, and individual problem-solving skills as coping resources

(Pearlin, 1999), coping resources include other types, such as financial resources and family-friendly workplace policies. Here again, sociologists focus on unequal distributions of coping resources across social locations. In general, parents with better resources, such as a higher level of education, higher earnings, and wealth, are more likely than those with limited resources to be able to better cope with challenges. For example, Cooper and colleagues (2009) found that the link between family structure transitions and parental strain are less pronounced among college educated mothers compared to mothers without college degrees. When balancing work and family life, higher-SES mothers have better resources to do so, including control over work schedules, which are related to less work–family conflict (Kelly et al., 2014). Higher-SES mothers can reduce housework hours through hiring cleaning services and ordering dinner from restaurants. Lower-SES mothers have limited options—they tend to drop out of the labor force in response to their children's needs and problems, which may result in financial strain (Budig & Hodges, 2010; Damaske, 2011; Gerstel & Clawson, 2015). Although having children with disabilities is stressful for any parent (Neece & Chan, in this volume), whether parents are economically and socially advantaged make a difference. For example, parents with more education are more likely than those with less education to easily interact with health professionals and educators, and thus receive more satisfying care for their children, which is a key factor reducing stressfulness and anxiety among parents raising children with disabilities (Hogan, 2012). It is important to note that research underscores that the same levels of parental strain could have different implications for different social groups.

Another reason for differential vulnerability to stressors in the parenting role by social groups is differences in the salience of the parenting role due to cultural ideology and structural factors. As mentioned earlier, women are more likely than men to be assumed to take the primary responsibility for raising children in the USA. These gendered cultural expectations may lead women to be more vulnerable to parental strain than men. Time strain with children has implications for mothers and fathers (Milkie et al., 2016); however, it may be more relevant for mothers' well-being as Nomaguchi, Milkie and Bianchi (2005) found that for mothers, time strain with children is associated with worse well-being, whereas for fathers, time strain for oneself, which could reflect role captivity in the parenting role, is a more important factor for life satisfaction. Salience of the parenting role may vary by race-ethnicity, too. The parenting role may be more important relative to other social roles, such as employment and marriage, for Blacks than for Whites because Blacks are more likely than Whites to face greater barriers and fewer opportunities to succeed in other social roles (Lee, Peek, & Coward, 1998). Milkie, Bierman, and Schieman (2008) found that the association between negative events experienced by adult children and aging parents' depressive symptoms was more likely to be found among Black parents than White parents, and among mothers more than fathers. Note that disparities in salience of the parenting role across different social groups change as the structured arrangements in the larger society change. For example, as gender inequality in the workplace and the mainstream culture diminishes, the gender gap in the salience of the parenting role should be narrowed, which may, in turn, lead to a narrowing gender gap in vulnerability to stressors in the parenting role.

Finally, the ability to mobilize care networks for children is a key resource, particularly in a culture which emphasizes individual or family responsibility rather than that of the larger community. Hansen (2005) found that some families were able to bolster their childrearing capacities by pulling in multiple hands to help care for their children, and creating interdependent networks to aid in their many responsibilities for their offspring. Small (2009) shows that social capital building for parents can be distinctly patterned by organizational practices that bring parents together (or do not). More research on how neighborhoods and social networks influence and may buffer parenting strain is crucial.

Other Key Factors in the Sociology of Parenting Stress

Comparisons Between Parents and Non-parents

Sociological studies on parenting stress and mental health have largely focused on the link between the parenting role and individuals' health and well-being (Umberson et al., 2010; Umberson, Thomeer, & Williams, 2013). Researchers investigate variations between parents and non-parents in various indicators such as depression (Evenson & Simon, 2005; Nomaguchi & Milkie, 2003), happiness or life satisfaction (Margolis & Myrskylä, 2011; Pollmann-Schult, 2014), loneliness (Koropeckyj-Cox, 2002), and emotions such as anger and guilt (Glavin, Schieman, & Reid, 2011; Ross & Van Willigen, 1996). Explanations for such effects lie in differences between parents and non-parents in exposure to social stressors in major life domains—work, marriage, and leisure. Major stressors include financial strains, relationship strains, and time strains (Nomaguchi & Milkie, 2003; Pollmann-Schult, 2014). These studies conceptualize that the demands of parenting proliferate into other domains, such as work or marriage and romantic partnership, increase work stress or relationship stress, and in turn may lead to poorer mental health.

Comparisons with non-parents are useful because results can reveal the social arrangements that are lacking in supports for adults who take care of dependents. The type of "non-parent" researchers compared to parents is vital—are those considered "non-parents" people who already reared children who are no longer in the household (and thus an age control is necessary)?; are they step-parents and/or perhaps have children living elsewhere?; or are they those who never had biological or step-children (in which issues of desirability and intentions for having children should be considered) (Nomauchi & Milkie, 2003)? Research using careful comparisons of parents and non-parents shows that parents fare worse in mental health and well-being by some, but not all measures, and this varies by social status (Nomaguchi & Milkie, 2003). In certain ways, parents may be better off, such as experiencing more meaning in life (Umberson et al., 2010).

To understand parents' well-being, it is important both to compare non-parents to parents and to expand our understanding of sources and mediators of stressors that parents experience uniquely and to greater extents or depths than non-parents. To better understand the mechanisms and variation by social contexts, it is important to examine specific forms of parental strain. One reason for focusing on more general mental health or well-being indicators, rather than parental strain, may be due to data limitations. Sociologists use national surveys that are designed to cover various issues and often include non-parents. Questions for everyone, not just parents, are more likely to be included in national surveys. We encourage researchers to include parental strain questions in ongoing large-scale data collections.

Cross-National Comparisons

Parenting experiences vary across different countries in part because the degree in which countries rely on individual family members to take care of the dependents—children and the elderly—varies. Several studies find cross-national variations in life satisfaction disparities by parental status (e.g., Aassve, Mencarini, & Sironi, 2015; Aassve, Goisis, & Sironi, 2012; Glass et al., 2016). Margolis and Myrskylä (2011) show that the link between the number of children and life satisfaction depends on life stage of the individuals and welfare regime of the county in which they live. Using data from the World Values Surveys (WVS), which include 86 countries, they found that overall the number of children is negatively related to happiness among those aged less than 30 years old, whereas it is positively related to happiness among those aged 40 or older. There is little association between the number of children and happiness among those aged 30–39. The negative association between the number of children and happiness among the youngest group is weakest in countries with high public support for families (e.g., Denmark and Sweden). The positive association between the number of children and happiness among the older age group is stronger in developing countries where support for the elderly depends mostly on the family. Similar patterns are found in a study by Aassve, Goisis, and Sironi (2012) that used the European Social Survey. Glass, Simon, and Andersson (2016) report that happiness disparities by parental status are larger for the USA than the other 21 OECD countries in part because of less generous policies such as subsidized childcare and paid leave. These studies indicate that institutional contexts in a larger society play a critical role in shaping the burdens and rewards of parenting.

In sum, the burden of being a parent is heavy. Parents must provide financially and socially for their children whereas, obviously, non-parents do not. They must provide enough monetary resources to invest in housing, clothing, food, health care, and so on, for these dependents, which can create financial strain, work overload, or both. While providing financially, they must figure out often complex childcare arrangements during work hours in the early years, and as children age, for after-school hours and summertime for many years. Simultaneously, parents must have the time, stamina, and energy to establish and maintain close ties with children as they manage and shape parent–child time and the child's independent social activities. They must plan and meet challenges related to the child's well-being. Non-parents simply do not have these incredibly extensive obligations in raising the next generation and are thus freed from the many and varied strains inherent in the parent role. While the work of parenting is heavy, it can be greatly supported, although public and workplace monetary and social supports in some countries, including the USA, are quite thin.

Conclusions

Parents face a multitude of pressures and difficulties that arise and are often sustained over the many years that children develop from helpless infants to mature adults. A sociological perspective is unique in that it "zooms out" to assess the "big picture" affecting parents—the social and economic statuses, the wider social and cultural milieu in which parents live—such as local communities, ethnic cultures, and nations—and the social changes which create new and different strains for parents. Knowing these structural and cultural factors can explain much variation in which parents experience strains, and thus potentially poorer mental health. Besides common stressors in parenting such as overload, parent–child relationship strain, caregiving strain or role captivity, financial strain, and work-family conflict, contemporary parents may be facing new types of challenges that parents from previous generations have not experienced. In addition to what we discussed above, there are several important venues for future research in sociological perspectives on parenting stress that will help advance the field.

First, more conceptual advancement in the study of the stress of parenting and their families is vital. The concept of *stress proliferation* in the stress process model would be useful to purse for parenting scholars. For example, we know that low-income parents may face a wide range of stressors, such as difficulties in unemployment, financial strain, arranging childcare, work–family conflict, major traumas and adversities, a history of intimate partner violence, incarceration, single parenthood, and ambient stressors reflecting neighborhood environments. Yet, we know less about the mechanisms through which these stressors proliferate from one to another arena for different groups of parents, as well as from one generation of parents to the next. As Pearlin (1999) noted, it is important to identify primary—or initial—stressors that are likely to lead to secondary stressors to understand why some people are more vulnerable than others, who hold similar social statuses and roles, to the same sets of stressors.

Additionally, understanding the stress process that involves multiple family members is warranted. As Milkie has written elsewhere (2010), stressful experiences confronting parents and families may be unequally shared, with mothers perhaps taking responsibility more often for trying to address "family" or children's problems as they arise. Examining how difficulties—large and small—such as financial setbacks, housing concerns, migration problems, and children's peer or health troubles come to be taken on as the burden of one parent, and how mothers and fathers may or may not share a sense of family togetherness or mastery in solving their problems may be fruitful venues for future research.

The poignant and profound moment that occurs when a mother or father holds a child for the first time signals that parenting is a life-long process. Life course scholars (Milkie et al., 2008; Umberson et al., 2010) contend that it is crucial to assess how parenting shapes life experiences and influences the well-being of adults over the life course. How different trajectories vary by the social statuses of parents is of central concern. For example, although many mothers experience disruptions of employment activities due to their children's schedules and needs, mothers with less education are more likely than mothers with a college degree to experience a greater number of disruptions, which is related to poorer health outcomes (Frech & Damaske, 2012). Avison (2010) urges researchers to investigate life course patterns of single mothers' exposures to a wide range of stressors in the broader scope of life span including their own childhood experiences.

Although studies tend to focus on strains and challenges, research suggests that parenthood also brings resources and facilitates adult's well-being. Sociological work assessing the contrasting costs and rewards of parenting can be expanded. For example, having children who are minors expands social networks with extended family members, other parents, and people who are engaged in carework such as childcare workers, teachers, and volunteers in the community (Gallagher & Gerstel, 2001; Nomaguchi & Milkie, 2003), although it may curtail social networks with adults without children (Munch, McPherson, & Smith-Lovin, 1997). Emotional gains from having children may include a sense of purpose, life meaning, responsibility, and direction in life (Edin & Kefalas, 2005; Umberson & Gove, 1989). Better relationship quality with their children leads to better psychological well-being (Nomaguchi, 2012a, b; Umberson, 1992). Some quantitative studies have considered both costs and benefits of parenting (Gove & Underson, 1989; Nomaguchi & Brown, 2011; Nomaguchi & Milkie, 2003; Pollmann-Schult, 2014). Children with special needs may strain parents' marriages and sibling relationships, but they also make their families have more family-centered lives, eating meals, playing games, or watching television together (Hogan, 2012). We need more research to investigate under which conditions and in which cultures parenting produces more stressors than resources. Similarly, studies investigating potential new supports as well as new stressors that parents today experience, compared to those in the past, will expand the field.

In all, mothers and fathers produce vital public goods—healthy children—and parents need a great deal of support to accomplish the ongoing and often arduous work of raising children. Along the life course, many potential roadblocks to successful parenting arise, particularly for those in society with less advantaged statuses, and with fewer social and economic resources. National and workplace policies can help alleviate some stressors of parenting, through help in providing paid leaves, tax relief, high-quality childcare and schooling, health care, university tuition support, and so on. Understanding the most important social factors supporting parents can go a long way in helping the multitudes of mothers and fathers on the front lines of the daily work of caring for the next generation of citizens.

References

Aassve, A., Goisis, A., & Sironi, M. (2012). Happiness and childbearing across Europe. *Social Indicators Research, 108*(1), 65–86.

Aassve, A., Mencarini, L., & Sironi, M. (2015). Institutional Change, Happiness, and Fertility. *European Sociological Review, 31*(6), 749–765.

Abidin, R. R. (2012). *Parenting stress index* (4th ed.). Lutz, FL: Psychological Assessment Resources.

Acker, J. (1992). From sex roles to gendered institutions. *Contemporary Sociology, 21*(5), 565–569.

Alwin, D. F. (1989). Changes in qualities valued in children in the United States, 1964 to 1984. *Social Science Research, 18*(3), 195–236.

Amato, P. R. (2010). Research on divorce: Continuing trends and new developments. *Journal of marriage and family, 72*(3), 650–666.

Aud, S., Fox, M., KewalRamani, A. (2010). Status and trends in the education of racial and ethnic groups. (NCES 2010–015). Washington, DC: U.S. Government Printing Office.

Avison, W.R. (2010). Family structure and women's lives: A life course perspective. In W.R. Avison et al. (eds.), *Advances in the conceptualization of the stress process: Essays in honor of Leonard I. Pearlin* (pp. 71–92). New York:Springer.

Avison, W. R., Ali, J., & Walters, D. (2007). Family structure, stress, and psychological distress: A demonstration of the impact of differential exposure. *Journal of Health and Social Behavior, 48*(3), 301–317.

Bakker, W., & Karsten, L. (2013). Balancing paid work, care and leisure in post-separation households: A comparison of single parents with co-parents. *Acta Sociologica, 56*(2), 173–187.

Beck, U., & Beck-Gernsheim, E. (1995). *The normal chaos of love*. Malden, MA: Polity Press.

Bianchi, S. M. (2011). Family change and time allocation in American families. *The ANNALS of the American Academy of Political and Social Science, 638*(1), 21–44.

Bianchi, S. M., & Milkie, M. A. (2010). Work and family research in the first decade of the 21st century. *Journal of Marriage and Family, 72*(3), 705–725.

Bianchi, S. M., Robinson, J. P., & Milke, M. A. (2006). *Changing rhythms of American family life*. New York: Russell Sage Foundation.

Bird, C. E. (1997). Gender differences in the social and economic burdens of parenting and psychological distress. *Journal of Marriage and the Family, 59*(4), 809–823.

Blum, L. M. (2015). *Raising generation Rx: Mothering kids with invisible disabilities in an age of inequality*. New York: New York University Press.

Brown, S. L. (2004). Family structure and child well-being: the significance of parental cohabitation. *Journal of Marriage and Family, 66*(2), 351–367.

Brown, T. N., Donato, K. M., Laske, M. T., & Duncan, E. M. (2013). Race, nativity, ethnicity, and cultural influences in the sociology of mental health. In *Handbook of the sociology of mental health* (pp. 255–276). Netherlands:Springer.

Budig, M. J., & Hodges, M. J. (2010). Differences in disadvantage variation in the motherhood penalty across white women's earnings distribution. *American Sociological Review, 75*(5), 705–728.

Carpenter, C., & Gates, G. J. (2008). Gay and lesbian partnership: Evidence from California. *Demography, 45*(3), 573–590.

Carson, E. A., & Golinelli, D. (2013). Prisoners in 2012. *Bureau of Justice Statistics, December, 2*(3).

Cassells, R. & Evans, G. (in this volume). Ethnic variation in poverty and parenting stress.
Chao, R., & Kanatsu, A. (2008). Beyond socioeconomics: Explaining ethnic group differences in parenting through cultural and immigration processes. *Applied Developmental Science, 12*(4), 181–187.
Cherlin, A. J. (2010). Demographic trends in the United States: A review of research in the 2000s. *Journal of Marriage and Family, 72*(3), 403–419.
Coles, R. L. (2009). Just Doing What They Gotta Do Single Black Custodial Fathers Coping With the Stresses and Reaping the Rewards of Parenting. *Journal of Family Issues, 30*(10), 1311–1338.
Conger, R. D., Ge, X., Elder, G. H., Lorenz, F. O., & Simons, R. L. (1994). Economic stress, coercive family process, and developmental problems of adolescents. *Child Development, 65* (2), 541–561.
Cooper, C. E., McLanahan, S. S., Meadows, S. O., & Brooks-Gunn, J. (2009). Family structure transitions and maternal parenting stress. *Journal of Marriage and Family, 71*(3), 558–574.
Copen CE, Daniels K, Mosher WD. (2013). First premarital cohabitation in the United States: 2006–2010 National Survey of Family Growth. National health statistics reports; no 64. Hyattsville, MD: National Center for Health Statistics.
Crnic, K. & Ross, E. (in this volume). Parenting stress and parental efficacy.
Damaske, S. (2011). *For the family? How class and gender shape women's work*. New York: Oxford University Press.
Deater-Deckard, K. D. (2004). *Parenting stress*. New Haven, CT: Yale University Press.
Denny, K., Brewton-Tiayon, S., Lykke, L. C., & Milkie, M. A. (2014). Admonished, then excused: portrayals of fathers' low levels of involvement with children across the 20th and 21st centuries. *Fathering, 12*(3), 221–241.
Dixon, S. V., Brooks-Gunn, J., & Graber, J. A. (2008). The roles of respect for parental authority and parenting practices in parent-child conflict among African American, Latino, and European American families. *Journal of Family Psychology, 22*(1), 1–10.
Dow, D. M. (2016). The Deadly Challenges of Raising African American Boys Navigating the Controlling Image of the "Thug". *Gender & Society, 30*(2), 161–188.
Doucet, A. (2006). *Do men mother? Fathering, care, and domestic responsibility*. Toronto, ON: University of Toronto Press.
Edin, K., & Kefalas, M. (2005). *Promises I can keep: Why poor women put motherhood before marriage*. Berkeley, CA: University of California Press.
Elder, G. H. (1999). *Children of the Great Depression: Social change in life experience, 25th* (anniversary ed.). Boulder, CO: Westview Press.
Elliott, S., Powell, R., & Brenton, J. (2015). Being a good mom: Low-income, black single mothers negotiate intensive mothering. *Journal of Family Issues, 36*(3), 351–370.
Evenson, R. J., & Simon, R. (2005). Clarifying the relationship between parenthood and depression. *Journal of Health and Social Behavior, 46*(4), 341–358.
Finegood, E. D., & Blair, C. (in this volume). Relating poverty and parenting stress to emergent executive functions in young children.
Fingerman, K. L., Pitzer, L., Lefkowitz, E. S., Birditt, K. S., & Mroczek, D. (2008). Ambivalent relationship qualities between adults and their parents: Implications for the well-being of both parties. *Journal of Gerontology B Series, 63,* P362–P371.
Fox, B. (2009). *When couples become parents: The creation of gender in the transition to parenthood*. University of Toronto Press.
Frech, A., & Damaske, S. (2012). The relationships between mothers' work pathways and physical and mental health. *Journal of Health and Social Behavior, 53*(4), 396–412.
Gallagher, S. K., & Gerstel, N. (2001). Connections and Constraints: The Effects of Children on Caregiving. *Journal of Marriage and Family, 63*(1), 265–275.
Gerstel, N., & Clawson, D. (2015). Class advantage and the gender divide: Flexibility on the job and at home. *American Journal of Sociology, 120*(2), 395–431.
Gibson-Davis, C. M. (2008). Family structure effects on maternal and paternal parenting in low-income families. *Journal of Marriage and Family, 70*(2), 452–465.

Glass, J., Simon, R. W., & Andersson, K. G. (2016). Parenthood and happiness: Effects of work-family reconciliation policies in 22 OECD countries. *American Journal of Sociology*. In press.

Glavin, P., Schieman, S., & Reid, S. (2011). Boundary-spanning work demands and their consequences for guilt and psychological distress. *Journal of Health and Social Behvaior, 52* (1), 43–57.

Glaze, L. E., & Maruschak, L. M. (2008). *Parents in prison and their minor children*. (Bureau of Justice Statistics Special Report). Washington, DC: Bureau of Justice Statistics.

Goode, W. J. (1960). A theory of role strain. *American Sociological Review, 25*(4), 483–496.

Green, K. M., Ensminger, M. E., Robertson, J. A., & Juon, H. S. (2006). Impact of adult sons' incarceration on African American mothers' psychological distress. *Journal of Marriage and Family, 68*(2), 430–441.

Greenfield, E., & Marks, N. (2006). Linked lives: Adult children's problems and their parents' psychological and relational well-being. *Journal of Marriage and Family, 68*(2), 442–454.

Grieco, E. (2010). Race and Hispanic origin of the foreign-born population in the United States: 2007. *American community survey reports*, ACS-11. Washington, DC: U.S. Census Bureau.

Guzzo, K. B. (2014). New partners, more kids multiple-partner fertility in the United States. *The ANNALS of the American Academy of Political and Social Science, 654*(1), 66–86.

Halpern-Meekin, S., & Turney, K. (2016). Relationship churning and parenting stress among mothers and fathers. *Journal of Marriage and Family, 78*(3), 715–729.

Hansen, K. V. (2005). *Not-so-nuclear families: Class, gender, and networks of care*. New Brunswick, NJ: Rutgers University Press.

Hays, S. (1996). *The cultural contradictions of motherhood*. New Haven and London: Yale University Press.

Hofferth, S. L. (2006). Residential father family type and child well-being: Investment versus selection. *Demography, 43*(1), 53–77.

Hogan, D. (2012). *Family consequences of children's disabilities*. New York: Russell Sage Foundation.

Hohmann-Marriot, B. E., & Amato, P. (2008). Relationship quality in interethnic marriages and cohabitations. *Social Forces, 87*(2), 825–855.

House, J. (1981). Social structure and personality. In M. Rosenberg & R. H. Turner (Eds.), *Social psychology: Social perspectives* (pp. 525–561). New Brunswick, NJ: Transaction Publishers.

Johansson, T., & Klinth, R. (2007). Caring fathers: The ideology of gender equality and masculine positions. *Men and masculinities, 11*(1), 42–62.

Kelly, E. L., Moen, P., Oakes, J. M., Fan, W., Okechukwu, C., Davis, K. D., et al. (2014). Changing work and work-family conflict evidence from the work, family, and health network. *American Sociological Review, 79*(3), 485–516.

Kirkpatrick Johnson, M. (2013). Parental Financial Assistance and Young Adults' Relationships With Parents and Well-being. *Journal of Marriage and Family, 75*(3), 713–733.

Koropeckyj-Cox, T. (2002). Beyond parental status: Psychological well-being in middle and old age. *Journal of Marriage and Family, 64*(4), 957–971.

Kurz, D. (2000). Work-family issues of mothers of teenage children. *Qualitative Sociology, 23*(4), 435–451.

Kurz, D. (2006). Keeping tabs on teenagers. In J. F. Gubruim & J. A. Holstein (Eds.), *Couples, kids, and family life* (pp. 84–103). New York: Oxford University Press.

Lamb, M. E. (2000). The history of research on father involvement: An overview. *Marriage & Family Review, 29*(2–3), 23–42.

Lanctôt, N., Cernkovich, S. A., & Giordano, P. C. (2007). Delinquent behavior, official delinquency, and gender: consequences for adulthood functioning and well-being. *Criminology, 45*(1), 131–157.

Lareau, A. (2003). *Unequal childhood: Class, race, and family life*. Berkeley, CA: University of California Press.

LaRossa, R., & LaRossa, M. M. (1981). *Transition to parenthood*. Sage Publications.

Lazarus, R. S., & Folkman, S. (1984). *Stress, appraisal, and coping*. New York: Springer.

LeBlanc, A. J., Frost, D. M., & Wight, R. G. (2015). Minority stress and stress proliferation among same-sex and other marginalized couples. *Journal of Marriage and Family, 77*(1), 40–59.
Lee, G. R., Peek, C. W., & Coward, R. T. (1998). Race differences in filial responsibility expectations among older parents. *Journal of Marriage and the Family, 60,* 404–412.
Lee, J., & Zhou, M. (2013). Frames of achievement and opportunity horizons: Second-generation Chinese, Vietnamese, and Mexicans in Los Angeles. In D. Card & S. Raphael (Eds.), *Immigration, poverty, and socioeconomic inequality* (pp. 206–231). New York: Russell Sage Foundation.
LeMoyne, T., & Buchanan, T. (2011). Does "hovering" matter? Helicopter parenting and its effect on well-being. *Sociological Spectrum, 31*(4), 399–418.
Lewis, Jamie M. and Rose M. Kreider. (2015). *Remarriage in the United States.* U.S. Census Bureau, Washington, DC. *American Community Survey Reports*, ACS-30.
MacPhee, D., Fritz, J., & Miller-Heyl, J. (1996). Ethnic variations in personal social networks and parenting. *Child Development, 67*(6), 3278–3295.
Manning, W. D. (2015). Remarriage is–and is not–what it used to be: new report outlines diverse trends. Brief Report, Council on Contemporary Families June 2. Retrieved from: https://contemporaryfamilies.org/remarriage-brief-report/.
Manning, W. D., Brown, S. L., & Stykes, B. (2015). Trends in births to single and cohabiting mothers, 1980 – 2013. National Center for Family & Marriage Research.
Manning, W. D., Fettro, M. N., & Lamidi, E. (2014). Child well-being in same-sex parent families: Review of research prepared for American Sociological Association Amicus Brief. *Population Research and Policy Review, 33*(4), 485–502.
Manning, W. D., & Stykes, B. (2015). Twenty-five years of changes in cohabitation in the U.S., 1987 – 2013. (FP-15–01). National Center for Family & Marriage Research.
Margolis, R., & Myrskylä, M. (2011). A global perspective on happiness and fertility. *Population and Development Review, 37*(1), 29–56.
Meezan, W., & Rauch, J. (2005). Gay marriage, same-sex parenting, and America's children. *The Future of Children, 15*(2), 97–113.
Milkie, M. A. (2010). The stress process model: Some family-level considerations. In W.R. Avison et al. (eds.), *Advances in the conceptualization of the stress process: Essays in honor of Leonard I. Pearlin* (pp. 93–108). New York:Springer.
Milkie, M. A., Bianchi, S. M., Mattingly, M. J., & Robinson, J. P. (2002). Gendered division of childrearing: Ideals, realities, and the relationship to parental well-being. *Sex Roles, 47*(1/2), 21–38.
Milkie, M. A., Bierman, A., & Schieman, S. (2008). How adult children influence older parents' mental health: Integrating stress-process and life-course perspectives. *Social Psychology Quarterly, 71*(1), 86–105.
Milkie, M. A., & Denny, K. E. (2014). Changes in the cultural model of father involvement: Descriptions of benefits to fathers, children and mothers in Parents' Magazine, 1926–2006. *Journal of Family Issues, 35*(2), 223–253.
Milkie, M. A., Kendig, S. M., Nomaguchi, K. M., & Denny, K. E. (2010). Time with children, children's well-being, and work-family balance among employed parents. *Journal of Marriage and Family, 72*(5), 1329–1343.
Milkie, M. A., Mattingly, M. J., Nomaguchi, K. M., Bianchi, S. M., & Robinson, J. P. (2004). The time squeeze: Parental statuses and feelings about time with children. *Journal of Marriage and Family, 66,* 739–761.
Milkie, M. A., Nomaguchi, K., & Schieman, S. (2016). Time deficits with children: The relationship to mothers' and fathers' mental and physical health. Paper presented at the 2016 Annual Meeting of the American Sociological Association, Seattle, WA.
Milkie, M. A., Norris, N., & Bierman, A. (2011). The long arm of offspring: Adult children's troubles as teenagers and elderly parents' mental health. *Research on Aging, 33*(3), 327–355.
Milkie, M. A., Raley, S. B., & Bianchi, S. M. (2009). Taking on the second shift: Time allocations and time pressures of US parents with preschoolers. *Social Forces, 88*(2), 487–517.

Milkie, M. A., & Warner, C. H. (2014). Status safeguarding: Mothering work as safety net. In L. Ennis (Ed.), *Intensive mothering: The cultural contradictions of modern motherhood* (pp. 66–85). Bradford, ON: Demeter Press.

Mirowsley, J., & Ross, C. E. (2003). *Social causes of psychological distress* (2nd ed.). Hawthorne, NY: Aldine de Gruyter.

Munch, A., McPherson, J. M., & Smith-Lovin, L. (1997). Gender, children, and social contact: The effects of childrearing for men and women. *American Sociological Review, 62*(4), 509–520.

Musick, K., England, P., Edgington, S., & Kangas, N. (2009). Education differences in intended and unintended fertility. *Social Forces, 88*(2), 543–572.

Neece, C. L., & Chan, N. (in this volume). The Stress of parenting children with developmental disabilities.

Nelson, M. K. (2010). *Parenting out of control: Anxious parents in uncertain times*. New York: New York University Press.

Nomaguchi, K. M. (2009). Change in work-family conflict among employed parents between 1977 and 1997. *Journal of Marriage and Family, 71*(1), 15–32.

Nomaguchi, K. M. (2012a). Parenthood and psychological well-being: Clarifying the role of child age and parent-child relationship quality. *Social Science Research, 41*(2), 489–498.

Nomaguchi, K. M. (2012b). Marital status, gender, and home-to-job conflict among employed parents. *Journal of Family Issues, 33*(3), 271–294.

Nomaguchi, K. M., & Brown, S. L. (2011). Parental strains and rewards among mothers: The role of education. *Journal of Marriage and Family, 73*(3), 621–636.

Nomaguchi, K., Brown, S.L., & Leyman, T. M. (2015). Father involvement and mothers' parenting stress: The role of relationship status. *Journal of Family Issues*. Published online, December 2015.

Nomaguchi, K., & Fettro, M. N. (2016). Mothers' employment patterns in early childhood and child outcomes at age 15. Paper presented at the 2016 Annual Meeting of the American Sociological Association, Seattle, WA.

Nomaguchi, K., & House, A. N. (2013). Racial-ethnic disparities in maternal parenting stress: The role of structural disadvantages and parenting values. *Journal of Health and Social Behavior, 54*(3), 386–404.

Nomaguchi, K., & Johnson, W. (2016). Parenting stress among low-income and working-class fathers: The role of employment. *Journal of Family Issues.* Forthcoming in August issue.

Nomaguchi, K., Johnson, W. L., Minter, M., & Aldrich, L. (2017) Clarifying the association between mother-father relationship aggression and parenting. *Journal of Marriage and Family*, *79*(1), 161–178.

Nomaguchi, K. M., & Milkie, M. (2003). Costs and rewards of children: The effects of becoming a parent on adults' lives. *Journal of Marriage and Family, 66*(2), 413–430.

Nomaguchi, K., & Milkie, M. A. (2016). "You must work hard": Changes in U.S. adults' values for children, 1986 – 2014. Paper presented at the 2016 Annual Meeting of American Sociological Association. Seattle, WA.

Nomaguchi, K. M., Milkie, M., & Bianchi, S. (2005). Time strains and psychological well-being: Do dual-earner mothers and fathers differ? *Journal of Family Issues, 26*(6), 756–792.

Patterson, C. J. (2006). Children of lesbian and gay parents. *Current Directions in Psychological Science, 15*(5), 241–244.

Pearlin, L. I. (1983). *Role strains and personal stress* (pp. 3–32). Psychosocial stress: Trends in theory and research.

Pearlin, L. I. (1989). The sociological study of stress. *Journal of Health and Social Behavior, 30* (3), 241–256.

Pearlin, L. I. (1999). The stress process revisited. In C. S. Aneshensel & J. C. Phelan (Eds.), *Handbook of the sociology of mental health* (pp. 395–415). New York: Kluwer Academic/Plenum Publishers.

Pearlin, L. I., & Bierman, A. (2013). Current issues and future directions in research into the stress process. In C. Aneshensel, J. C. Phelan, & A. Bierman (Eds.), *Handbook of the sociology of mental health* (pp. 325–340). Netherlands: Springer.

Pearlin, L. I., Menaghan, E. G., Lieberman, M. A., & Mullan, J. T. (1981). The stress process. *Journal of Health and Social behavior*, 337–356.

Pillemer, K., & Suitor, J. J. (1991). Will I ever escape my child's problems? Effects of adult children's problems on elderly parents. *Journal of Marriage and Family, 53*(3), 585–594.

Pollmann-Schult, M. (2014). Parenthood and Life Satisfaction: Why Don't Children Make People Happy? *Journal of Marriage and Family, 76*(2), 319–336.

Presser, H. B. (2000). Nonstandard work schedules and marital instability. *Journal of Marriage and Family, 62*(1), 93–110.

Putnam, R. D. (2015). *Our kids: The American dream in crisis*. New York, NY: Simon & Schuster.

Qian, Z., & Lichter, D. T. (2011). Changing patterns of interracial marriage in a multiracial society. *Journal of Marriage and Family, 73*(5), 1065–1084.

Ross, C. E., & Mirowsky, J. (1988). Child care and emotional adjustment to wives' employment. *Journal of Health and Social Behavior, 29*(2), 127–138.

Ross, C. E., & Van Willigen, M. (1996). Gender, Parenthood, and Anger. *Journal of Marriage and the Family, 58*(3), 572–584.

Ross, C. E., & Van Willigen, M. (1997). Education and the subjective quality of life. *Journal of Health and Social Behavior, 38*(3), 275–297.

Rutherford, M. B. (2011). *Adult Supervision Required: Private Freedom and Public Constraints for Parents and Children*. New Brunswick, NJ: Rutgers University Press.

Schieman, S., & Glavin, P. (2011). Education and work-family conflict: Explanations, contingencies and mental health consequences. *Social Forces, 89*(4), 1341–1362.

Schieman, S., Milkie, M. A., & Glavin, P. (2009). When work interferes with life: Work-nonwork interference and the influence of work-related demands and resources. *American Sociological Review, 74*(6), 966–988.

Simon, R. W. (1992). Parental role strains, salience of parental identity and gender differences in psychologial distress. *Journal of Health and Social Behavior, 33*(1), 25–35.

Small, M. L. (2009). *Unanticipated gains: Origins of network inequality in everyday life*. New York: Oxford University Press.

Spitze, G., Logan, J. R., Deane, G., & Zerger, S. (1994). Adult children's divorce and intergenerational relationships. *Journal of Marriage and Family, 56*(2), 279–293.

Stavrova, O., & Fetchenhauer, D. (2015). Married and cohabiting parents' well-being: The effects of a cultural normative context across countries. *Journal of Social and Personal Relationships, 32*(5), 601–632.

Strazdins, L., Clements, M. S., Korda, R. J., Broom, D. H., & D'Souza, R. M. (2006). Unsociable work? Nonstandard work schedules, family relationships, and children's well-being. *Journal of Marriage and Family, 68*(2), 394–410.

Su, J. H. (2012). Pregnancy Intentions and Parents' Psychological Well-Being. *Journal of Marriage and Family, 74*(5), 1182–1196.

Swisher, R. R., & Waller, M. R. (2008). Confining fatherhood incarceration and paternal involvement among nonresident white, African American, and Latino fathers. *Journal of Family Issues, 29*(8), 1067–1088.

Turney, K., & Carlson, M. J. (2011). Multipartnered fertility and depression among Fragile Families. *Journal of Marriage and Family, 73,* 570–587.

Turney, K., & Wildeman, C. (2013). Redefining Relationships Explaining the Countervailing Consequences of Paternal Incarceration for Parenting. *American Sociological Review, 78*(6), 949–979.

Umberson, D. (1992). Relationships between adult children and their parents: Psychological consequences for both generations. *Journal of Marriage and the Family, 54*(3), 664–674.

Umberson, D., & Gove, W. R. (1989). Parenthood and psychological well-being theory, measurement, and stage in the family life course. *Journal of Family Issues, 10*(4), 440–462.

Umberson, D., Pudrovska, T., & Reczek, C. (2010). Parenthood, childlessness, and well-being: A life course perspective. *Journal of Marriage and Family, 72*(3), 612–629.
Umberson, D., Thomeer, M., & Williams, K. (2013). Family status and mental health: Recent advances and future directions. In C. S. Aneshensel & J. C. Phelan (Eds.), *Handbook of the Sociology of mental health* (2nd ed., pp. 405–431). United States: Springer Publishing.
van der Heijden, F., Poortman, A.-R., & Van der Lippe, T. (2016). Children's Postdivorce Residence Arrangements and Parental Experienced Time Pressure. *Journal of Marriage and Family, 78*(2), 468–481.
Villalobos, A. (2014). *Motherload: Making it all better in insecure times*. Berkeley: University of California Press.
Ward, R. (2008). Multiple parent-adult child relations and well-being in middle and later life. *Journal of Gerontology Series B, 63,* S239–S247.
Warner, C. H. (2010). Emotional safeguarding: Exploring the nature of middle-class parents' school involvement. *Sociological Forum, 25*(4), 703–724.
Wheaton, B., Young, M/. Montazer, S., & Stuart-Lahman, K. (2013). Social stress in the twenty-first century. In C. Aneshensel, J. C. Phelan, & A. Bierman (Eds.), *Handbook of sociology of mental health* (2nd ed., pp. 299–323). Springer.
Wildeman, C., Schnittker, J., & Turney, K. (2012). Despair by association? The mental health of mothers with children and recently incarcerated fathers. *American Sociological Review, 77*(2), 216–243.
Williams, K. (2003). Has the future of marriage arrived? A contemporary examination of gender, marriage, and psychological well-being. *Journal of Health and Social Behavior, 44*(4), 470–487.

Chapter 4
Parental Stress and Child Temperament

Maureen E. McQuillan and John E. Bates

Parental stress is generally associated with poor adjustment outcomes in children, including insecure attachment and behavior problems (Jarvis & Creasy, 1991; Cummings & El-Sheikh, 1991; Thompson, Merritt, Keith, Bennett, & Johndrow, 1993). Some prevention and intervention efforts focus on this association (Kaaresen, Rønning, Ulvund, & Dahl, 2006; Nair, Schuler, Black, Kettinger, & Harrington, 2003; Piquero, Farrington, Welsh, Tremblay, & Jennings, 2009; Sanders, 1999; Turner & Sanders, 2006; Wolfe, Edwards, Manion, & Koverola, 1988; Zubrick et al., 2005). However, at this point, the processes explaining the association between parental stress and child adjustment have not been clearly established. Consideration of mediating and moderating processes underlying the link between stress and child functioning will aid the development of prevention and intervention efforts. Research does suggest that highly stressed parents tend to use harsh or otherwise ineffective parenting practices (Belsky, Woodworth, & Crnic, 1996; Rodgers, 1993). At extreme levels, parental stress can even result in child abuse and neglect (Chan, 1994; Holden & Banez, 1996). Further, parental stress can negatively affect parent adjustment, specifically physical health and psychological well-being (DeLongis, Coyne, Dakof, Folkman, & Lazarus, 1982; Gelfand, Teti, & Fox, 1992).

Parental stress can be further exacerbated by challenges due to child temperament. Temperament refers to individual differences in reactivity and self-regulation that are biologically based and shaped over time, at least at the phenotypic level of expression, by maturation and experience (Rothbart & Bates, 2006). Several dimensions of child temperament, including fearfulness, effortful self-regulation,

M.E. McQuillan (✉) · J.E. Bates
Department of Psychological and Brain Sciences, Indiana University, Bloomington, IN, USA
e-mail: memcquil@umail.iu.edu

J.E. Bates
e-mail: batesj@indiana.edu

K. Deater-Deckard and R. Panneton (eds.), *Parental Stress and Early Child Development*, DOI 10.1007/978-3-319-55376-4_4

and difficultness, are associated with child adjustment outcomes and can also influence parental stress. Early fearfulness is associated with later internalizing behavior problems, such as anxiety, more so than with externalizing problems, such as aggression. Early effortful self-regulation deficits are associated with later externalizing problems more so than internalizing problems. Difficultness, which is here defined as a disposition to constitutionally based negative emotional reactivity, predicts both internalizing and externalizing equally (Rothbart & Bates, 2006; Bates, Schermerhorn, & Petersen, 2012). Behavior problems and their temperamental underpinnings can create challenges for parents, including disruption in the family system, increased time demands, and parent feelings of frustration, worry, guilt, and/or embarrassment regarding their child's behavior (Bussing et al., 2003). In addition, parent stress and its consequences for parenting may affect child experiences, and children's response to parental stress and behavior may depend on their temperament. Some children develop negative adjustment outcomes when exposed to high levels of parental stress, while others demonstrate more resilience (Barton & Zeanah, 1990). As a further complication, to the extent that these temperament dimensions are separable, there is also the possibility of interactions between the various temperament dimensions and their effects on child problem behavior and parent stress (Bates, Schermerhorn, & Petersen, 2014). For example, a negatively reactive child who has good effortful control will not create as many hassles for a parent as a reactive child with low effortful control. An emotionally reactive child with good regulation can be less affected by the parents' stress than a similarly reactive but less well-regulated child (Schermerhorn et al., 2013). One illustration of this is the finding that children who are highly reactive and poorly regulated have a greater likelihood of developing behavior problems when exposed to maternal negativity and a stressful home environment compared to their reactive but better regulated peers (Chen, Deater-Deckard, & Bell, 2014).

Parent stress is multifaceted, just as temperament (Rothbart & Bates, 2006) and parenting (Bugental & Grusec, 1998) are. The processes underlying the link between stress and parent–child functioning likely involve complex interactions between multiple dimensions of stress. This chapter has five main objectives: 1. Consider multiple possible aspects of parental stress, including sleep deficits, and their influence on parent–child relations; 2. describe connections between child temperament and parental stress; 3. examine the additive and interactive effects of parental stress and child temperament on parent–child relations; 4. consider theoretically plausible risk and protective factors that could moderate the processes underlying links between stress and functioning; and 5. building from the recent literature on these questions, offer suggestions for future research.

To achieve these aims, we primarily focus on parental stress and sleep deficits experienced when rearing typically developing children during early childhood. We recognize the significant stress associated with children who have intellectual and developmental disabilities (Deater-Deckard, 2004; Neece and Chan, this volume, Chap. 5), and there is a literature on sleep disruptions in parents of children with chronic health issues (Cottrell & Khan, 2005; Ikeda, Nagai, Kato-Nishimura, Mohri, & Taniike, 2012; Meltzer & Mindell, 2006; Mörelius and Hemmingsson, 2014; Shaki,

Goldbart, Daniel, Fraser, & Shorer, 2011). However, in the interest of space and because of our own research focus, this chapter focuses only on parenting stress, sleep, and temperament in families with typically developing children.

This chapter puts emphasis on parental stress and sleep deficits during toddlerhood, preschool, and school-age eras, even though existing research on parental sleep has emphasized the postpartum and infancy periods. We note that between the ages of 3 and 6, child self-regulation grows markedly and daytime naps decline (Iglowstein, Jenni, Molinari, & Largo, 2003; Dahl, 1996). For a number of parents, especially those with children whose self-regulation develops more slowly than expected or whose sleep patterns fail to mature, parent stress and sleep could be affected during this time period. Impulsive, noncompliant, and aggressive behavior is relatively common during early preschool years and can contribute to parent stress (Campbell, 1995; Crnic, Gaze, & Hoffman, 2005). At the transition to school, most children have developed self-regulation skills and have reduced misbehavior (Tremblay, 2000), and social expectations for child behavior increase markedly, so children with continued externalizing behavior could elicit negative feedback from teachers and other parents, further adding to parent distress (Gross, Shaw, & Moilanen, 2008).

Defining Parental Stress and Moderating Factors

Stress is a popular concept with a variety of definitions. One general definition states that stress involves a stimulus or demand (a stressor), which results in distress and/or strain (pressure to adapt to address the stressor), and a physiological reaction, such as elevated norepinephrine or, when adaptive resources are strained, elevated cortisol (Rutter, 1981; Selye, 1979). Stress, as conceptualized here, can have adaptive functions. Moderate levels of stress can help the body remain alert for overcoming challenges, but too much stress can impair functioning (Selye, 1979). Different degrees of stress may vary in their impact, depending on an individual's interpretation of and response to stress. Parents' personality characteristics, cognitive resources, and social supports may explain individual differences in stress response. We consider high parental stress to include the effects of general stressors such as shortage of money, employment changes, relocation, death of a loved one, or marital conflict, as well as effects of stressors specifically related to child-rearing, such as daily demands of raising a young child, household chaos with busy schedules, disorganization, crowding, and noise, and subsequent feelings of frustration, worry, and incompetence.

Daily hassles of raising a child. Parents commonly experience irritating and distressing everyday demands, such as needing to clean messes, resolve sibling conflicts, and prepare children for outings (Crnic & Greenberg, 1990). Such events, often referred to as hassles, are predictive of parental psychological distress above and beyond the effect of stressful life events (Quittner, Glueckauf, & Jackson, 1990; Kanner, Coyne, Schaefer, & Lazarus, 1981; Lazarus & Folkman, 1984). Although stressful life events increase the likelihood of negative outcomes, such as negative parenting attitudes and parent–child interactions (Crnic, Greenberg, Ragozin, Robinson, & Basham, 1983), these events tend to be rare, time-limited occurrences for most families (Crnic & Greenberg, 1987). Stressful life events may indirectly affect family functioning because stressful life events tend to increase the frequency and intensity of everyday hassles. These everyday hassles can subsequently lead to diminished health and well-being and have a greater cumulative impact on family functioning (Compas, Howell, Phares, Williams, & Ledoux, 1989; Farber, Primavera, & Felner, 1983; Crnic & Greenberg, 1990; Crnic et al., 2005).

Observational studies have shown that on days when mothers reported a higher frequency of parenting hassles, they tended to show more irritability in interactions with their child, compared to days on which they reported minimal daily hassles (Patterson, 1983). It is unclear whether daily hassles leave mothers feeling distressed and behaving irritably, or whether maternal distress and irritability increase challenging child behaviors, such as a child resisting preparation for going out, which may make parenting tasks more difficult and increase the parent's perception of tasks as upsetting. Of course, both processes could operate, even within the same time periods. However, an experimental manipulation has provided evidence that with increased parent demands (e.g., needing to prepare a meal or complete paperwork), mothers have been observed to pay less attention to their children, show less positive affect, and use more directive or intrusive parenting strategies in interactions (Miller, Shim, & Holden, 1998). Parents with lower emotional and cognitive control capacities may be more likely to experience highly frequent and intense daily hassles. Limited cognitive control capacities are associated with less parental monitoring, involvement, and consistency (Crandall, Deater-Deckard, & Riley, 2015), and this may intensify child misbehavior and make parenting tasks especially challenging and demanding.

Parental feelings of incompetence. Subjective impact of a stressor depends on cognitive appraisal or interpretation of the stressor (Lazarus, DeLongis, Folkman, & Gruen, 1985). Some parents may interpret challenging child behavior and parenting demands as problems that can be solved and challenges that can be overcome, but other parents may interpret them as evidence that they are ineffectual parents, thus feeling incompetent, hopeless, and dissatisfied as parents, and further stressed. Parents reporting more intense and frequent child behavior problems consistently tend to report lower levels of self-esteem, suggesting that they may interpret the stress of challenging child behavior as a personal failure and sign of their own incompetence (Patterson, 1980; Wolf & Acton, 1968). This is more thoroughly illustrated in Crnic and Ross' consideration of child influences on parents' sense of self-efficacy (this volume, Chap. 11). Crnic and Ross importantly emphasize the bidirectional nature of parenting stress and parental self-efficacy, noting how various sources of parental stress can make parents feel less efficacious, which in turn makes parenting more stressful.

Interparental conflict. Difficult child behavior and overwhelming parenting demands can also lead to disagreements between parents about parenting responsibilities and decisions, which can then exacerbate child emotional reactivity and difficult child behavior (Belsky et al., 1996). Interparental conflict has also been shown to disrupt child sleep, especially in low-income minority families, and these sleep problems are associated with subsequent increases in marital conflict, perpetuating a negative cycle (Kelly & El-Sheikh, 2011; Peterson & Zill, 1986). Interparental conflict therefore serves as an additional parental stressor, which could result in worsening child sleep and behavior and more negative parenting.

Single parenting and social isolation. Some single parents may have escaped, at least mostly, the stress of interparental conflict, but they could still experience the stress (in effect, at least) of limited social support and possible social isolation. Single parents are especially likely to use ineffective and inconsistent parenting practices (Bank, Forgatch, Patterson, & Fetrow, 1993), but this is less likely if they have social support (Adamakos et al., 1986; Cohen & Wills, 1985). Parents who have and use a social support system tend to report less stress (Mulsow, Caldera, Pursley, Reifman, & Huston, 2002) and use less ineffective and more positive parenting behaviors (Crnic et al., 1983). Additionally, social support can reduce the risk of disturbed sleep resulting from psychosocial stressors (Akerstedt et al., 2002). In short, single parents who do not have another adult in the home to provide social support, and who do not use or have other resources for social support, may experience additional stress and be especially likely to parent ineffectively.

Even with some social support, a single mother can end up feeling inadequate, isolated, or distressed (Hobfoll & Lerman, 1988). For example, one study found that increased use of community resources was associated with more maternal distress (Podolski & Nigg, 2001), although its cross-sectional nature prevented conclusions about whether mothers who were more distressed sought out more social support or whether mothers found social support to be unhelpful or rejecting, and thus were left feeling distressed. Nevertheless, on average, single parents, compared with partnered parents, tend to experience more aversive and fewer positive social events, limited social support in the home, and the risk of unhelpful social support in the community, which can leave single parents feeling incompetent, embarrassed, and even more stressed (Wahler & Dumas, 1989, 1984).

Role overload. When parents' workload and perceived demands exceed their time and energy, they may experience an additional stress of role overload (Reilly, 1982). Workload in the home, including non-child-rearing tasks, such as needing to cook, wash, clean, garden, shop, and manage family finances, significantly contributes to an overarching parental stress construct (Östberg & Hagekull, 2000). Domestic workload was directly and indirectly associated with parent stress through difficult child temperament, such that parents who perceived their household responsibilities as pressing and demanding tended to also perceive their child as more difficult and reported higher levels of stress.

Parents who also work outside of the home may experience further role overload. Working parents, despite not having to do many of the day's childcare tasks, must do many other important tasks. Moreover, in some instances, working parents may be too tired themselves to fully enjoy warm, responsive interactions with their child. For example, when mothers returned home from work on days in which they reported higher levels of job stress, they tended to be more withdrawn in interactions with their children, showing fewer expressions of affection and speaking less compared to days when they reported less job stress (Repetti & Wood, 1997). Working parents may also be more likely to perceive their household as rushed and chaotic and may experience conflicting home and work obligations. For instance, mothers who reported high levels of satisfaction with their career positions also tended to report higher levels of parental stress, which may be a direct result of role conflict and overload (Mulsow et al., 2002). Alternatively, a stable career outside of the home could provide parents with life satisfaction, sense of purpose, and financial resources that can aid parenting ability. Employment status could reflect parents' personality trait of conscientiousness, a trait that could help parents lead well-organized households (Weinstein et al., 1998). Despite these varying hypotheses with theoretical plausibility and preliminary empirical support, additional research is needed to clarify the influence of parental employment status on parent functioning.

Home chaos. Families facing numerous parenting tasks, interparental conflict, limited social support, and role overload may be especially likely to also experience what is hyperbolically but commonly called chaos in the home. Home chaos can be defined as confusion, rush, and disorganization in the home, due to little order, few routines, and high levels of crowding, home traffic (i.e., people coming and going in the home), and background noise (Corapci & Wachs, 2002; Dumas, Nissley, Nordstrom, Smith, Prinz, & Levine, 2005; Matheny, Wachs, Ludwig, & Phillips, 1995).

Cross-sectional research has demonstrated a link between home chaos and more ineffective parenting practices, including laxness, verbosity, over-reactivity, and intrusiveness, and less effective practices, including responsiveness and involvement (Dumas et al., 2005; Matheny et al., 1995; Evans, Lepore, Shejwal, & Palsane, 1998; Wachs, 1993; Evans, Maxwell, & Hart, 1999; Wachs & Camli, 1991; Valiente, Lemery-Chalfant, & Reiser, 2007). Parents with limited cognitive and emotional control capacities may be more susceptible to parenting hassles (Crandall et al., 2015), so it is understandable that parents with ADHD symptoms, showing similar deficits in cognitive control, also tend to report more household chaos, even when demographic factors and child ADHD symptoms are controlled (Mokrova, O'Brien, Calkins, & Keane, 2010). Again, longitudinal designs are critical for distinguishing whether parent characteristics and ineffective parenting practices lead to disorganized, poorly managed, chaotic homes, or whether home chaos leads to less supportive and more ineffective parenting practices. Chaotic homes may, through some yet unidentified process, cause parents to use ineffective and inconsistent parenting practices, further adding to chaos in the home and parental stress. Parental sleep deficits, for example, could be involved in this cycle, mediating the association between home chaos and parenting practices.

Sleep deficits. Household chaos may partially result from and contribute to inconsistent routines, including bedtime routines. Few or inconsistent routines could precipitate a sense of disorder and haste in the home, and inconsistent bedtime routines, in particular, are associated with child sleep difficulties, including frequent night wakings and variability in the timing and duration of sleep (Sadeh, Mindell, Luedtke, & Wiegand, 2009), which of course are often notable stressors for parents. Regular use of an effective bedtime routine is associated with less frequent and prolonged child night wakings and increased child sleep duration in clinical (Mindell, Telofski, Wiegand, & Kurtz, 2009) and nonclinical contexts (Staples, Bates, & Petersen, 2015). A dose-dependent relationship between regular bedtime routines and child sleep outcomes has even been established in a large global sample of mother–child pairs from over ten different countries (Mindell, Li, Sadeh, Kwon, & Goh, 2015). Parents facing high levels of chaos and other stressors may be unable to implement consistent routines and thus may be more likely to experience child sleep difficulties, which are robustly associated with parent sleep difficulties. Parent sleep timing (i.e., bedtime and wake time) and total sleep duration are significantly related to the concurrent timing and duration of child sleep (Gau & Merikangas, 2004), and parent night wakings are tightly linked with child night wakings, as parents often attend to their child when they wake in the night (Meltzer & Mindell, 2007; Mindell, Sadeh, Kwon, & Goh, 2015). Child sleep difficulties, which can at least partially result from inconsistent routines, are associated not only with parent sleep deficits, but also with parental stress in general, including feelings of exhaustion, depression, incompetence, and less positive perceptions of parenting (Thunstrom, 1999; Martin, Hiscock, Hardy, Davey, & Wake, 2007).

The association between parental sleep deficits and stress is likely to be bidirectional. For example, stress in the home (e.g., lack of routines and child sleep difficulties) could result in parent night wakings, which are in turn associated with increased negative affect, daytime sleepiness, and perceived role overload, as well as increased morning cortisol and cholesterol levels relative to those with fewer night wakings, which reflects a physical stress response (Meltzer & Mindell, 2007; Ekstedt, Akerstedt, & Soderstrom, 2004). Stress, through experimental manipulations such as informing subjects that they must perform a speech after the sleep period (Gross & Borkovec, 1982), and real-world daily stressors such as high work demands and physical effort at work (Kim & Dimsdale, 2007; Akerstedt et al., 2002), can reduce the total duration and quality of sleep, as evidenced by both subjective self-reports and objective measures (i.e., actigraphy and polysomnography) (Akerstedt, 2006; Akerstedt, Kecklund, & Axelsson, 2007). Sleep deficits in turn limit the regulatory functioning of the prefrontal cortex and therefore can increase one's negative emotionality, impulsivity, and sensitivity to low-level stressors (Minkel et al., 2012; Pilcher & Huffcutt, 1996; Horne, 1985; Motomura et al., 2013; Anderson & Platten, 2011). Sleep deficits result in poorer performance on tasks requiring flexible thinking, management of competing demands, and impulse control (Harrison & Horne, 2000). Therefore, it would be reasonable to expect that sleep-deprived parents may struggle to flexibly respond to their child's changing needs and interests, manage competing demands in a chaotic household, and inhibit their frustrated or impulsive responses to child behavior.

Sleep deficits may have a more proximal influence on parent functioning compared to other stressors. Sleep deficits could make ineffectual or negative parenting more likely, which could maintain or even worsen child misbehavior, thereby adding to parent stress. Nevertheless, not all families would experience such sequences, because parent–child interactions do not just depend on sleep deficits and other stressors, but also upon the temperament, or basic personality, of family members. Next, we consider child temperament and how it may influence the process underlying stress and functioning, levels of parental stress and sleep difficulties, and parent–child dyadic interaction. Parent temperament (Putnam, Sanson, & Rothbart, 2002) will be discussed in a later section.

Parental Stress in Relation to Child Temperament

Children have dispositional tendencies to respond to situations with differing levels of positive and negative reactivity and effortful self-regulation (Rothbart & Bates, 2006). These individual traits are biologically rooted and appear relatively early in development. There is growing evidence that temperament can be summarized by three main constructs: (1) positive emotionality, usually manifested as high approach tendencies, reward-seeking behaviors, and positive affects such as smiling and laughter; (2) negative emotionality, typically manifested through negative affects, such as fear, anger, or sadness, in response to a particular stimulus (this dimension can separate into fear and anger tendencies with development); and (3) effortful control, or the volitional regulation of emotional and other kinds of responses to inhibit a dominant response in favor of a socially preferred, subdominant response. Based on both conceptual arguments and empirical findings, these three constructs are not only related but also substantially independent from one another. Temperament is relatively stable over the life span, but mean-level and rank-order (between-person) change in temperament can be observed during early childhood (Bates et al., 2012).

The child behavior traits that operationally define temperament can be affected by socialization through day-to-day parent–child interactions (Maccoby & Martin, 1983), which gradually contribute to the multiply determined behavioral phenotypes of temperament (Bates et al., 2012). Parental stress and parent behavior can affect the formation and manifestation of early child temperament (Pesonen et al., 2008), and child temperament can moderate child reactivity to stressors and parent behavior. For example, divorce and remarriage are common stressors faced by families, but the effect of these stressors on child adjustment depends on child temperament, among other factors. In Hetherington's (1989) study, three groups of children were identified based on their characteristics and ultimate adjustment following parental divorce. One group of children had negative adjustment outcomes after experiencing parental divorce, while the later two groups adapted and functioned well after parental divorce, with age-typical social development, prosocial behavior, and academic achievement. A key difference between these groups was child temperament. The two resilient groups comprised children who were competent and caring, with high self-esteem, flexibility, and persistence, while the first group was comprised of temperamentally irritable and impulsive children.

In another example of the moderating role of child temperament, children with low reactivity (as measured by cortisol reactivity) were more likely to show externalizing behavior problems when their mother reported high levels of stress, but this association between parental stress and externalizing behavior problems was not found for highly reactive children (Buodo, Moscardino, Scrimin, Altoè, & Palomba, 2013). A possible explanation for this finding is that these children inherited "hypo-responsiveness" that could develop into externalizing behavior problems, depending on environmental input (Beauchaine, Katkin, Strassberg, & Snarr, 2001; Raine, 1996). In other words, these children are constitutionally less reactive to stress, but when they have highly stressed parents they seem to be more likely to show externalizing behavior problems, potentially because they have less developed emotion regulation skills. It is also possible this happens due to fewer regulatory responses by parents to child misbehavior, as suggested by the longitudinal findings of Bates, Pettit, Dodge, & Ridge (1998). Underdeveloped child self-regulation could come from highly stressed mothers' failures to socialize and monitor the child sufficiently due to the child's early, hypo-reactive temperament and the mothers' preoccupation with high levels of stress. This parallels Havighurst and Kehoe's discussion of parental emotional awareness (this volume, Chap. 12), which suggests that some parents may only respond to escalated displays of child emotion due to limited emotional awareness. A more reactive child may elicit more parent responsiveness and be more responsive to parent control, such that parent responses could scaffold the child's self-regulatory abilities and prevent development of externalizing behavior problems. In short, there is probably not a simple link between stressors and child adjustment. Instead, temperamentally different children may show differential susceptibility or sensitivity to stressful experiences and environmental contexts in the development of behavior problems (Belsky, 1997; Boyce & Ellis, 2005).

Parental stress and parent behavior can gradually contribute to the multiply determined behavioral phenotypes of child temperament (Bates et al., 2012; Pesonen et al., 2008), but the reverse is also plausible. Child temperament can contribute to parental stress through challenging child behavior and sleep difficulties. Difficult child temperament, defined in various ways but usually centering on negative emotionality, is positively associated with parental stress (Gelfand et al., 1992; Östberg & Hagekull, 2000) and with negative parent reactions to child behavior (Barron & Earls, 1984; Thomas & Chess, 1977)—at least with children past infancy (Lee & Bates, 1985).

Child temperament can also interact with other parent stressors to affect parent functioning. For example, mothers raising a temperamentally difficult infant are at an increased likelihood of developing postpartum depression, and this is especially true for mothers who have limited social support (Cutrona, 1986; Cutrona & Troutman, 1986; Terry, Mayocchi, & Hynes, 1996). Further, the association between stressors of difficult child temperament and limited social support and parent depression seems to be mediated by parental feelings of self-efficacy.

Mothers facing limited social support when raising a difficult infant tend to feel less confident in their parenting abilities, which can subsequently result in the development of postpartum depression (Cutrona, 1986; Cutrona & Troutman, 1986; Gross, Conrad, Fogg, & Wothke, 1994). The interacting effect of difficult child temperament and limited social support on maternal depressive symptoms was replicated by Terry and colleagues (1996), providing further evidence to suggest that child temperament interacts with other stressors to affect parent functioning. Similarly, mothers raising a difficult child and reporting low levels of perceived power show greater cortisol reactivity and, as a result, use harsh parenting practices, such as spanking (Martorell & Bugental, 2006). This means that stressors such as limited social support and feelings of incompetence are especially likely to lead to negative parental adjustment in the context of difficult child temperament and challenging child behavior.

Children who are temperamentally difficult are also more likely to have sleep difficulties (Thunstrom, 1999), which could further contribute to parental sleep deficits and stress. For example, children rated by their mothers as highly reactive, distractible, and demanding tend to have frequent night wakings (Sadeh, Lavie, & Scher, 1994). Additionally, early low levels of self-regulation and high negative emotionality are associated with later externalizing problems (Rothbart & Bates, 2006; Martel & Nigg, 2006), which, in turn, are linked with sleep problems (Stein, Mendelsohn, Obermeyer, Amromin, & Benca, 2001; Aronen, Lampenius, Fontell, & Simola, 2014). Approximately half of all parents of children with ADHD, for example, report that their child resists bedtime, has settling difficulties, or wakes frequently in the night (Corkum, Tannock, & Moldofsky, 1998; Owens, 2005; Crabtree, Ivanenko, & Gozal, 2003; Bullock & Schall, 2005; Cohen-Zion & Ancoli-Israel, 2004; Bartholomew & Owens, 2006). Objective measures of sleep (i.e., polysomnography, actigraphy, and video monitoring) support evidence from studies using parent reports, demonstrating that children with ADHD take more time to fall asleep and have more sleep activity and night wakings (Bullock & Schall, 2005; Konofal, Lecendreux, Bouvard, & Mouren-Simeoni, 2001). Difficult child temperament is therefore associated with challenging child behavior and child sleep problems, both of which could contribute to parental sleep deficits and additional parental stress.

Stress Within the Parent–Child Process

Theories of social learning suggest that child behavior problems can arise from repeated, coercive parent–child interactions (Patterson, 1982; Patterson, DeBaryshe, & Ramsey, 1989; Loeber & Dishion, 1983; Snyder & Patterson, 1986), and such problematic parent–child interactions may be especially likely when the parent–child dyad is characterized by child temperamental resistance and high levels of parental stress. In Patterson's (1982) coercive family process model, a parent makes a request of a temperamentally resistant child, and the child ignores, denies, or protests the

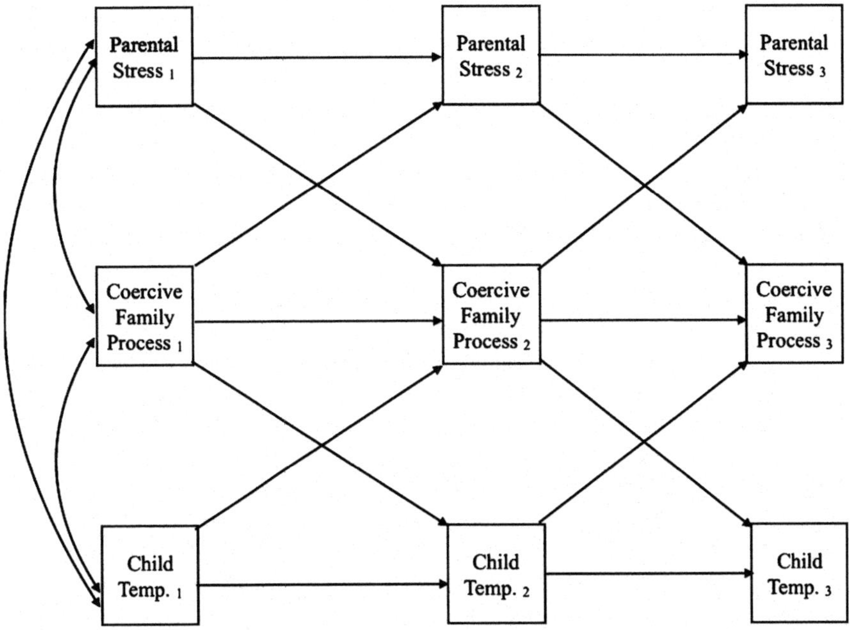

Fig. 4.1 Cross-lagged panel model to test longitudinal mediation for parental stress, coercive family process, and child temperament (abbreviated as temp.)

parent's request. When confronting the stress of this resistant child, the parent may abandon their request, which reinforces both the child (who no longer must complete the requested and unwelcomed task) and the parent (who no longer faces the child's resistance) so that the cycle repeats. This perpetuates a pattern of coercive child behavior and ineffective parental responses, which ultimately adds to parental stress and maintains adverse child temperament and behavior (see Fig. 4.1). Children who are high on the dimension of temperamental resistance tend to be impulsive and relatively unresponsive to adult management attempts (Bates et al., 1998). Temperamentally difficult (high negative emotionality) and fearful children challenge parents in similar ways, often coercing ineffectual parent responses to dysregulated displays of negative emotion (Patterson, Reid, & Dishion, 1992).

A stressful environment could increase the likelihood of parents responding to resistant, fearful, or difficult child behavior ineffectively. Parents could show high levels of harsh responses, overly lax or dismissive responses, as well as inconsistent responses, such as when they occasionally remain firm, but more often give into the child's demands. Stressed parents may be more likely to make in-the-moment, impulsive decisions in response to child misbehavior due to depletion of their own cognitive and emotional self-regulation resources. With heightened arousal caused by stress, decision-making is accelerated (Mendl, 1999) and processing capacity is limited, resulting in narrowed attention, focused on salient negative cues perceived as threats (Easterbrook, 1959; Eysenck, 1976; Mandler, 1975). Accelerated decision-making and selective attention to negative information could contribute to impulsive harsh responses to child misbehavior and dismissal of positive bids for attention. A parent operating under stressful conditions, such as feelings of incompetence and role overload, home chaos, and sleep deficits, could respond to a child's positive bids for attention in a negative or ineffective manner, such as by failing to attend to the child's positive behavior or by responding in ways that elicit fear and anger from a child, further diminishing the child's own regulatory function by failing to reinforce the child's positive behavior. Stressed parents may be too distracted to attend to positive child behavior and may thus primarily attend to and reinforce negative child behavior. Poorly regulated parents, such as those with ADHD symptoms, appear to be especially prone to inconsistent responses to child behavior, wavering between over-reactions and dismissal of child-directed attempts at interaction (Johnston, Mash, Miller, & Ninowski, 2012), and this inconsistency may result from the influence of stress on already limited cognitive control capacity. Less stressed (or more well-regulated) parents may be better able to consider the long-term consequences of their responses to child misbehavior and consistently select and implement a behavioral response to child behavior that can break the coercive pattern. We further discuss such protective factors in a subsequent section.

The mechanisms by which parental stress results in ineffectual parenting and coercive child behavior in moment-to-moment parent–child interactions remain relatively unclear. We nominate sleep as a potential conduit, at least for some people. Poor sleep is an outcome of stress as well as a contributor; it is intertwined with metabolic and physiological components of stress because stress activates the hypothalamic–pituitary–adrenal axis, which contributes to the regulation of the sleep–wake cycle (Van Reeth et al., 2000). Sleep deficits, potentially resulting from a stressful environment, may deplete parents' resources and amplify the stressful context within which they must operate. We have worked in our clinic with several families exemplifying this sequence. In one case, 5-year-old "Daniel" and his father, "Patrick", had frequent negative interactions with each other. Daniel often did annoying, attention-seeking behaviors, which elicited frustration and impulsive, harsh responses from Patrick, such as spanking or sending Daniel to his room for the rest of the night. Patrick's responses often escalated Daniel's misbehavior into a spiral with a dramatic, prolonged tantrum, with crying, screaming, and even hitting his head against the wall. Patrick was more likely to respond to Daniel's low-level, annoying misbehaviors in a harsh manner when he was sleep deprived than when he was well-rested. Patrick was adjusting to a new job, working late hours, and regularly disrupted at night by Daniel's frequent night wakings. Due to Patrick's busy schedule and disorganized tendencies, he failed to implement a consistent bedtime routine for Daniel. Daniel frequently awoke at night, which Patrick often attended to and reinforced. Cycles such as this are probably not uncommon and could involve sleep deficits in both parent and child, along with impulsive, ineffectual, or even exacerbating attempts by parent and child to resolve their conflicts.

Processes like the ones we have sketched take place over multiple timescales. They unfold moment-to-moment when parents attempt to manage stressful contexts and respond to low-level child misbehavior. Repeated aversive and minimally rewarding interactions with bickering, criticism, irritability, vague commands, and noncompliance can be gradually undermining and corrosive to the parent–child relationship (Snyder, 2015). Both parent and child can form habits of behavior that may have short-term functionality in the relationship, but fail to teach the child relationship skills and attitudes that will be adaptive in society. On a longer timescale, some processes in the parent–child relationship and child behavioral adjustment involve infrequent, but high impact, memorable events, such as a parent's major explosion of anger toward the child or a child's highly destructive act (Patterson, Reid, & Dishion, 1992; Snyder, 2015). Such events can lead parents to form habits and draw conclusions about how to parent in future interactions. The conclusions are most likely not only at the level of a strong emotional association, but also perhaps at a social cognitive level, too, such as hostile attributions for ambiguous behavior by a social partner (Dodge, Bates, & Pettit, 1990).

Both corrosive daily occurrences and intermittent explosions can strengthen response tendencies to become deeply entrenched over an even longer timescale. However, as development proceeds, parents may hold developmentally advanced expectations for the child, so child misbehavior may be seen as more offensive and lead to harsher parental responses. Higher expectations may help children mature, but when poorly related to a child's actual developmental level, they can create unproductive conflict. Patrick often had such developmentally inappropriate expectations for Daniel. With each new developmental transition, parents also face new kinds of conflicts to resolve with their children, and thus new stressors. Parents must master age-appropriate forms of discipline balanced with support for autonomy, which becomes especially salient in adolescence and can create new stressors (Conger, Patterson, & Ge, 1995; Kazdin, 2010).

Characteristics That Moderate Parental Stress

Although there are common patterns in how parents respond to stress, sleep deficits, and challenging child behavior, we would not expect all parents to respond in the same way. Just as child temperament can moderate child response to stress and parent behavior (Bates & Pettit, 2014; Schermerhorn et al., 2013), parent characteristics may moderate the effect of stress on functioning. We briefly discuss a few variables that could plausibly attenuate or intensify the "typical" negative association between parental stress and adaptive functioning, including parent gender, economic and cultural background, temperament, intelligence, and specific parenting skills.

Parent gender. During early childhood, mothers, compared to fathers, tend to be more directly involved in their children's caregiving (McBride & Mills, 1994). For example, when mothers and fathers estimated the percent of time they spent on twelve childcare tasks, including making snacks and running errands, mothers spent up to 60% of their time, while fathers, on average, spent up to 40% of their time on these activities (Ehrenberg, Gearing-Small, Hunter, & Small, 2001). Paternal involvement with children tends to increase as mothers work more hours outside of the home (Almeida, Maggs, & Galambos, 1993; Bonney, Kelley, & Levant, 1999), and fathers in dual-earner couples spend more time on childcare activities compared to fathers in single-earner families (Crouter, Perry-Jenkins, Huston, & McHale, 1987). Nevertheless, even when both parents work full-time outside of the home, fathers tend to interact less frequently with children, while mothers remain primarily responsible for childcare (Scarr, Phillips, & McCartney, 1990, Kotila, Schoppe-Sullivan, & Kamp Dush, 2013). Moreover, although paternal involvement has increased with increases in maternal employment, mothers are still more likely to attend to child sleep difficulties, compared to fathers, whose sleep is less strongly associated with child sleep (Mindell, Li, Sadeh, Kwon, & Goh, 2015; Zhang, Li, Fok, & Wing, 2010). Despite the primacy of mothers in the early lives of their children, both parents' stress can be important, although perhaps in different ways.

McBride, Schoppe, and Rane (2002) found that both mothers and fathers reported high levels of stress when their children were perceived as emotionally intense, but mothers' and fathers' reported correlates of child temperamental sociability differed: Fathers reported more parental involvement when children were rated as more sociable, whereas mothers did not. This suggests that paternal involvement may be more influenced by child characteristics, compared to the involvement of mothers who tend to play a more active role in raising their children regardless of child characteristics. In contrast to the McBride et al. (2002) finding about the possible role of child characteristics influencing paternal involvement, several studies have demonstrated that the experience of parenting stress, such as in the form of feelings of incompetence and perceived demands of parenting, is common in both mothers and fathers, and mothers' and fathers' average stress ratings tend to be more similar than different (Deater-Deckard & Scarr, 1996; Baker, 1994; Creasey & Reese, 1996). This is consistent with findings suggesting that mothers and fathers experience similar levels of work–family conflict (Nomaguchi, 2009; Winslow, 2005) and parenting stress due to inflexible work schedules (Nomaguchi & Johnson, 2014; see also Nomaguchi & Milkie, Chap. 3). Crnic and Ross discuss co-parenting processes in Chap. 11 of this book and call for future research on the effect of mothers' stress on fathers and fathers' stress on mothers, which could significantly advance understanding of interparental dynamics and parent gender in the broader family system.

Economic and cultural background. Economic circumstances and background can include additional forms of chronic stress, such as low income, unstable employment, and indebtedness, which, along with low education attainment, are all associated with ineffective parenting practices (Conger et al., 1992; Longfellow, Zelkowitz, & Saunders, 1982). This negative association between socioeconomic stress and effective parenting may be explained by two factors. First, according to the family stress model, parents with these stressful background characteristics are at increased risk of experiencing other stressors, such as marital discord, intimate partner violence, and negative life events, as described by Finegood and Blair (this volume, Chap. 8) and by Cassells and Evans (this volume, Chap. 2). By extension, economically disadvantaged parents may also face higher levels of stress specific to the parenting role, including demanding parenting tasks, challenging child behavior, and home chaos—the latter having a more direct impact on parenting practices. Cassells and Evans also discuss the disproportionate number of economically disadvantaged parents working nonstandard hours, which could result in additional stress, including time away from children, difficulties scheduling childcare, and strained sleep schedules. Such stressors may at least partially explain the relatively more frequent use of ineffective parenting practices among low-income parents (Conger & Donnellan, 2007; Deater-Deckard, Chen, Wang, & Bell, 2012).

Second, ethnic and racial minority families tend to experience additional stressors beyond those specific to the parenting role and economic disadvantage, such as discrimination and acculturation difficulties. The link between minority status and effective parenting remains when socioeconomic status is taken into account (Berlin, Brady-Smith, & Brooks-Gunn, 2002; Yaman, Mesman, Van IJzendoorn, Bakermans-Kranenburg, & Linting, 2010), which suggests that other stress processes may be operating to explain this association, such as the minority-specific stress of acculturation (Emmen et al., 2013). With the added stressors of discrimination and acculturation found among low-income minority parents, it would be expected that they might relatively often use ineffective parenting practices.

Parent temperament. Temperament can operate as a risk or protective factor, either heightening one's response to stressors, or providing a buffer or compensatory resource to draw from when stressed (Rothbart & Bates, 1998). Temperament can influence how one internally responds to external events, and this influence of temperament may be most apparent under stressful conditions (Strelau, 2001). For example, parents high in positive emotionality tend to be warmer and more responsive to their child (Prinzie, Stams, Deković, Reijntjes, & Belsky, 2009; Clark, Kochanska, & Ready, 2000), helping to form a habit of sharing warm, mutually enjoyed parent–child interactions (Kochanska, Friesenborg, Lange, & Martel, 2004). When a parent high in positive emotionality faces stress, such as child negativity, his or her default phenotype is likely to still be positive, refraining from harsh parenting practices, like power assertion (Clark et al., 2000). And of course, the parent's temperament can also predict the child's. A child with a biologically inherited disposition for positive emotionality and a history of repeated positive transactions with their parent may tend to behave positively toward the parent, offering little resistance, and thus little opportunity for the stressed parent to respond out of impulsive frustration.

Another protective temperament trait for parents is effortful control. Well-regulated parents may be able to rely on their effortful control when sleep deprived or faced with other sources of stress, helping them implement effective responses to child behavior rather than impulsive, emotionally reactive responses. In contrast, parents who are lower in effortful control and/or high in negative emotionality may be especially sensitive to stressors and especially prone to and affected by sleep deficits. When stressed and sleep deprived, these temperamentally negative parents may be more likely to respond with irritability and over-reaction to even mild stressors compared to parents who are lower in negative affect or more well-regulated. For example, mothers high in negative emotionality and disagreeableness tend to use more power assertion and less nurturance in observed interactions with their child, compared to their more positive and well-regulated counterparts (Kochanska, Clark, & Goldman, 1997). Additionally, adults with high negative affect and low positive affect tend to report low-quality sleep (Norlander, Johansoon, & Bood, 2005), as do individuals who are higher in neuroticism, which is comparable to high negative emotionality (Soehner, Kennedy, & Monk, 2007). Highly neurotic adults not only tend to experience poorer sleep, but also are more affected by low-quality sleep, as evidenced by worsened performance on a variety of cognitive tasks, including delayed recall, digit span, and Stroop color-word tasks (Taylor & McFatter, 2003).

Because temperament has important biological components, including, for most psychological traits, a substantial heritability, shared genetic factors between parent and child may help to explain similarity of parent and child temperament, associated qualities of parent–child interaction, and, ultimately, parent and child self-regulation skills and sensitivity to stress (Fischer, 1990). The many associations observed between parental stress, child temperament, and parenting practices (e.g., Östberg and Hagekull, 2000; Mash & Johnston, 1983a, b; Pinderhughes, Dodge, Bates, Pettit, & Zelli, 2000) may thus be driven by or better explained by an additional variable—parent temperament. Parent temperament could drive a parent's sensitivity or susceptibility to stress, regulation in a stressful context, failure to prevent recurring stressors, susceptibility to sleep difficulties, and in-the-moment behavioral responses to child behavior, as well as child temperament, through the hereditary influence of the parent's temperament (see Fig. 4.2). We are not saying

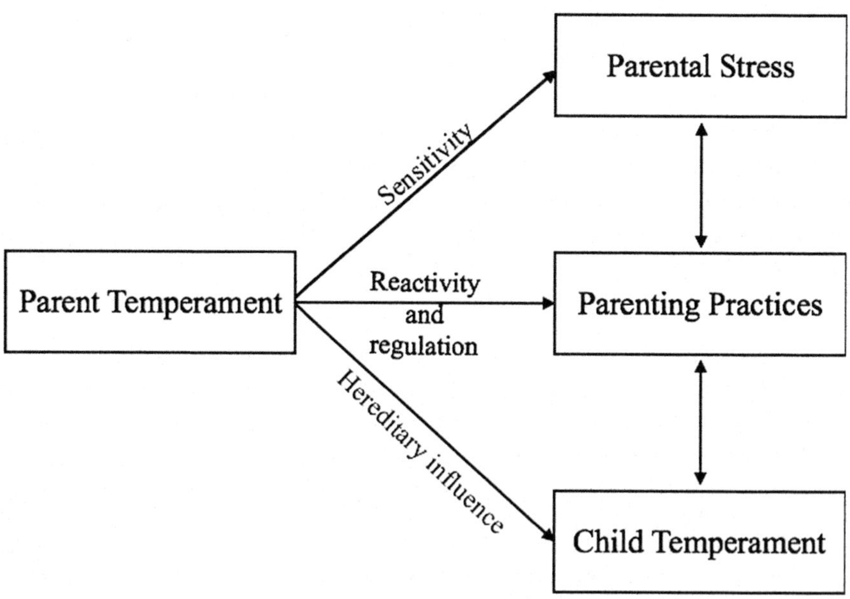

Fig. 4.2 Conceptual model of how the links between parental stress, parenting practices, and child temperament could be partially explained by parent temperament

that children's experiences in interaction with their parents do not matter. In fact, there are studies with genetically informative samples that suggest that parenting does matter (Goldsmith, Buss, & Lemery, 1997; Kochanska, Philibert, & Barry, 2009), and there are also many experiments in which parenting has effects (e.g., Scott & O'Connor, 2012). However, there has been too little developmental research on the implications of parent temperament variables as explanatory factors in the associations between the stress and parenting concepts for us to conclude how useful parent temperament and shared genetic factors are in the account of child-rearing processes.

Cognitive skills and capacities. As with parents who have strong effortful control, parents with strong cognitive abilities may be able to overcome the effects of sleep deficits, using higher processing speed, memory capacity, and vocabulary as compensatory resources to accurately and efficiently process information in interactions with their child (Durmer & Dinges, 2005). Social information, such as a conflict with one's child, is processed through a series of steps, including encoding relevant information, forming a representation of this information, accessing a behavioral response to this representation, evaluating the suitability of the response, and then behaviorally implementing the response (Dodge, 1993; Deater-Deckard & Dodge, 1997). Efficient and accurate processing could benefit from advanced cognitive abilities in complex social situations, such as those contexts in which parents are burdened and distracted by various stressors. Cognitive abilities could aid in efficiently and effectively encoding and interpreting social information and selecting and implementing an appropriate behavioral response, buffering parents from using ineffective parenting practices in the face of challenging child behavior, sleep deficits, and other sources of parental stress. When stressed by challenging child behaviors, such as oppositionality or distractibility, mothers with low levels of working memory are especially likely to react negatively, while mothers with high working memory capacity refrain from negative reactivity (Deater-Deckard, Sewell, Petrill, & Thompson, 2010). Maternal working memory also moderates the link between mothers' negative attributions for child behavior and harsh parenting: Negative attributions result in harsh parenting, but only for mothers with lower working memory capacity (Sturge-Apple, Suor, & Skibo, 2014). Maternal executive function (measured by attention, inhibition, and working memory tasks) similarly moderates the link between child conduct problems and harsh parenting: Child conduct problems are associated with harsher parenting when mothers have lower executive functioning (Deater-Deckard et al., 2012).

The role of parental cognitive abilities may depend on the kind of stress being considered. In one study, maternal executive function did not operate in a protective way under circumstances of high home chaos, as child conduct problems were positively associated with harsh parenting in this context, regardless of maternal executive function capacity (Deater-Deckard et al., 2012b). However, in another study, maternal working memory was protective in families with high economic disadvantage, such that mothers with low working memory capacity were especially likely to respond to negative attributions of child behavior with harsh parenting when economically stressed (Sturge-Apple et al., 2014). Taken together, these findings highlight a need for more research on the role of parental cognitive abilities, especially in stressful contexts, to advance understanding of the link between parental stress and parent–child functioning.

Specific parenting knowledge and skills. An additional protective factor that could temper the effect of parental stress on parent functioning is parental knowledge and use of specific parenting skills. One illustration of the power of knowledge might be the finding showing that parents who participate in parent management training programs can learn to respond to child behavior in more effective ways, terminating coercive parent–child cycles and helping child behavior to improve. Parents can improve their effectiveness with formal behavioral interventions (Eyberg, 1988; Kazdin, 2010). Such programs can help parents learn to increase positive interactions with their children and reduce ineffective practices and inconsistency. With consistent, mild, and predictable consequences for child behavior, impulsive, hyperactive, or aggressive children can learn to inhibit inappropriate responses. And when children become less oppositional, they can receive fewer negative parent responses, reducing the negativity of parent–child interactions and motivating continued positive child behavior (Bor, Sanders, Markie-Dadds, 2002). Parents can also make improvements independent of psychoeducational treatments, engaging in what we call "campaigns"—self-initiated attempts to change interactions with their child. In a study of this, parents who reported campaigns to increase their positive involvement and management later saw reduced growth of child conduct problems, and this was especially true for those with temperamentally resistant children (Goodnight, Bates, Pettit, & Dodge, 2008). Parents' successful acquisition and use of effective parenting skills, at least through formal interventions, increase parents' feelings of competency and self-esteem (Wolfson, Lacks, & Futterman, 1992; Deković et al., 2010), and reduce stress (Feldman & Werner, 2002; Kaaresen et al., 2006; Pisterman et al., 1992).

Key Questions and Research Directions

A large body of research has established that child adjustment can be affected by parent stress and parenting practices. However, less research has explored the plausibly bidirectional relation between parent stress and parenting practices. Research is needed to identify processes that explain how parental stress affects parent and child functioning and vice versa. This chapter has considered parental stress as a multidimensional construct, comprised of stressful life events as well as chronic stressors, such as daily parenting tasks, interparental conflict, limited social support, role overload, feelings of incompetence, home chaos, sleep deficits, and challenging child behavior. Future research is needed to determine how these dimensions of stress dynamically interrelate at timescales from narrow—minutes to days—slices of time to multi-year sequences. Future research is also needed on how parental sleep deficits affect parenting practices, perhaps through impaired executive function, decreased positive emotionality, and increased negative emotionality.

This chapter has also considered potential moderators of stress–parenting relationships, including parent temperament, intelligence, and parenting knowledge and skills, all of which could help parents avoid over-reliance on ineffective parenting practices when stressed. Well-designed longitudinal studies using complex statistical techniques for testing multi-factor models, including both direct, main transactional effects and mediator and moderator effects, will be important.

For example, with structural equation modeling (SEM), research could determine how parent sleep deficits relate to other sources of parental stress. This research could advance understanding of whether sleep difficulties and other parental stressors converge to form an overall stress construct or whether they have separable influences on parenting practices and the family system. When SEM was used to test a theoretical model of parenting stress in a large sample of Swedish mothers, parenting stress was primarily predicted by stressful life events, lack of social support, domestic workload, difficult child temperament, and caretaking demands (Östberg & Hagekull, 2000). This model accounted for 48% of the variance in parenting stress, and potentially more variance could be explained in future studies if parent sleep deficits are also taken into account. Alternatively, experimental manipulations of parent sleep, by sleep restriction or added naps, could advance understanding of how sleep variations relate to parenting stress and functioning.

Future research is also still needed on how parent, child, family, and environmental/contextual factors interact with each other and influence parental stress and functioning. Studies assessing cumulative stress in families, along with measures of parental involvement, education, marital status, socioeconomic status, home crowding, availability and use of social support resources, and neighborhood qualities, have shown that a higher level of risk is associated with more negative outcomes for parent and child functioning (e.g., Furstenberg, Cook, Eccles, Elder, & Sameroff, 1999; Sameroff, 2006; Valiente et al., 2007; Goyal, Gay, & Lee, 2009). However, as important as they have been, such studies are limited because they fail to "unpack the processes by which each individual is impacted" by various stressors (Sameroff, 2010, p. 14). Hierarchical linear modeling (HLM) can be used in longitudinal designs to model initial levels of parental stress, as well as change in parental stress, to understand which factors are associated with increases in stress and which factors are associated with reduction in parental stress. Williford, Calkins, and Keane (2007) employed HLM to study the stability of parenting stress across the preschool period (ages 2, 4, and 5) and to determine which maternal and child characteristics would be predictive of initial levels and change in stress. They found that overall, parenting stress decreased during this developmental period. Single mothers and mothers of children with more disruptive behavior problems had higher initial levels of stress, and mothers of children who consistently showed high levels of externalizing behavior problems did not show the overall decline in parenting stress over time. Instead, the high stress level of these mothers was stable across time, demonstrating the developmentally important association between child behavior problems and parental stress in a longitudinal design.

Longitudinal and intervention studies will also be critical to determine whether ineffective parenting practices lead to greater frequency and intensity of stressors and poorer sleep quality, or whether parent stressors indirectly predict change in parenting practices through maternal sleep and executive function, or whether bidirectional relationships exist. The direction of these effects can be explicitly tested using longitudinal, cross-lagged panel analyses and experimental manipulations of sleep. Using longitudinal, cross-lagged panel analyses, Neece and colleagues tested the association between parent-reported child behavior problems from age 3 to 9 and parent-reported family stress (Neece, Green, & Baker, 2012). They found bidirectional effects, but not at every age. In another study, Mackler et al. (2015) used a cross-lagged panel model to test the directionality of the associations between parent-reported child externalizing behavior, parenting stress, and negative parental reactions to child behavior at ages 4, 5, 7, and 10, while controlling for the cross-time continuity in externalizing behavior. They found bidirectional effects between externalizing behavior and parental stress at each age, but these associations were not mediated by parenting practices (i.e., negative parental reactions to child behavior). They consistently found that parental stress was predictive of more intense and frequent negative parental reactions to child behavior, but these reactions were not subsequently predictive of later externalizing behavior problems over and beyond earlier problems (Mackler et al., 2015). Despite the fact that the latter nonfinding fails to support our conceptual model, at this very early stage of research on a very complex theoretical model, further studies still seem appropriate.

In our collaboration with the Deater-Deckard laboratory, we have been collecting maternal reports on stressful life events, background demographic information, parenting demands, challenging child behavior, and home chaos along with observer reports, avoiding some of the single informant bias so prevalent in the parenting stress literature (Crnic & Greenberg, 1990). Observers report on challenging child behavior in the laboratory and the home, and rate home crowding, noise, and other markers of chaos. We have also been collecting measures of maternal sleep, for one of the few times in research on parenting stress, using actigraphs to provide objective measures of naturally occurring short sleep, fragmented sleep, late sleep, and variable sleep to complement subjective reports of parents' bedtimes, wake times, night wakings, and sleep problems.

If after statistically accounting for other stressors, we learn that parental sleep deficits have a significant effect on parenting practices, parental sleep could be designated as a useful intervention target. We would hypothesize that improved parental sleep would help mitigate the effects of other forms of parenting stress on parenting practices. We also think it will be interesting to learn which particular dimensions of sleep deficits are most impactful—sleep timing, duration, fragmentation, or, our favorite candidate, variability (Bates et al., 2002). It is possible that improving the duration, quality, and regularity of parental sleep would make parents' response to stressors less negative and their executive functioning less impaired. Interventions highlighting sleep and consistent bedtime routines may benefit the broader family system by reducing home chaos, improving parents' cognitive and emotional processing, and improving parents' management of child behavior and the home. However, as theoretically appealing as these concepts are, clinical use of them should be guided by concrete empirical evidence demonstrating the role of parental sleep in its relation to other stressors, executive function, and parenting behaviors.

We also advocate and are pursuing tests of probable moderators of the relationship between parental stress and parent functioning. It seems unlikely that all parents will respond to stressors, including sleep deficits, in the same way. We would find it practically useful to learn which families are most at risk of using ineffective parenting practices. Treatments could then be individualized to best meet the needs of each family. Perhaps it would even be possible to offer treatments in a graded way to give only as much treatment as a given family needs. Moderator analyses could also test how the relation between parental stress and family functioning depends on child temperament. This research could then be used to design interventions that could be tailored to best meet the individual child's needs. Assessment of child temperament could uncover motivating factors and strengths, which could be used and highlighted in treatment. For example, children with high reward-seeking tendencies may respond best to consistent discipline in the context of a mutually responsive, socially rewarding parent–child relationship (Kochanska, 1997; Kochanska & Murray, 2000). Future research on child and parent temperament should also include genetically informed designs, because shared genetic factors between parent and child may help to explain similarity of parent and child temperament, associated qualities of parent–child interaction, and, ultimately, parent and child self-regulation skills and sensitivity to stress.

Conclusion

To summarize, we have considered the multifaceted nature of temperament, parenting, and parental stress along with potential mediating and moderating processes that connect these constructs at different timescales. Ordinary, but unpleasant parenting tasks, harder challenges from children who are temperamentally or environmentally conditioned to be high in negative emotionality, and ineffectual parental responses to child behavior challenges could contribute to daily hassles, feelings of incompetence and dissatisfaction with the parenting role, interparental conflict, social isolation, role overload, home chaos, and sleep deficits. Evidence suggests that chronic psychosocial stressors can reduce the duration and quality of sleep. Moreover, parents of young children, especially those with difficult temperament, frequently experience sleep disruptions. Low quality and quantity of sleep could increase parents' negative emotionality and decrease their executive function capacity, resulting in impulsive decision-making and inflexible thinking. Research is needed to evaluate the hypothesis that poor sleep, especially in interaction with other risk factors and stressors, could set the stage for ineffectual and negative parental reactions to challenging child behavior, which could result in continued child misbehavior and hostility, exacerbating parent stress. Such research could help to identify proximal targets for intervention, such as sleep hygiene or home decluttering, and clarify for whom and under which circumstances these targets may be most effective to successfully translate this research into practice.

References

Adamakos, H., Ryan, K., Ullman, D. G., Pascoe, J., Diaz, R., & Chessare, J. (1986). Maternal social support as a predictor of mother-child stress and stimulation. *Child Abuse and Neglect, 10*(4), 463–470. doi:10.1016/0145-2134(86)90050-5.

Akerstedt, T. (2006). Psychosocial stress and impaired sleep. *Scandinavian Journal of Work, Environment and Health, 32,* 493–501.

Akerstedt, T., Kecklund, G., & Axelsson, J. (2007). Impaired sleep after bedtime stress and worries. *Biological Psychology, 76,* 170–173. doi:10.1016/j.biopsycho.2007.07.010.

Akerstedt, T., Knutsson, A., Westerholm, P., Theorell, T., Alfredsson, L., & Kecklund, G. (2002). Sleep disturbances, work stress and work hours: A cross-sectional study. *Journal of Psychosomatic Research, 53,* 741–748. doi:10.1016/S0022-3999(02)00333-1.

Almeida, D. M., Maggs, J. L., & Galambos, N. L. (1993). Wives' employment hours and spousal participation in family work. *Journal of Family Psychology, 7,* 233–244. doi:10.1037/0893-3200.7.2.233.

Anderson, C., & Platten, C. R. (2011). Sleep deprivation lowers inhibition and enhances impulsivity to negative stimuli. *Behavioural Brain Research, 217*(2), 463–466. doi:10.1016/j.bbr.2010.09.020.

Aronen, E. T., Lampenius, T., Fontell, T., & Simola, P. (2014). Sleep in children with disruptive behavioral disorders. *Behavioral Sleep Medicine, 12*(5), 373–388. doi:10.1080/15402002.2013.821653.

Baker, D. B. (1994). Parenting stress and ADHD a comparison of mothers and fathers. *Journal of Emotional and Behavioral Disorders, 2*(1), 46–50.

Bank, L., Forgatch, M. S., Patterson, G. R., & Fetrow, R. A. (1993). Parenting practices of single mothers: Mediators of negative contextual factors. *Journal of Marriage and the Family, 55,* 371–384. doi:10.2307/352808.

Barron, A. P., & Earls, F. (1984). The relation of temperament and social factors to behavior problems in three-year-old children. *Journal of Child Psychology and Psychiatry, 25*(1), 23–33. doi:10.1111/j.1469-7610.1984.tb01716.x.

Bartholomew, K., & Owens, J. (2006). Sleep and ADHD: A review. *Medicine and Health Rhode Island, 89*(3), 91–93.

Barton, M. L., & Zeanah, C. H. (1990). Stress in the preschool years. *Childhood Stress*, 193–221.

Bates, J. E., & Pettit, G. S. (2014). Temperament, parenting, and social development. In J. E. Grusec & P. D. Hastings (Eds.), *Handbook of Socialization: Theory and Research* (pp. 372–397). New York: Guilford.

Bates, J. E., Pettit, G. S., Dodge, K. A., & Ridge, B. (1998). Interaction of temperamental resistance to control and restrictive parenting in the development of externalizing behavior. *Developmental Psychology, 34*(5), 982–995. doi:10.1037/0012-1649.34.5.982.

Bates, J. E., Schermerhorn, A. C., & Petersen, I. T. (2012). Temperament and parenting in developmental perspective. In M. Zentner & R. L. Shiner (Eds.), *Handbook of temperament* (pp. 425–441). New York: Guilford.

Bates, J. E., Schermerhorn, A. C., & Petersen, I. T. (2014). Temperament concepts in developmental psychopathology. In M. Lewis & K.D. Rudolph (Eds)., *Handbook of developmental psychopathology* (pp. 311–329). US:Springer. doi:10.1007/978-1-4614-9608-3_16.

Bates, J. E., Viken, R. J., Alexander, D. B., Beyers, J., & Stockton, L. (2002). Sleep and adjustment in preschool children: Sleep diary reports by mothers relate to behavior reports by teachers. *Child Development, 73*(1), 62–75. doi:10.1111/1467-8624.00392.

Beauchaine, T. P., Katkin, E. S., Strassberg, Z., & Snarr, J. (2001). Disinhibitory psychopathology in male adolescents: Discriminating conduct disorder from attention-deficit/hyperactivity disorder through concurrent assessment of multiple autonomic states. *Journal of Abnormal Psychology, 110,* 610–624.

Belsky, J. (1997). Variation in susceptibility to rearing influences: An evolutionary argument. *Psychological Inquiry, 8,* 182–186.

Belsky, J., Woodworth, S., & Crnic, K. (1996). Troubled family interaction during childhood. *Development and Psychopathology, 8,* 477–495. doi:10.1017/S0954579400007227.

Berlin, L. J., Brady-Smith, C., & Brooks-Gunn, J. (2002). Links between childbearing age and observed maternal behaviors with 14-month-olds in the early head start research and evaluation project. *Infant Mental Health Journal, 23,* 104–129. doi:10.1002/imhj.10007.

Bonney, J. F., Kelley, M. L., & Levant, R. F. (1999). A model of fathers' behavioral involvement in childcare in dual-earner families. *Journal of Family Psychology, 13,* 401–415. doi:10.1037/0893-3200.13.3.401.

Bor, W., Sanders, M. R., & Markie-Dadds, C. (2002). The effects of the Triple P Positive Parenting Program on preschool children with co-occurring disruptive behavior and attentional/hyperactive difficulties. *Journal of Abnormal Child Psychology, 30,* 571–587. doi:10.1023/A:1020807613155.

Boyce, W. T., & Ellis, B. J. (2005). Biological sensitivity to context: I. An evolutionary-developmental theory of the origins and functions of stress reactivity. *Development and Psychopathology, 17,* 271–301. doi:10.1017/S0954579405050145.

Bugental, D. B., & Grusec, J. E. (1998). *Socialization processes.* Handbook of Child Psychology: Wiley. doi:10.1002/9780470147658.chpsy0307.

Bullock, G. L., & Schall, U. (2005). Dyssomnia in children diagnosed with attention deficit hyperactivity disorder: A critical review. *Australian and New Zealand Journal of Psychiatry, 39*(5), 373–377. doi:10.1080/j.1440-1614.2005.01584.x.

Buodo, G., Moscardino, U., Scrimin, S., Altoè, G., & Palomba, D. (2013). Parenting stress and externalizing behavior symptoms in children: The impact of emotional reactivity. *Child Psychiatry and Human Development, 44*(6), 786–797.

Bussing, R., Zima, B. T., Gary, F. A., Mason, D. M., Leon, C. E., Sinha, K., et al. (2003). Social networks, caregiver strain, and utilization of mental health services among elementary school students at high risk for ADHD. *Journal of the American Academy of Child and Adolescent Psychiatry, 42*(7), 842–850. doi:10.1097/01.CHI.0000046876.27264.BF.

Campbell, S. B. (1995). Behavior problems in preschool children: A review of recent research. *Journal of Child Psychology and Psychiatry, 36*(1), 113–149. doi:10.1111/j.1469-7610.1995.tb01657.x.

Chan, Y. C. (1994). Parenting stress and social support of mothers who physically abuse their children in Hong Kong. *Child Abuse and Neglect, 18*(3), 261–269. doi:10.1016/0145-2134(94)90110-4.

Chen, N., Deater-Deckard, K., & Bell, M. A. (2014). The role of temperament by family environment interactions in child maladjustment. *Journal of Abnormal Child Psychology, 42* (8), 1251–1262. doi:10.1007/s10802-014-9872-y.

Clark, L. A., Kochanska, G., & Ready, R. (2000). Mothers' personality and its interaction with child temperament as predictors of parenting behavior. *Journal of Personality and Social Psychology, 79*(2), 274–285. doi:10.1037/0022-3514.79.2.274.

Cohen, S., & Wills, T. A. (1985). Stress, social support, and the buffering hypothesis. *Psychological Bulletin, 98*(2), 310–357. doi:10.1037/0033-2909.98.2.310.

Cohen-Zion, M., & Ancoli-Israel, S. (2004). Sleep in children with attention-deficit hyperactivity disorder (ADHD): A review of naturalistic and stimulant intervention studies. *Sleep Medicine Reviews, 8*(5), 379–402. doi:10.1016/j.smrv.2004.06.002.

Compas, B. E., Howell, D. C., Phares, V., Williams, R. A., & Ledoux, N. (1989). Parent and child stress and symptoms: An integrative analysis. *Developmental Psychology, 25*(4), 550–559. doi:10.1037/0012-1649.25.4.550.

Conger, R. D., Conger, K. J., Elder, G. H., Lorenz, F. O., Simons, R. L., & Whitbeck, L. B. (1992). A family process model of economic hardship and adjustment in early adolescent boys. *Child Development, 62,* 525–541. doi:10.1111/j.1467-8624.1992.tb01644.x.

Conger, R. D., & Donnellan, M. B. (2007). An interactionist perspective on the socioeconomic context of human development. *Annual Review of Psychology, 58,* 175–199.

Conger, R. D., Patterson, G. R., & Ge, X. (1995). It takes two to replicate: A mediational model for the impact of parents' stress on adolescent adjustment. *Child Development, 66*(1), 80–97. doi:10.1111/j.1467-8624.1995.tb00857.x.

Corapci, F., & Wachs, T. D. (2002). Does parental mood or efficacy mediate the influence of environmental chaos upon parenting behavior? *Merrill-Palmer Quarterly, 48*(2), 182–201. doi:10.1353/mpq.2002.0006.

Corkum, P., Tannock, R., & Moldofsky, H. (1998). Sleep disturbances in children with attention-deficit/hyperactivity disorder. *Journal of American Academy of Child and Adolescent Psychiatry, 37*(6), 637–646. doi:10.1097/00004583-199806000-00014.

Cottrell, L., & Khan, A. (2005). Impact of childhood epilepsy on maternal sleep and socioemotional functioning. *Clinical Pediatrics, 44,* 613–616. doi:10.1177/000992280504400709.

Crabtree, V. M., Ivanenko, A., & Gozal, D. (2003). Clinical and parental assessment of sleep in children with attention-deficit/hyperactivity disorder referred to a pediatric sleep medicine center. *Clinical Pediatrics, 42*(9), 807–813. doi:10.1177/000992280304200906.

Crandall, A., Deater-Deckard, K., & Riley, A. W. (2015). Maternal emotion and cognitive control capacities and parenting: A conceptual framework. *Developmental Review, 36,* 105–126. doi:10.1016/j.dr.2015.01.004.

Creasey, G., & Reese, M. (1996). Mothers' and fathers' perceptions of parenting hassles: Associations with psychological symptoms, nonparenting hassles, and child behavior problems. *Journal of Applied Developmental Psychology, 17*(3), 393–406.

Crnic, K. A., Gaze, C., & Hoffman, C. (2005). Cumulative parenting stress across the preschool period: Relations to maternal parenting and child behavior at age 5. *Infant and Child Development, 14*(2), 117–132. doi:10.1002/icd.384.

Crnic, K. A., & Greenberg, M. T. (1987). Transactional relationships between perceived family style, risk status, and mother-child interactions in two year olds. *Journal of Pediatric Psychology, 12,* 343–362. doi:10.1093/jpepsy/12.3.343.

Crnic, K. A., & Greenberg, M. T. (1990). Minor parenting stresses with young children. *Child Development, 61*(5), 1628–1637. doi:10.1111/j.1467-8624.1990.tb02889.x.

Crnic, K. A., Greenberg, M. T., Ragozin, A. S., Robinson, N. M., & Basham, R. B. (1983). Effects of stress and social support on mothers and premature and full-term infants. *Child Development*, 209–217. doi:10.2307/1129878.

Crouter, A. C., Perry-Jenkins, M., Huston, T. L., & McHale, S. M. (1987). Processes underlying father involvement in dual-earner and single-earner families. *Developmental Psychology, 23,* 431–440. doi:10.1037/0012-1649.23.3.431.

Cummings, E. M., & El-Sheikh, M. (1991). Children's coping with angry environments: A process oriented approach. In E. M. Cummings, A. Greene, & K. Karraker (Eds.), *Life-span developmental psychology: Perspectives on stress and coping* (pp. 131–150). Hillsdale, NJ: Erlbaum.

Cutrona, C. E. (1986). Behavioral manifestations of social support: A microanalytic investigation. *Journal of Personality and Social Psychology, 51*(1), 201–208. doi:10.1037/0022-3514.51.1.201.

Cutrona, C. E., & Troutman, B. R. (1986). Social support, infant temperament, and parenting self-efficacy: A mediational model of postpartum depression. *Child Development*, 1507–1518. doi:10.2307/1130428.

Dahl, R. E. (1996). The regulation of sleep and arousal: Development and psychopathology. *Development and Psychopathology, 8*(1), 3–27. doi:10.1017/S0954579400006945.

Deater-Deckard, K. (2004). *Parenting stress*. New Haven: Yale University Press.

Deater–Deckard, K., Chen, N., Wang, Z., & Bell, M. A. (2012a). Socioeconomic risk moderates the link between household chaos and maternal executive function. *Journal of Family Psychology*, 26(3), 391–399. doi:10.1037/a0028331.

Deater-Deckard, K., & Dodge, K. A. (1997). Externalizing behavior problems and discipline revisited: Nonlinear effects and variation by culture, context, and gender. *Psychological Inquiry, 8*(3), 161–175. doi:10.1207/s15327965pli0803_1.

Deater-Deckard, K., & Scarr, S. (1996). Parenting stress among dual-earner mothers and fathers: Are there gender differences? *Journal of Family Psychology, 10,* 45–59. doi:10.1037/0893-3200.10.1.45.

Deater-Deckard, K., Sewell, M. D., Petrill, S. A., & Thompson, L. A. (2010). Maternal working memory and reactive negativity in parenting. *Psychological Science, 21,* 75–79. doi:10.1177/0956797609354073.

Deater-Deckard, K., Wang, Z., Chen, N., & Bell, M. A. (2012). Maternal executive function, harsh parenting, and child conduct problems. *Journal of Child Psychology and Psychiatry, 53*(10), 1084–1091. doi:10.1111/j.1469-7610.2012.02582.x.

Deković, M., Asscher, J. J., Hermanns, J., Reitz, E., Prinzie, P., & Van Den Akker, A. L. (2010). Tracing changes in families who participated in the home-start parenting program: Parental sense of competence as mechanism of change. *Prevention Science, 11*(3), 263–274. doi:10.1007/s11121-009-0166-5.

DeLongis, A., Coyne, J., Dakof, G., Folkman, S., & Lazarus, R. (1982). Relationship of daily hassles, uplifts, and major life events to health status. *Health Psychology, I,* 119–136. doi:10.1037/0278-6133.1.2.119.

Dodge, K. A. (1993). Social-cognitive mechanisms in the development of conduct disorder and depression. *Annual Review of Psychology, 44*(1), 559–584. doi:10.1146/annurev.ps.44.020193.003015.

Dodge, K. A., Bates, J. E., & Pettit, G. S. (1990). Mechanisms in the cycle of violence. *Science, 250*(4988), 1678–1683. doi:10.1126/science.2270481.

Dumas, J. E., Nissley, J., Nordstrom, A., Smith, E. P., Prinz, R. J., & Levine, D. W. (2005). Home chaos: Sociodemographic, parenting, interactional, and child correlates. *Journal of Clinical Child and Adolescent Psychology, 34*(1), 93–104. doi:10.1207/s15374424jccp3401_9.

Durmer, J. S., & Dinges, D. F. (2005). Neurocognitive consequences of sleep deprivation. *Seminars in Neurology*, 25 (1). 117–129.

Easterbrook, J. A. (1959). The effect of emotion on cue utilization and the organization of behavior. *Psychological Review, 66,* 183–201.

Ehrenberg, M. F., Gearing-Small, M., Hunter, M. A., & Small, B. J. (2001). Childcare task division and shared parenting attitudes in dual-earner families with young children. *Family Relations, 50*(2), 143–153.

Ekstedt, M., Akerstedt, T., & Soderstrom, M. (2004). Microarousals during sleep are associated with increased levels of lipids, cortisol, and blood pressure. *Psychosomatic Medicine, 66*(6), 925–931.

Emmen, R. A., Malda, M., Mesman, J., van IJzendoorn, M. H., Prevoo, M. J., & Yeniad, N. (2013). Socioeconomic status and parenting in ethnic minority families: Testing a minority family stress model. *Journal of Family Psychology, 27*(6), 896–904. doi:10.1037/a0034693.

Evans, G. W., Lepore, S. J., Shejwal, B., & Palsane, M. N. (1998). Chronic residential crowding and children's well-being. *Child Development, 69,* 1514–1523. doi:10.2307/1132129.

Evans, G. W., Maxwell, L. E., & Hart, B. (1999). Parental language and verbal responsiveness to children in crowded homes. *Developmental Psychology, 35,* 1020–1023. doi:10.1037/0012-1649.35.4.1020.

Eyberg, S. M. (1988). PCIT: Integration of traditional and behavioral concerns. *Child and Family Behavior Therapy, 10,* 33–46. doi:10.1300/J019v10n01_04.

Eysenck, M. W. (1976). Arousal, learning, and memory. *Psychological Bulletin, 83,* 389–404.

Farber, S. S., Primavera, J., & Felner, R. D. (1983). Older adolescents and parental divorce: Adjustment problems and mediators of coping. *Journal of Divorce, 7*(2), 59–75.
Feldman, M. A., & Werner, S. E. (2002). Collateral effects of behavioral parent training on families of children with developmental disabilities and behavior disorders. *Behavioral Interventions, 17*(2), 75–83. doi:10.1002/bin.111.
Fischer, M. (1990). Parenting stress and the child with attention deficit hyperactivity disorder. *Journal of Clinical Child Psychology, 19*(4), 337–346. doi:10.1207/s15374424jccp1904_5.
Furstenberg, F. F., Jr., Cook, T. D., Eccles, J., Elder, G. H., Jr., & Sameroff, A. (1999). *Managing to make it: Urban families and adolescent success*. Chicago: University of Chicago Press.
Gau, S. S., & Merikangas, K. R. (2004). Similarities and differences in sleep–wake patterns among adults and their children. *Sleep, 27,* 299–304.
Gelfand, D. M., Teti, D. M., & Fox, C. E. (1992). Sources of parenting stress for depressed and nondepressed mothers of infants. *Journal of Clinical Child and Adolescent Psychology, 21*(3), 262–272. doi:10.1207/s15374424jccp2103_8.
Goldsmith, H. H., Buss, K. A., & Lemery, K. S. (1997). Toddler and childhood temperament: Expanded content, stronger genetic evidence, new evidence for the importance of environment. *Developmental Psychology, 33*(6), 891–905. doi:10.1037/0012-1649.33.6.891.
Goodnight, J. A., Bates, J. E., Pettit, G. S., & Dodge, K. A. (2008). Parents' campaigns to reduce their children's conduct problems: Interactions with temperamental resistance to control. *International Journal of Developmental Science, 2*(1–2), 100–119. doi:10.3233/DEV-2008-21207.
Goyal, D., Gay, C., & Lee, K. (2009). Fragmented maternal sleep is more strongly correlated with depressive symptoms than infant temperament at three months postpartum. *Archives of Women's Mental Health, 12*(4), 229–237. doi:10.1007/s00737-009-0070-9.
Gross, R. T., & Borkovec, T. D. (1982). Effects of a cognitive intrusion manipulation on the sleep-onset latency of good sleepers. *Behavior Therapy, 13*(1), 112–116. doi:10.1016/S0005-7894(82)80054-3.
Gross, D., Conrad, B., Fogg, L., & Wothke, W. (1994). A longitudinal model of maternal self-efficacy, depression, and difficult temperament during toddlerhood. *Research in Nursing & Health, 17*(3), 207–215. doi:10.1002/nur.4770170308.
Gross, H. E., Shaw, D. S., & Moilanen, K. L. (2008). Reciprocal associations between boys' externalizing problems and mothers' depressive symptoms. *Journal of Abnormal Child Psychology, 36,* 693–709. doi:10.1007/s10802-008-9224-x.
Harrison, Y., & Horne, J. A. (2000). The impact of sleep deprivation on decision-making: A review. Journal of Experimental Psychology: Applied, 6(3), 236. doi:10.I037// 1076-898X.6.3.236
Hetherington, E. M. (1989). Coping with family transitions: Winners, losers, and survivors. *Child Development, 60*(1), 1–14. doi:10.2307/1131066.
Hobfoll, S. E., & Lerman, M. (1988). Personal relationships, personal attributes, and stress resistance: Mothers' reactions to their child's illness. *American Journal of Community Psychology, 16*(4), 565–589.
Holden, E. W., & Banez, G. A. (1996). Child abuse potential and parenting stress within maltreating families. *Journal of Family Violence, 11*(1), 1–12. doi:10.1007/BF02333337.
Horne, J. A. (1985). Sleep function, with particular reference to sleep deprivation. *Annals of Clinical Research, 17*(5), 199–208.
Iglowstein, I., Jenni, O. G., Molinari, L., & Largo, R. H. (2003). Sleep duration from infancy to adolescence: Reference values and generational trends. *Pediatrics, 111*(2), 302–307.
Ikeda, T., Nagai, T., Kato-Nishimura, K., Mohri, I., & Taniike, M. (2012). Sleep problems in physically disabled children and burden on caregivers. *Brain and Development, 34*(3), 223–229. doi:10.1016/j.braindev.2011.04.011.
Jarvis, P. A., & Creasy, G. L. (1991). Parental stress, coping, and attachment in families with an 18-month-old infant. *Infant Behavior and Development, 14,* 383–395. doi:10.1016/0163-6383 (91)90029-R.

Johnston, C., Mash, E. J., Miller, N., & Ninowski, J. E. (2012). Parenting in adults with attention-deficit/hyperactivity disorder (ADHD). *Clinical Psychology Review, 32*(4), 215–228. doi:10.1016/j.cpr.2012.01.007.

Kaaresen, P. I., Rønning, J. A., Ulvund, S. E., & Dahl, L. B. (2006). A randomized, controlled trial of the effectiveness of an early-intervention program in reducing parenting stress after preterm birth. *Pediatrics, 118*(1), e9–e19.

Kanner, A. D., Coyne, J. C., Schaefer, C., & Lazarus, R. S. (1981). Comparison of two modes of stress measurement: Daily hassles and uplifts versus major life events. *Journal of Behavioral Medicine, 4*(1), 1–39. doi:10.1007/BF00844845.

Kazdin, A. E. (2010). Problem-solving skills training and parent management training for oppositional defiant disorder and conduct disorder. *Evidence-based psychotherapies for children and adolescents*, 211–226.

Kelly, R. J., & El-Sheikh, M. (2011). Marital conflict and children's sleep: Reciprocal relations and socioeconomic effects. *Journal of Family Psychology, 25*(3), 412–422. doi:10.1037/a0023789.

Kim, E. J., & Dimsdale, J. E. (2007). The effect of psychosocial stress on sleep: A review of polysomnographic evidence. *Behavioral Sleep Medicine, 5*(4), 256–278. doi:10.1080/15402000701557383.

Kochanska, G. (1997). Mutually responsive orientation between mothers and their young children: Implications for early socialization. *Child Development, 68*(1), 94–112. doi:10.1111/j.1467-8624.1997.tb01928.x.

Kochanska, G., Clark, A., & Goldman, M. S. (1997). Implications of mothers' personality for their parenting and their young children's developmental outcomes. *Journal of Personality, 65*(2), 387–420. doi:10.1111/1467-6494.ep9708305699.

Kochanska, G., Friesenborg, A. E., Lange, L. A., & Martel, M. M. (2004). Parents' personality and infants' temperament as contributors to their emerging relationship. *Journal of Personality and Social Psychology, 86*(5), 744–759. doi:10.1037/0022-3514.86.5.744.

Kochanska, G., & Murray, K. T. (2000). Mother–child mutually responsive orientation and conscience development: From toddler to early school age. *Child Development, 71*(2), 417–431. doi:10.1111/1467-8624.00154.

Kochanska, G., Philibert, R. A., & Barry, R. A. (2009). Interplay of genes and early mother-child relationship in the development of self-regulation from toddler to preschool age. *Journal of Child Psychology and Psychiatry, 50*(11), 1331–1338. doi:10.1111/j.1469-7610.2008.02050.x.

Konofal, E., Lecendreux, M., Bouvard, M. P., & Mouren-Simeoni, M. C. (2001). High levels of nocturnal activity in children with attention-deficit hyperactivity disorder: A video analysis. *Psychiatry and Clinical Neurosciences, 55*(2), 97–103. doi:10.1046/j.1440-1819.2001.00808.x.

Kotila, L. E., Schoppe-Sullivan, S. J., & Kamp Dush, C. M. (2013). Time in parenting activities in dual-earner families at the transition to parenthood. *Family Relations, 62*(5), 795–807. doi:10.1111/fare.12037.

Lazarus, R. S., DeLongis, A., Folkman, S., & Gruen, R. (1985). Stress and adaptational outcomes: The problem of confounded measures. *American Psychologist, 40,* 70–779. doi:10.1037/0003-066X.40.7.770.

Lazarus, R. S., & Folkman, S. (1984). *Stress, appraisal, and coping*. New York: Springer.

Lee, C. L., & Bates, J. E. (1985). Mother-child interaction at age two years and perceived difficult temperament. *Child Development, 56*(5), 1314–1325. doi:10.2307/1130246.

Loeber, R., & Dishion, T. (1983). Early predictors of male delinquency: A review. *Psychological Bulletin, 94*(1), 68–99. doi:10.1037/0033-2909.94.1.68.

Longfellow, C., Zelkowitz, P., & Saunders, E. (1982). The quality of mother-child relationships. In D. Belle (Ed.), *Lives in stress: Women and depression* (pp. 163–176). Beverly Hills, CA: Sage.

Maccoby, E. E., & Martin, J. A. (1983). Socialization in the context of the family: Parent-child interaction. *Handbook of child psychology: formerly Carmichael's Manual of child psychology/Paul H. Mussen, editor.*

Mackler, J. S., Kelleher, R. T., Shanahan, L., Calkins, S. D., Keane, S. P., & O'Brien, M. (2015). Parenting stress, parental reactions, and externalizing behavior from ages 4 to 10. *Journal of Marriage and Family, 77*(2), 388–406.

Mandler, G. (1975). *Mind and emotion*. New York: Wiley.

Martel, M. M., & Nigg, J. T. (2006). Child ADHD and personality/temperament traits of reactive and effortful control, resiliency, and emotionality. *Journal of Child Psychology and Psychiatry, 47*(11), 1175–1183. doi:10.1111/j.1469-7610.2006.01629.x.

Martin, J., Hiscock, H., Hardy, P., Davey, B., & Wake, M. (2007). Adverse associations of infant and child sleep problems and parent health: An Australian population study. *Pediatrics, 119*(5), 947–955.

Martorell, G. A., & Bugental, D. B. (2006). Maternal variations in stress reactivity: Implications for harsh parenting practices with very young children. *Journal of Family Psychology, 20,* 641–647. doi:10.1037/0893-3200.20.4.641.

Mash, E. J., & Johnston, C. (1983a). Parental perceptions of child behavior problems, parenting self-esteem, and mothers' reported stress in younger and older hyperactive and normal children. *Journal of Consulting and Clinical Psychology, 51*(1), 86. doi:10.1037/0022-006X.51.1.86.

Mash, E. J., & Johnston, C. (1983b). Sibling interactions of hyperactive and normal children and their relationship to reports of maternal stress and self-esteem. *Journal of Clinical Child & Adolescent Psychology, 12*(1), 91–99. doi:10.1080/15374418309533116.

Matheny, A. P., Wachs, T. D., Ludwig, J. L., & Phillips, K. (1995). Bringing order out of chaos: Psychometric characteristics of the confusion, hubbub, and order scale. *Journal of Applied Developmental Psychology, 16*(3), 429–444. doi:10.1016/0193-3973(95)90028-4.

McBride, B. A., & Mills, G. (1994). A comparison of mother and father involvement with their preschool age children. *Early Childhood Research Quarterly, 8,* 457–477. doi:10.1016/S0885-2006(05)80080-8.

McBride, B. A., Schoppe, S. J., & Rane, T. R. (2002). Child characteristics, parenting stress, and parental involvement: Fathers versus mothers. *Journal of Marriage and Family, 64*(4), 998–1011.

Meltzer, L. J., & Mindell, J. A. (2006). Impact of a child's chronic illness on maternal sleep and daytime functioning. *Archives of Internal Medicine, 166*(16), 1749–1755. doi:10.1001/archinte.166.16.1749.

Meltzer, L. J., & Mindell, J. A. (2007). Relationship between child sleep disturbances and maternal sleep, mood, and parenting stress: A pilot study. *Journal of Family Psychology, 21*(1), 67–73. doi:10.1037/0893-3200.21.1.67.

Mendl, M. (1999). Performing under pressure: Atress and cognitive function. *Applied Animal Behaviour Science, 65*(3), 221–244. doi:10.1016/S0168-1591(99)00088-X.

Miller, P. C., Shim, J. E., & Holden, G. W. (1998). Immediate contextual influences on maternal behavior: Environmental affordances and demands. *Journal of Environmental Psychology, 18* (4), 387–398. doi:10.1006/jevp.1998.0111.

Mindell, J. A., Li, A. M., Sadeh, A., Kwon, R., & Goh, D. Y. (2015a). Bedtime routines for young children: A dose-dependent association with sleep outcomes. *Sleep, 38*(5), 717–722. doi:10.5665/sleep.4662.

Mindell, J. A., Sadeh, A., Kwon, R., & Goh, D. Y. (2015b). Relationship between child and maternal sleep: A developmental and cross-cultural comparison. *Journal of Pediatric Psychology*. doi:10.1093/jpepsy/jsv008.

Mindell, J. A., Telofski, L. S., Wiegand, B., & Kurtz, E. S. (2009). A nightly bedtime routine: Impact on sleep in young children and maternal mood. *Sleep, 32*(5), 599–606.

Minkel, J. D., Banks, S., Htaik, O., Moreta, M. C., Jones, C. W., McGlinchey, E. L., et al. (2012). Sleep deprivation and stressors: Evidence for elevated negative affect in response to mild stressors when sleep deprived. *Emotion, 12*(5), 1015–1020. doi:10.1037/a0026871.

Mokrova, I., O'Brien, M., Calkins, S., & Keane, S. (2010). Parental ADHD symptomology and ineffective parenting: The connecting link of home chaos. *Parenting: Science and Practice*, 10 (2), 119–135. doi:10.1080/15295190903212844.

Mörelius, E., & Hemmingsson, H. (2014). Parents of children with physical disabilities–perceived health in parents related to the child's sleep problems and need for attention at night. *Child: Care, Health and Development, 40*(3), 412–418. doi:10.1111/cch.12079.

Motomura, Y., Kitamura, S., Oba, K., Terasawa, Y., Enomoto, M., Katayose, Y., et al. (2013). Sleep debt elicits negative emotional reaction through diminished amygdala-anterior cingulate functional connectivity. *PLoS ONE, 8*(2), e56578. doi:10.1371/journal.pone.0056578.

Mulsow, M., Caldera, Y. M., Pursley, M., Reifman, A., & Huston, A. C. (2002). Multilevel factors influencing maternal stress during the first three years. *Journal of Marriage and Family, 64*(4), 944–956. doi:10.1111/j.1741-3737.2002.00944.x.

Nair, P., Schuler, M. E., Black, M. M., Kettinger, L., & Harrington, D. (2003). Cumulative environmental risk in substance abusing women: Early intervention, parenting stress, child abuse potential and child development. *Child Abuse and Neglect, 27*(9), 997–1017. doi:10.1016/S0145-2134(03)00169-8.

Neece, C. L., Green, S. A., & Baker, B. L. (2012). Parenting stress and child behavior problems: A transactional relationship across time. *American Journal on Intellectual and Developmental Disabilities, 117*(1), 48–66. doi:10.1352/1944-7558-117.1.48.

Nomaguchi, K. M. (2009). Change in work-family conflict among employed parents between 1977 and 1997. *Journal of Marriage and Family, 71*(1), 15–32. doi:10.1111/j.1741-3737.2008.00577.x.

Nomaguchi, K.M., & Johnson, W. (2014). Parenting stress among low-income and working-class fathers: The role of employment. *Journal of Family Issues*, 1–23. doi:10.1177/0192513X14560642.

Norlander, T., Johansson, Å., & Bood, S. Å. (2005). The affective personality: Its relation to quality of sleep, well-being and stress. *Social Behavior and Personality: An international journal, 33*(7), 709–722.

Östberg, M., & Hagekull, B. (2000). A structural modeling approach to the understanding of parenting stress. *Journal of Clinical Child Psychology, 29*(4), 615–625. doi:10.1207/S15374424JCCP2904_13.

Owens, J. A. (2005). The ADHD and sleep conundrum: A review. *Journal of Developmental Behavioral Pediatrics, 26*(4), 312–322.

Patterson, G. R. (1980). Mothers: The unacknowledged victims. *Monographs of the Society for Research in Child Development,* 1980, 45(5).

Patterson, G. R. (1982). *Coercive family process* (Vol. 3). Castalia Publishing Company.

Patterson, G. R. (1983). Stress: A change agent for family process. In N. Garmezy & M. Rutter (Eds.), *Stress, coping, and development in children* (pp. 235–264). New York: McGraw-Hill.

Patterson, G. R., DeBaryshe, B. D., & Ramsey, E. (1989). *A developmental perspective on antisocial behavior* (Vol. 44, No. 2, p. 329). American Psychological Association.

Patterson, G. R., Reid, J. B., & Dishion, T. J. (1992). *Antisocial boys: A social interactional approach.* Eugene, OR: Castalia.

Pesonen, A. K., Räikkönen, K., Heinonen, K., Komsi, N., Järvenpää, A. L., & Strandberg, T. (2008). A transactional model of temperamental development: Evidence of a relationship between child temperament and maternal stress over five years. *Social Development, 17*(2), 326–340. doi:10.1111/j.1467-9507.2007.00427.x.

Peterson, J. L., & Zill, N. (1986). Marital disruption, parent-child relationships, and behavior problems in children. *Journal of Marriage and the Family*, 295–307. doi:10.2307/352397.

Pilcher, J. J., & Huffcutt, A. J. (1996). Effects of sleep deprivation on performance: A meta-analysis. *Sleep: Journal of Sleep Research & Sleep Medicine, 19* (4), 318–326.

Pinderhughes, E. E., Dodge, K. A., Bates, J. E., Pettit, G. S., & Zelli, A. (2000). Discipline responses: Influences of parents' socioeconomic status, ethnicity, beliefs about parenting, stress, and cognitive-emotional processes. *Journal of Family Psychology, 14*(3), 380–400. doi:10.1037/0893-3200.14.3.380.

Piquero, A. R., Farrington, D. P., Welsh, B. C., Tremblay, R., & Jennings, W. G. (2009). Effects of early family/parent training programs on antisocial behavior and delinquency. *Journal of Experimental Criminology, 5*(2), 83–120. doi:10.1007/s11292-009-9072-x.

Pisterman, S., Firestone, P., McGrath, P., Goodman, J. T., Webster, I., Mallory, R., et al. (1992). The effects of parent training on parenting stress and sense of competence. *Canadian Journal of Behavioral Science, 24*(1), 41–58. doi:10.1037/h0078699.

Podolski, C. L., & Nigg, J. T. (2001). Parent stress and coping in relation to child ADHD severity and associated child disruptive behavior problems. *Journal of Clinical Child Psychology, 30* (4), 503–513. doi:10.1207/S15374424JCCP3004_07.

Prinzie, P., Stams, G. J. J., Deković, M., Reijntjes, A. H., & Belsky, J. (2009). The relations between parents' Big Five personality factors and parenting: A meta-analytic review. *Journal of Personality and Social Psychology, 97*(2), 351–362. doi:10.1037/a0015823.

Putnam, S. P., Sanson, A. V., & Rothbart, M. K. (2002). Child temperament and parenting. *Handbook of Parenting, 1,* 255–277.

Quittner, A. L., Glueckauf, R. L., & Jackson, D. N. (1990). Chronic parenting stress: Moderating versus mediating effects of social support. *Journal of Personality and Social Psychology, 59* (6), 1266–1278. doi:10.1037/0022-3514.59.6.1266.

Raine, A. (1996). Autonomic nervous system factors underlying disinhibited, antisocial, and violent behavior biosocial perspectives and treatment implications. *Annals of the New York Academy of Science, 794,* 46–59.

Reilly, M. D. (1982). Working wives and convenience consumption. *Journal of Consumer Research, 8,* 407–418.

Repetti, R., & Wood, J. (1997). Effects of daily stress at work on mothers' interactions with preschoolers. *Journal of Family Psychology, 11,* 90–108. doi:10.1037/0893-3200.11.1.90.

Rodgers, A. Y. (1993). The assessment of variables related to the parenting behavior of mothers with young children. *Children and Youth Services Review, 15*(5), 385–402. doi:10.1016/0190-7409(93)90011-W.

Rothbart, M.K., & Bates, J. E. (1998). Temperament. In Diamond & N. Eisenberg, Handbook of Child Psychology: Social, emotional and personality development (Vol. 3, pp. 105–162). New York: Wiley.

Rothbart, M. K., & Bates, J. E. (2006). Handbook of Child Psychology (6th ed.). In W. Damon, R. Lerner & N. Eisenberg (Eds.), *Social, emotional, and personality development* (Vol. 3, pp. 99–166). New York: Wiley.

Rutter, M. (1981). Stress, coping and development: Some issues and some questions. *Journal of Child Psychology and Psychiatry, 22*(4), 323–356. doi:10.1111/j.1469-7610.1981.tb00560.x.

Sadeh, A., Lavie, P., & Scher, A. (1994). Sleep and temperament: Maternal perceptions of temperament of sleep-disturbed toddlers. *Early Education and Development, 5*(4), 311–322. doi:10.1207/s15566935eed0504_6.

Sadeh, A., Mindell, J. A., Luedtke, K., & Wiegand, B. (2009). Sleep and sleep ecology in the first 3 years: A web-based study. *Journal of Sleep Research, 18*(1), 60–73. doi:10.1111/j.1365-2869.2008.00699.x.

Sameroff, A. J. (2006). Identifying risk and protective factors for healthy youth development. In A. ClarkeStewart & J. Dunn (Eds.), *Families count: Effects on child and adolescent development* (pp. 53–76). Cambridge, UK: Cambridge University Press.

Sameroff, A. (2010). A unified theory of development: A dialectic integration of nature and nurture. *Child Development, 81*(1), 6–22. doi:10.1111/j.1467-8624.2009.01378.x.

Sanders, M. R. (1999). Triple P-Positive Parenting Program: Towards an empirically validated multilevel parenting and family support strategy for the prevention of behavior and emotional problems in children. *Clinical Child and Family Psychology Review, 2*(2), 71–90.

Scarr, S., Phillips, D., & McCartney, K. (1990). Facts, fantasies and the future of child care in the United States. *Psychological Science, 1*(1), 26–35.

Schermerhorn, A. C., Bates, J. E., Goodnight, J. A., Lansford, J. E., Dodge, K. A., & Pettit, G. S. (2013). Temperament moderates associations between exposure to stress and children's externalizing problems. *Child Development, 84*(5), 1579–1593. doi:10.1111/cdev.12076.

Scott, S., & O'Connor, T. G. (2012). An experimental test of differential susceptibility to parenting among emotionally-dysregulated children in a randomized controlled trial for oppositional behavior. *Journal of Child Psychology and Psychiatry*. doi:10.1111/j.1469-7610.2012.02586.x.

Selye, H. (1979). *The stress of my life: A scientist's memoirs*. New York: Toronto; Van Nostrand Reinhold.

Shaki, D., Goldbart, A., Daniel, S., Fraser, D., & Shorer, Z. (2011). Pediatric epilepsy and parental sleep quality. *Journal of Clinical Sleep Medicine, 7*(5), 502–506. doi:10.5664/JCSM.1318.

Snyder, J. (2015). Coercive family processes and the development of child social behavior and self-regulation. In T. J. Dishion & J. Snyder (Eds.), *The Oxford handbook of coercive relationship dynamics* (pp. 101–114). New York: Oxford University Press.

Snyder, J., & Patterson, G. R. (1986). The effects of consequences on patterns of social interaction: A quasi-experimental approach to reinforcement in natural interaction. *Child Development*, 1257–1268. doi:10.2307/1130448.

Soehner, A. M., Kennedy, K. S., & Monk, T. H. (2007). Personality correlates with sleep-wake variables. *Chronobiology International, 24*(5), 889–903.

Staples, A. D., Bates, J. E., & Petersen, I. T. (2015). IX. Bedtime routines in early childhood: Prevalence, consistency, and associations with nighttime sleep. *Monographs of the Society for Research in Child Development, 80*(1), 141–159. doi:10.1111/mono.12149.

Stein, M. A., Mendelsohn, J., Obermeyer, W. H., Amromin, J., & Benca, R. (2001). Sleep and behavior problems in school-aged children. *Pediatrics, 107*(4), e60–e69.

Strelau, J. (2001). The concept and status of trait in research on temperament. *European Journal of Personality, 15*(4), 311–325.

Sturge-Apple, M. L., Suor, J. H., & Skibo, M. A. (2014). Maternal child-centered attributions and harsh discipline: The moderating role of maternal working memory across socioeconomic contexts. *Journal of Family Psychology, 28*(5), 645–654. doi:10.1037/fam0000023.

Taylor, D. J., & McFatter, R. M. (2003). Cognitive performance after sleep deprivation: Does personality make a difference? *Personality and Individual Differences, 34*(7), 1179–1193. doi:10.1016/S0191-8869(02)00108-3.

Terry, D. J., Mayocchi, L., & Hynes, G. J. (1996). Depressive symptomatology in new mothers: A stress and coping perspective. *Journal of Abnormal Psychology, 105*(2), 220–231. doi:10.1037/0021-843X.105.2.220.

Thomas, A., & Chess, S. (1977). *Temperament and development*. Brunner/Mazel.

Thompson, R. J., Merritt, K. A., Keith, B. R., Bennett, L., & Johndrow, D. A. (1993). The role of maternal stress and family functioning in maternal distress and mother-reported psychological adjustment of non-referred children. *Journal of Clinical Child Psychology, 22,* 78–84. doi:10.1207/s15374424jccp2201_8.

Thunstrom, M. (1999). Severe sleep problems among infants: Family and infant characteristics. *Ambulatory Child Health, 5*(1), 27–41.

Tremblay, R. E. (2000). The development of aggressive behavior during childhood: What have we learned in the past century? *International Journal of Behavioral Development, 24,* 129–141. doi:10.1080/016502500383232.

Turner, K. M., & Sanders, M. R. (2006). Help when it's needed first: A controlled evaluation of brief, preventive behavioral family intervention in a primary care setting. *Behavior Therapy, 37* (2), 131–142. doi:10.1016/j.beth.2005.05.004.

Valiente, C., Lemery-Chalfant, K., & Reiser, M. (2007). Pathways to problem behaviors: Chaotic homes, parent and child effortful control, and parenting. *Social Development, 16*(2), 249–267. doi:10.1111/j.1467-9507.2007.00383.x.

Van Reeth, O., Weibel, L., Spiegel, K., Leproult, R., Dugovic, C., & Maccari, S. (2000). Physiology of sleep (review)–interactions between stress and sleep: From basic research to clinical situations. *Sleep Medicine Reviews, 4*(2), 201–219. doi:10.1053/smrv.1999.0097.

Wachs, T. D. (1993). Nature of relations between the physical and social microenvironment of the two-year-old child. *Early Development and Parenting, 2,* 81–87. doi:10.1002/edp.2430020202.

Wachs, T. D., & Camli, O. (1991). Do ecological or individual characteristics mediate the influence of the physical environment upon maternal behavior? *Journal of Environmental Psychology, 11,* 249–264. doi:10.1016/S0272-4944(05)80186-0.

Wahler, R. G., & Dumas, J. E. (1984). *Changing the observational coding styles of insular and noninsular mothers: A step toward maintenance of parent training effects* (pp. 379–416). Parent training: Foundations of research and practice.

Wahler, R. G., & Dumas, J. E. (1989). Attentional problems in dysfunctional mother-child interactions: An interbehavioral model. *Psychological Bulletin, 105*(1), 116–130. doi:10.1037/0033-2909.105.1.116.

Weinstein, C. S., Apfel, R. J., & Weinstein, S. R. (1998). Description of mothers with ADHD with children with ADHD. *Psychiatry, 61*(1), 12–19. doi:10.1521/00332747.1998.11024815.

Williford, A. P., Calkins, S. D., & Keane, S. P. (2007). Predicting change in parenting stress across early childhood: Child and maternal factors. *Journal of Abnormal Child Psychology, 35*(2), 251–263. doi:10.1007/s10802-006-9082-3.

Winslow, S. (2005). Work-family conflict, gender, and parenthood, 1977–1997. *Journal of Family Issues, 26,* 727–755. doi:10.1177/0192513X05277522.

Wolf, S., & Acton, W. P. (1968). Characteristics of parents of disturbed children. *British Journal of Psychiatry, 114,* 593–601.

Wolfe, D. A., Edwards, B., Manion, I., & Koverola, C. (1988). Early intervention for parents at risk of child abuse and neglect: A preliminary investigation. *Journal of Consulting and Clinical Psychology, 56*(1), 40–47. doi:10.1037/0022-006X.56.1.40.

Wolfson, A., Lacks, P., & Futterman, A. (1992). Effects of parent training on infant sleeping patterns, parents' stress, and perceived parental competence. *Journal of Consulting and Clinical Psychology, 60*(1), 41–48. doi:10.1037/0022-006X.60.1.41.

Yaman, A., Mesman, J., Van IJzendoorn, M. H., Bakermans-Kranenburg, M. J., & Linting, M. (2010). Parenting in an individualistic culture with a collectivistic cultural background: The case of Turkish immigrant families with toddlers in the Netherlands. *Journal of Child and Family Studies, 19,* 617–628. doi:10.1007/s10826-009-9346-y.

Zhang, J., Li, A. M., Fok, T. F., & Wing, Y. K. (2010). Roles of parental sleep/wake patterns, socioeconomic status, and daytime activities in the sleep/wake patterns of children. *Journal of Pediatrics, 156*(4), 606–612. doi:10.1016/j.jpeds.2009.10.036.

Zubrick, S. R., Ward, K. A., Silburn, S. R., Lawrence, D., Williams, A. A., Blair, E., et al. (2005). Prevention of child behavior problems through universal implementation of a group behavioral family intervention. *Prevention Science, 6*(4), 287–304. doi:10.1007/s11121-005-0013-2.

Chapter 5
The Stress of Parenting Children with Developmental Disabilities

Cameron L. Neece and Neilson Chan

The Stress of Parenting Children with Developmental Disabilities

Parenting stress is one family-level attribute that has consistently been implicated in the creation of risk for families of children with intellectual and developmental disabilities (IDD; Baker et al., 2003; Woodman, Mawdsley, & Hauser-Cram, 2015), and may be the catalyst for many of the other risks that these families and children experience. Parents of children with IDD generally report higher levels of stress than do parents of typically developing children (Baker et al., 2003; Hauser-Cram, Warfield, Shonkoff, & Kraus, 2001). Stress processes, however, are mutable and interventions for parenting stress may be especially beneficial for these families given the noted adverse correlates of their obstacles and challenges.

Stress has long played an integral role in understanding parenting processes. Yet, despite the volume of work on parenting stress, no single, clear, conceptualization of parenting stress has emerged (see Chap. 11 by Crnic and Ross for an overview of conceptualizations of parenting stress). In general, research on stress among parents of children with IDD has focused on three types of stress: general distress, stress specific to the child's condition, and daily parenting hassles. General parenting distress is defined as the extent to which the parent perceives stress in his/her role as a parent (Abidin, 1990). Stress specific to the child with IDD has been assessed using measures that ask about the child's impact on the family compared to the impact other children his/her age have on their families (e.g., Family Impact Questionnaire; Donenberg & Baker, 1993). Studies have also examined parents'

C.L. Neece (✉) · N. Chan
Department of Psychology, Loma Linda University, Loma Linda, CA, USA
e-mail: cneece@llu.edu

N. Chan
e-mail: nechan@llu.edu

K. Deater-Deckard and R. Panneton (eds.), *Parental Stress and Early Child Development*, DOI 10.1007/978-3-319-55376-4_5

daily stressors and everyday challenges and caregiving demands that characterize their routine childrearing responsibilities (Crnic & Greenberg, 1990). Research indicates that the degree of stress experienced by parents of children with developmental disabilities may vary by type of stress, with some studies indicating parents of young children with developmental delays experience similar levels of parenting daily hassles to parents of typically developing children (Crnic, Arbona, Baker, & Blacher, 2009), but greater parenting stress related to the impact of the child on the family (Baker et al., 2003). Thus, disability-specific stresses may well be at play and should be further differentiated from more general stress contexts experienced by all families. Parents of children with IDD may experience stress associated with increased caregiving demands and coordination of care (Crnic, Greenberg, Ragozin, Robinson, & Basham, 1983) as well as the presence of co-occurring behavioral or medical conditions (e.g., Baker et al., 2003). These stressors, coupled with additional financial strain (e.g., Parish, Seltzer, Greenberg, & Floyd, 2004) and feelings of isolation and lack of social support (e.g., Weiss, 2002), may place parents of children with IDD at risk for psychological distress.

Although studies consistently find heightened levels of various stressors among parents of children with IDD, such findings are not universal, and there can be marked individual variation in the trajectory of experienced stress over the developmental period being considered (Glidden & Schoolcraft, 2003; Pai et al., 2007). For parents of children with IDD, average levels of stress are higher across all developmental periods from infancy through adolescence (Baker et al., 2003; Lopez, Clifford, Minnes, & Ouellette-Kuntz, 2008), and there is some evidence to suggest that parenting stress increases over time (Gerstein, Crnic, Blacher, & Baker, 2009; Hauser-Cram & Warfield, 2001; Neece, Green, & Baker, 2012). Other studies indicate parental stress generally appears to peak around the preschool period and decreases over time as a function of reductions in child behavior problems, although stresses not accounted for by the child actually increase over time (Crnic et al., 2009; Neece et al., 2012). Parents of children with IDD may be more likely to have recurrent and new stressors that maintain and even increase stress levels across time. Transitions, including school entry and reintegrations (Canter & Roberts, 2012; DuPaul, Weyandt, O'Dell, & Varejao, 2009; Madan-Swain, Katz, & LaGory, 2004), may be particularly difficult times for parents of children with IDD as these are often when parents make peer comparisons and realize how far their children are behind other children, or have to help their children to cope with challenging social situations. It is clear that parents of children with IDD are faced with multiple challenges across their children's lives, including overcoming the disappointments and fears associated with the original diagnoses, securing appropriate medical interventions and school placements, and learning to navigate the complex health and educational systems (DuPaul et al., 2009). Effects may vary depending on the type of parental stress and be different for fathers and mothers, and highlight the necessity for multidimensional longitudinal studies addressing the experience of these families.

Among parents of children with disabilities, those who have children with autism spectrum disorders (ASD) typically report the highest levels of stress

(Blacher & McIntyre, 2006; Dabrowska & Pisula, 2010; Eisenhower, Baker, & Blacher, 2005; Estes et al., 2009; Pisula, 2007; Sanders & Morgan, 1997), whereas those with genetic syndromes of intellectual disability (e.g., Down syndrome) typically reporting lower levels of parenting stress (Dabrowska & Pisula, 2010; Smith, Romski, Sevcik, Adamson, & Barker, 2014). In fact, in studies examining the clinical profiles of these parents, approximately one-third to two-thirds of both mothers and fathers reported clinical levels of parental stress (greater than 85th percentile on the Parenting Stress Index; Abidin, 1990) indicating they should be referred for professional consultation (Davis & Carter, 2008; Tomanik, Harris, & Hawkins, 2004). Furthermore, while parents of children with ADHD report higher levels of child-related stress compared to parents of children with IDD, no significant difference exists in stress derived from the parenting role between parents of children with ADHD or IDD (Theule, Wiener, Tannock, & Jenkins, 2013). Parents of children with IDD also report higher levels of parenting stress than those of children with medical disabilities (e.g., HIV and asthma) but no IDD (Gupta, 2007).

Predictors and Consequences of Parenting Stress Among Families of Children with IDD

High levels of parental stress are concerning given their association with numerous undesirable outcomes including parent depression (Anastopoulos & Guevremont, 1992; Deater-Deckard, 1998; Hastings, Daley, Burns, & Beck, 2006), marital conflict (Kersh, Hedvat, Warfield, Hauser-Cram, & Warfield, 2006; Suárez & Baker, 1997), poorer physical health (Eisenhower, Baker, & Blacher, 2009; Oelofsen & Richardson, 2006), and less effective parenting (Coldwell, Pike, & Dunn, 2006; Crnic, Gaze, & Hoffman, 2005). Further, families of children with IDD, who experienced high levels of stress on average, reported more family problems, lower parental satisfaction and well-being, and less parental competence and social support (Pisula, 2007; Rodrigue, Morgan, & Geffken, 1990; Sanders & Morgan, 1997). See Chap. 11 by Crnic and Ross (2016) for further discussion on how parenting stress impacts parental efficacy and competence. These studies highlight the salience of parental stress as an environmental risk factor for the development of children with IDD.

Child behavior problems have been found to be the most consistent predictor of parenting stress among families of children with IDD. Persons with IDD are at high risk for behavior problems, and studies have found heightened externalizing and internalizing behavior problems relative to typically developing children (Baker, Blacher, Crnic, & Edelbrock, 2002; Emerson & Einfeld, 2010; Merrell & Holland, 1997). These elevated levels of behavior problems are associated with heightened risk for developing comorbid mental disorders later in life (Baker, Neece, Fenning, Crnic, & Blacher, 2010). Further, studies have shown that both the frequency and severity of externalizing and internalizing child behavior problems have been found to predict elevated levels of parenting stress above and beyond the influence of other child and parent factors, such as child's adaptive behavior (Hodapp, Fidler, & Smith, 1998; Woodman, 2014), autism symptoms (Osborne & Reed, 2009), family socioeconomic status, and parent social support (Quine & Pahl, 1991; Sloper, Knussen, Turner, & Cunningham, 1991; Woodman, 2014). Interestingly, the relationship between child developmental status and parenting stress appears to be mediated by child behavior problems such that once behavior problems are accounted for, there is no longer a significant relationship between child cognitive delay and parenting stress (Baker et al., 2002; Hauser-Cram & Warfield, 2001; Herring et al., 2006). In other words, these studies indicate that the child's behavioral functioning, rather than his or her cognitive functioning, is a more salient predictor of parent stress.

Importantly, research has indicated that the relationship between parenting stress and child behavior problems is bidirectional and transactional over time. Thus, while child behavior problems are a robust and consistent predictor of parenting stress, parenting stress has also been found to predict increases in child behavior problems over time (Baker et al., 2003; Donenberg & Baker, 1993; Neece et al., 2012). Further, early elevations in parenting stress have been associated with poorer social skills in children later in development (Neece & Baker, 2008) and a subsequent ADHD diagnosis (Baker et al., 2010). Thus, increasing parental stress acts as a predictor of multiple negative outcomes for children with IDD. Moreover, the literature on typically developing children provides additional evidence of negative child outcomes associated with elevated parenting stress to which children with IDD may also be susceptible, including higher levels of emotion dysregulation (Anthony et al., 2005; Mathis & Bierman, 2015), more depressive symptoms (Anthony, Bromberg, Gil, & Schanberg, 2011), poorer peer competence (Guralnick, Neville, Connor, & Hammond, 2003), and an overall poorer quality of life (Moreira, Gouveia, Carona, Silva, & Canavarro, 2014).

As mentioned above, research indicates that the relationship between parental stress and behavior problems in children is reciprocal such that child behavior problems lead to increases in parental stress, which further exacerbate the development of child behavior problems. Longitudinal studies indicate that high behavior problems lead to increases in parenting stress over time, and high parenting stress leads to increases in behavior problems in children (Baker et al., 2003; Neece et al., 2012) as well as adults (Orsmond, Seltzer, Krauss, & Hong, 2003). We conducted a study investigating the relationship between parenting stress and child behavior problems at seven time points from child ages 3 to 9 using a sample of 237 children, 144 who were typically developing and 93 who were identified as developmentally delayed (Neece et al., 2012). Results indicated that behavior problems and parenting stress covaried significantly across development, and that child developmental status in general did not moderate the relationship between behavior problems and stress over time. These findings are congruent with past studies showing cognitive functioning has an indirect effect on parenting stress that is accounted for by child behavior problems (e.g., Baker et al., 2003). We investigated the *direction* of the relationship between child behavior problems and parenting stress across early and middle childhood (ages 3–9), using cross-lagged panel analyses. These analyses supported a bidirectional relationship between parenting stress and child behavior problems for both mothers and fathers, after controlling for the child's developmental status.

Recently, Woodman, Mawdsley, and Hauser-Cram (2015) expanded these findings by investigating the transactional relationship between parenting stress and child behavior problems among families of children with IDD at five time points from early childhood (age 3) through late adolescence (age 18), examining the unique contributions of internalizing and externalizing child behavior problems to parental stress. Consistent with earlier findings (e.g., Neece et al., 2012), cross-lagged panel analyses supported a bidirectional relationship between parenting stress and internalizing child behavior problems in early childhood (ages 3–5), but not between parenting stress and externalizing behavior problems.

Interestingly, the Neece et al. (2012) study found the effect of early parental stress on later child behavior problems was more consistent over time than the effect of early behavior problems on later parental stress. This is consistent with studies investigating families of children with ASD which indicate that parenting stress is associated with child behavior problems over time, even after controlling for prior child behavior problems, severity of child ASD symptoms, intellectual functioning, and adaptive behavior (Osborne & Reed, 2009; Lecavalier, Leone, & Wiltz, 2006). Further, parenting stress appears to predict future child behavior problems more strongly than child behavior problems predict subsequent parenting stress (Lecavalier et al., 2006; Osborne & Reed, 2009).

Intervention studies provide a more controlled test of the transactional relationship between parenting stress and child behavior problems (see also Chap. 12 by Havighurst & Kehoe). When participants are randomly assigned to an intervention group, and the intervention successfully reduces child behavior problems (or parenting stress), researchers can examine the collateral effects on parenting stress (or child behavior problems). For example, some studies have found that parent stress-reduction interventions have led to improvements in child behavior problems with no child-specific intervention (Neece, 2013; Singh et al., 2007), whereas other studies have found that behavioral parent training interventions aimed at reducing child behavior problems also resulted in reductions in parenting stress (Feldman & Werner, 2002; Nieter, Thornberry, & Brestan-Knight, 2013; Painter, Cook, & Silverman, 1999; Singh et al., 2014; Wainberg, 1999). However, behavioral parent training approaches do not consistently result in reductions of parenting stress (Singer, Ethridge, & Aldana, 2007), and stress-reduction interventions for parents of children with IDD do not always lead to reductions in child behavior problems (Dykens, Fisher, & Taylor, 2014). Thus, an integrated intervention model that directly targets parenting stress within the context of building parenting skills that promote more positive parent-child interactions and reduce behavior problems may be optimally effective.

Nevertheless, findings generally provide converging evidence of a transactional relationship between parenting stress and child behavior problems among families of children with IDD. In general, results indicate that parenting stress is both an antecedent and consequence of child behavior problems. Simultaneously, child behavior problems are an antecedent and consequence of parenting stress, and both appear to have a mutually escalating, or de-escalating, effect on each other over time. As such, both appear critical targets for intervention.

Intervention Implications and Mindfulness-Based Strategies

Given the negative consequences associated with parenting stress for both the parent and the child with IDD, parenting stress is a clear target for intervention. Interventions that target parental stress offer the opportunity to ameliorate and ideally prevent the development of psychopathology among youth with IDD. Surprisingly, parenting stress is rarely directly addressed in interventions targeting child problems. Most of these interventions are child-focused, teaching parents skills to manage their children's behavior problems and assume that by reducing behavior problems parenting stress will decline. However, in light of findings showing that parenting stress has an impact on the development of children's behavior problems, it seems logical that parenting stress should be a target for interventions aiming to reduce child behavior problems. This is reasonable not only because parental stress has been shown to affect the development of children's emotional and behavior problems over time, but also because parenting stress has been associated with poor outcomes for interventions focused on children with IDD and other developmental disabilities. More specifically, high parental stress predicts less beneficial outcomes for children in early intervention programs (Brinker, Seifer, & Sameroff, 1994; Osborne, McHugh, Saunders, & Reed, 2008; Robbins, Dunlap, & Plienis, 1991; Strauss et al., 2012) and fewer gains in parenting skills in behavioral parenting training interventions (e.g., Baker, Landen, & Kashima, 1991).

Consistent with transactional models of family process in which ongoing parental stress can serve to promote later child behavior problems (Neece et al., 2012; see also Chap. 4 by McQuillan & Bates), emerging research indicates that interventions focused on reducing parental stress in families of young children with IDD benefits not only parents (e.g., significant reduction in stress and depression as well as improved life satisfaction) but also children with IDD who showed a reduction in behavior problems following intervention (Neece, 2013). While behavioral parent training focuses on the acquisition of specific parenting skills that promote positive child behavior, mindfulness-based strategies directly target stressors that may be associated with the presence of problematic child behavior (Bazzano et al., 2015; Neece, 2013). Mindfulness is the awareness that emerges through paying attention on purpose and nonjudgmentally to the unfolding of experience moment by moment (Kabat-Zinn, 2003). Mindfulness training involves teaching individuals to use strategies to disengage attention from internal thoughts and feelings that elicit distress and to focus on their present experience directly without appraisals or interpretations (Singh et al., 2014)

Although still in its infancy, research examining mindfulness-based interventions for parents of children with intellectual and developmental disabilities is growing rapidly. During the past decade, the feasibility and preliminary efficacy of mindfulness-based interventions have been tested in pilot studies (Bazzano et al., 2015; Minor, Carlson, Mackenzie, Zernicke, & Jones, 2006; Roberts & Neece, 2015) and in larger, well-controlled studies that consisted of methodologically rigorous, single-case designs (Singh et al., 2006, 2007, 2014); waitlist-control randomized trials (Neece, 2013); and large-scale randomized, controlled trials with an active comparison group (Dykens et al., 2014). Currently, the majority of the literature about mindfulness interventions for parents consists of studies of parents with children who have developmental disabilities. This indicates that researchers are increasingly recognizing the need for stress-reduction and parenting interventions among this population.

Two types of mindfulness-based interventions have been used primarily with parents of children with IDD. First is mindfulness-based stress reduction (MBSR), which is an evidence-based stress-reduction intervention program supported by more than two decades of extensive research that has revealed its effectiveness for reducing stress, anxiety, and depression and for promoting overall well-being (Chiesa & Serretti, 2009). However, only recently has MBSR been used to address parenting stress specifically (Bazzano et al., 2015; Dykens et al., 2014; Minor et al., 2006; Neece, 2013). Again, mindfulness interventions like MBSR train individuals to use strategies to disengage attention from internal thoughts and feelings that elicit distress and to focus on their present experience directly without appraisals or interpretations (Singh et al., 2014). By focusing on the immediate experience, individuals are able to become more aware of which aspects of the experience are worth responding to, ignoring, or simply observing. It is thought that mindfulness training improves participants' emotion regulation skills through enhancing their attention monitoring abilities and facilitating nonjudgmental awareness of emotions, allowing people to genuinely experience and express their emotions without underengagement (e.g., avoidance) or overengagement (e.g., rumination; Chambers, Gullone, & Allen, 2009). In the MBSR program, parents learn to cope more effectively with both short- and long-term stressful situations. These coping skills are critical for parents of children with IDD. MBSR may also help improve one's parenting experience in that mindfulness may help parents slow down, notice impulses before they act, truly listen to their children, and come to a more relaxed and peaceful state of mind, which in turn may have a positive effect on their children with IDD.

The second kind of mindfulness-based parenting intervention, mindful parenting, has also been used with parents of children with IDD and other developmental disabilities, and initial findings are promising (Singh et al., 2006, 2014). Mindful parenting differs from MBSR in that the focus of mindful parenting is on using mindfulness specifically in the context of parent–child interactions and identifying interactions that result in relational disconnectedness (Altmaier & Maloney, 2007), rather than on applying mindfulness techniques to parental stress more broadly, regardless of the source of stress. These interventions incorporate mindfulness, self-awareness, and intentionality into the parent–child relationship. As a result, parent–child interactions are less reactive and are characterized by more relaxed communication and problem solving, which are ultimately thought to result in the reduction of children's challenging behavior (Singh et al., 2014). Findings indicate that mindful parenting interventions are effective for reducing children's externalizing behavior and attention problems and for improving children's self-control, compliance, and attunement to others (Bögels, Hoogstad, van Dun, de Schutter, & Restifo, 2008; Singh et al., 2009; Singh, Singh, & Lancioni, 2010).

Other Stress-Reduction Interventions

Other interventions aimed at reducing stress of parents of children with IDD range from respite interventions, to peer support interventions, to more structured psycho-educational group interventions (Hastings & Beck, 2004). Respite care generally involves short-term care of an individual with disabilities in order to bring relief to the primary caregiver or family of the individual (Warren & Cohen, 1985). Cowen and Reed (2002) describe different types of respite services that typically range between either primary or secondary sources of relief. Primary respite care services generally provide relief to the primary caregiver from the intense care demands of the child with disabilities. Secondary respite care services more specifically target the needs of those with developmental disabilities and may provide educational training programs in addition to services such as speech-, occupational-, and physical-therapy.

Not surprisingly, among families of children with IDD, parents who report greater psychological distress and lower levels of optimism about their coping abilities are more likely to use respite care services (Hoare, Harris, Jackson, & Kerley, 1998). Researchers have found that families that used respite care services generally reported lower levels of parenting stress as well as a greater ability to cope with stressors of having a child with IDD. These parents also reported lower levels of psychological distress, including lower levels of anxiety, depression, and a higher overall quality of life (Chan & Sigafoos, 2001; Cowen & Reed, 2002; Rimmerman, Kramer, Levy, & Levy, 1989). In a longitudinal study examining whether the effects of respite care services persisted six months after services ceased, Mullins, Aniol, Boyd, Page, and Chaney (2002) found that while lowered levels of general psychological distress were maintained in the long-term, reduced levels of parenting stress returned back to baseline levels at the six-month follow-up. These studies demonstrate that while respite care services may diminish the general distress parents of IDD experience, the specific stress related to parenting a child with IDD may only be temporarily ameliorated.

Peer support interventions, such as the Parent-to-Parent Movement (Davidson & Dosser Jr, 1982), have a growing research base supporting their effectiveness in reducing parenting stress among parents of children with IDD. The parent-to-parent model involves matching a parent with a parent supporter based on the following features: (1) the parent supporter with experience in caring for children with IDD must have had training in providing support techniques; (2) referrals to this service come from a range of sources, including both professional and informal contacts; (3) the parent supporter is matched to the parent based on the parent's needs, typically based on the child's diagnosis; and (4) the parent and parent supporter self-manage the extent of contact between one another (Hastings & Beck, 2004). In a controlled study by Singer et al. (1999) examining the impact of the parent-to-parent support model, results suggested a decrease in parenting stress among parents involved in the parent-support model. Specifically, parents reported more positive perceptions of their child and their impact on the family, as well as a marked improvement in their progress toward the resolution of their primary needs. However, when the four criteria above were not met (e.g., children's needs were not comparable), the parent-to-parent model of support was less effective (Ainbinder et al., 1998).

The literature also supports the potential efficacy of group-based interventions focused on improving parental well-being. The majority of structured group interventions aimed at reducing parenting stress among families of children with IDD incorporate some aspects of cognitive behavioral therapy (CBT), including problem solving, cognitive restructuring, and monitoring thoughts and feelings (Gammon & Rose, 1991; Greaves, 1997; Kirkham & Schilling, 1990; Kirkham, 1993; Wong & Poon, 2010). While these studies examining interventions incorporating elements of CBT report optimistic results in reducing parenting stress, certain limitation should be considered. First, because these interventions operate in a group setting in which CBT elements are only a part of the intervention, we cannot isolate the CBT aspects as the sole active ingredient responsible for reducing parenting stress, especially in studies utilizing a waitlist-control design (Nixon & Singer, 1993; Singer, Irvin, & Hawkins, 1988). It is likely that other therapeutic aspects of simply being in a group, such as receiving support from others with a shared experience, may have contributed to reductions in stress (Hastings & Beck, 2004). Second, there were limited follow-up data collected in these studies, and limiting conclusions we can draw about the effectiveness of the interventions in the long-term.

Directions for Future Research

Although parenting stress has been a significant focus of research among families of children with IDD over the last few decades, there are still a number of avenues for future research. Perhaps most importantly, it is critical that future investigations examine the mechanisms through which parental stress may influence child behavior problems and other child outcomes. Parenting behavior is one possible mediating variable that may partially account for this relationship. Parenting stress has been linked to less responsive, more authoritarian, and more neglectful parenting (Belsky, Woodworth, & Crnic, 1996; Conger, Patterson, & Ge, 1995; Crnic et al., 2005; Deater-Deckard & Scarr, 1996), which, in turn, has been associated with poorer developmental outcomes for the child (NICHD Early Child Care Research Network, 2004; Rothbaum & Weisz, 1994). It is possible, and probably likely, that parenting behavior is also linked to parenting stress such that parents who exhibit less effective parenting experience more stress. However, very few studies have examined the impact of parenting behavior on subsequent stress (Mackler et al., 2015). Additionally, these parents may not model good self-regulation for their children, which may lead to higher behavior problems. With regard to the opposite direction of effect (child behavior to parenting stress), child behavior problems may create more stress in the broader ecological environment (e.g., school and neighborhood) leading to augmented parental stress (Bronfenbrenner, 1979). However, despite multiple studies supporting the associations between parental stress, parenting behavior, and child outcomes, little research has explicitly tested bidirectional, meditational models based on theory that attempt to capture the complexity of these families processes across development (Deater-Deckard & Scarr, 1996), especially among families of children with IDD (Crnic & Neece, 2015).

Beyond identifying intermediate factors that account for the impact of parenting stress on child outcomes, moderators of the relationship between these variables must also be explored. Much of the research on the trajectories of these variables over time examines mean changes in child behavior problems and parent stress across development (Neece et al., 2012). However, it is likely that there are families for which these patterns diverge, and future research should identify moderators of changes in these variables over time. For example studies indicated that parents' coping styles may reduce or exacerbate the impact of various stressors on parent outcomes such that emotion-oriented coping styles may exacerbate the impact of child symptom severity and behavior problems on parenting stress (Lyons et al., 2010) while problem-focused coping may reduce the impact of child behavior concerns on parental distress (Woodman & Hauser-Cram, 2013). Further, social support may also reduce the impact of stressors on parent psychological outcomes (Dunn et al., 2001). Studies should continue ascertain the primary risk and protective factors that change the strength of this relationship over time. Further, little is known about the sources of stress among parents of children with IDD and the relative contribution of individual sources to overall parenting stress. The literature focuses on the child with IDD and his or her associated behavior problems as the primary source of stress. However, after spending many years interviewing families about their stress, it is clear that the child with IDD is one of many sources of stress that contribute to parents' overall well-being. Researchers need to identify these additional sources of stress and characterize how other related factors (e.g., financial stress, sibling stress, and family support stress) interact with the stress associated with the child with IDD in predicting parents' overall stress. McQuillian and Bates (Chap. 4) in this volume outline key moderators of parenting stress (e.g., parent gender, economic and cultural background, parent temperament, cognitive skills and capacities, and specific parenting knowledge and skills) that may be important to consider in future research. Finally, the parenting stress literature would benefit from a more refined definition of "parenting stress." We all use this term with the assumption that there is a shared understanding of the construct. However, there are many definitions of parenting stress, and there has been little differentiation between parenting stress and stressed parenting.

Turning to intervention research, given the rapidly growing literature supporting the efficacy of mindfulness-based interventions for adults in general and parents of children with IDD specifically, future research should continue to focus on these interventions. Research examining the mechanisms by which mindfulness interventions operate indicates that mindfulness training leads to improvements in self-regulation, values clarification, cognitive, emotional, and behavioral flexibility, and exposure to anxiety stimuli, which account for a wide range of positive outcomes, including stress reduction.

However, it behooves future researchers investigating mindfulness interventions for parents and children with IDD to use common intervention protocols and measures in order to compare and perhaps collapse findings across studies. Broadly speaking, one of the most significant problems in mindfulness intervention research is that nearly every study uses a different interventions and a different set of outcome measures, making it difficult for readers to synthesize this literature and identify what treatment works best and for whom. When researchers choose to apply mindfulness interventions to a new population, it would be advantageous to first determine whether standard manualized intervention protocols (e.g., MBSR and MBCT) are effective before making adaptations for the group; if adaptations are made before the standard protocol is tested, one cannot determine whether the observed effects are a result of the mindfulness intervention or the adaptations made. In addition, the literature base for mindfulness interventions with parents of children with IDD would greatly benefit from systematic dismantling of studies to identify which aspects of the intervention are related to the observed benefits. Standard mindfulness interventions are quite intensive, requiring several hours of intervention each week and daily homework for several weeks. Preliminary data indicate that adaptations to interventions that are less time intensive may be worthwhile for people seeking to reduce psychological distress (Carmody & Baer, 2009). Studies to systematically examine each of these individual concerns identified above are needed.

Examination of the possible benefits of integrating behavioral parent training and mindfulness-based interventions is a key area for future research on interventions for parents of children with IDD. Research indicates that parent emotion and cognitive control capacities (ECCCs) influence parenting practices (e.g., ability to be perceptive, responsive, and flexible), and that mindfulness training can improve ECCCs (Crandall, Deater-Deckard & Riley, 2015). Therefore, incorporating mindfulness training into parenting interventions may optimize outcomes. There is small but growing literature supporting the use of adding a mindfulness component to interventions or approaches (e.g., Kazdin & Whitley, 2003; Singh et al., 2006, 2014). Future investigation is needed to determine whether adding a parental stress reduction module that uses mindfulness-based techniques to existing evidence-based treatments for child behavioral issues (Bagner & Eyberg, 2007; McIntyre & Abbeduto, 2008) maximizes the efficacy of parent training and behavior interventions that target challenging behavior among children with IDD. Given that elevated parental stress has been associated with decreased efficacy of behavioral interventions for children (Baker et al., 1991; Brinker et al., 1994; Osborne et al., 2008; Robbins et al., 1991; Strauss et al., 2012), we predict that addressing parental stress would improve the impact of interventions commonly used with children with IDD. The challenge lies in identifying what aspects of mindfulness-based interventions for parents are most effective for reducing stress and the intensity of the intervention, so the desired outcome is achieved, which further underscores the critical need for identifying the "active ingredients" of the interventions.

Nevertheless, parenting stress is a highly prevalent and deeply concerning problem among parents of children with IDD. Designing and implementing effective stress-reduction interventions for these families is critical in optimizing parent *and* child outcomes. We know from scientific studies as well as professional experience that families matter in determining outcomes for children, especially for children with IDD. Parent stress has a significant impact on children's development and, therefore, in any attempt to intervene and help children we must also consider and intervene with families.

References

Abidin, R. R. (1990). *Parenting stress index manual* (3rd ed.). Charlottesville, VA: Pediatric Psychology Press.

Ainbinder, J., Blanchard, L. W., Singer, G. H., Sullivan, M. E., Powers, L., K., Marquis, J. G., & Santelli, B. (1998). A qualitative study of parent to parent support for parents of children with special needs. *Journal of Pediatric Psychology, 23*(2), 99–109.

Altmaier, E., & Maloney, R. (2007). An initial evaluation of a mindful parenting program. *Journal of Clinical Psychology, 63*(12), 1231–1238.

Anastopoulos, A., & Guevremont, D. (1992). Parenting stress among families of children with attention deficit hyperactivity disorder. *Journal of Abnormal Child Psychology, 20*(5), 503–520.

Anthony, K., Bromberg, M., Gil, K., & Schanberg, L. (2011). Parental perceptions of child vulnerability and parent stress as predictors of pain and adjustment in children with chronic arthritis. *Children's Health Care, 40*(1), 53–69.

Anthony, L., Anthony, B., Glanville, D., Naiman, D., Waanders, C., & Shaffer, S. (2005). The relationships between parenting stress, parenting behavior and preschoolers' social competence and behavior problems in the classroom. *Infant and Child Development, 14*(2), 133–154.

Bagner, D., & Eyberg, S. (2007). Parent–child interaction therapy for disruptive behavior in children with mental retardation: A randomized controlled trial. *Journal of Clinical Child and Adolescent Psychology, 36*(3), 418–429.

Baker, B. L., Blacher, J., Crnic, K. A., & Edelbrock, C. (2002). Behavior problems and parenting stress in families of three-year-old children with and without developmental delays. *American Journal of Mental Retardation, 107*(6), 433–444.

Baker, B. L., Landen, S., & Kashima, K. (1991). Effects of parent training on families of children with mental retardation: Increased burden or generalized benefit? *American Journal on Mental Retardation.*

Baker, B. L., McIntyre, L. L., Blacher, J., Crnic, K., Edelbrock, C., & Low, C. (2003). Pre-school children with and without developmental delay: Behaviour problems and parenting stress over time. *Journal of Intellectual Disability Research, 47*(4), 217–230.

Baker, B. L., Neece, C. L., Fenning, R. M., Crnic, K. A., & Blacher, J. (2010). Mental disorders in five-year-old children with or without developmental delay: Focus on ADHD. *Journal of Clinical Child & Adolescent Psychology, 39*(4), 492–505.

Bazzano, A., Wolfe, C., Zylowska, L., Wang, S., Schuster, E., Barrett, C., et al. (2015). Mindfulness based stress reduction (MBSR) for parents and caregivers of individuals with developmental disabilities: a community-based approach. *Journal of Child and Family Studies, 24*(2), 298–308.

Belsky, J., Woodworth, S., & Crnic, K. (1996). Trouble in the second year: Three questions about family interaction. *Child Development, 67*(2), 556–578.

Blacher, J., & McIntyre, L. L. (2006). Syndrome specificity and behavioural disorders in young adults with intellectual disability: Cultural differences in family impact. *Journal of Intellectual Disability Research, 50*(3), 184–198.

Bögels, S., Hoogstad, B., van Dun, L., de Schutter, S., & Restifo, K. (2008). Mindfulness training for adolescents with externalizing disorders and their parents. *Behavioural and Cognitive Psychotherapy, 36*(02), 193–209.

Brinker, R., Seifer, R., & Sameroff, A. (1994). Relations among maternal stress, cognitive development, and early intervention in middle-and low-SES infants with developmental disabilities. *American Journal on Mental Retardation.*

Bronfenbrenner, U. (1979). Contexts of child rearing: Problems and prospects. *American Psychologist, 34*(10), 844.

Canter, K. S., & Roberts, M. C. (2012). A systematic and quantitative review of interventions to facilitate school reentry for children with chronic health conditions. *Journal of Pediatric Psychology, 37*(10), 1065–1075.

Carmody, J., & Baer, R. (2009). How long does a mindfulness-based stress reduction program need to be? A review of class contact hours and effect sizes for psychological distress. *Journal of Clinical Psychology, 65*(6), 627–638.

Chambers, R., Gullone, E., & Allen, N. B. (2009). Mindful emotion regulation: An integrative review. *Clinical Psychology Review, 29*(6), 560–572.

Chan, J. B., & Sigafoos, J. (2001). Does respite care reduce parental stress in families with developmentally disabled children? *Child & Youth Care Forum, 30*(5), 253–263.

Chiesa, A., & Serretti, A. (2009). Mindfulness-based stress reduction for stress management in healthy people: A review and meta-analysis. *The Journal of Alternative and Complementary Medicine, 15*(5), 593–600.

Coldwell, J., Pike, A., & Dunn, J. (2006). Household chaos—Links with parenting and child behaviour. *Journal of Child Psychology and Psychiatry and Allied Disciplines, 47*(11), 1116–1122.

Conger, R. D., Patterson, G. R., & Ge, X. (1995). It takes two to replicate: A mediational model for the impact of parents' stress on adolescent adjustment. *Child Development, 66*(1), 80–97.

Cowen, P. S., & Reed, D. A. (2002). Effects of respite care for children with developmental disabilities: Evaluation of an intervention for at risk families. *Public Health Nursing, 19*(4), 272–83.

Crandall, A., Deater-Deckard, K., & Riley, A. W. (2015). Maternal emotion and cognitive control capacities and parenting: A conceptual framework. *Developmental Review, 36,* 105–126.

Crnic, K., Arbona, A. P., Baker, B., & Blacher, J. (2009). Mothers and fathers together: Contrasts in parenting across preschool to early school age in children with developmental delays. *International Review of Research in Mental Retardation, 37,* 3–30.

Crnic, K., Gaze, C., & Hoffman, C. (2005). Cumulative parenting stress across the preschool period: Relations to maternal parenting and child behaviour at age 5. *Infant and Child Development, 14*(2), 117–132.

Crnic, K. A., & Greenberg, M. T. (1990). Minor parenting stresses with young children. *Child Development, 61*(5), 1628–1637.

Crnic, K. A., Greenberg, M. T., Ragozin, A. S., Robinson, N. M., & Basham, R. B. (1983). Effects of stress and social support on mothers and premature and full-term infants. *Child development,* 209–217.

Crnic, K., & Neece, C. (2015). Socioemotional consequences of illness and disability. *Handbook of Child Psychology and Developmental Science, 3*(8), 1–37.

Dabrowska, A., & Pisula, E. (2010). Parenting stress and coping styles in mothers and fathers of pre-school children with autism and Down syndrome. *Journal of Intellectual Disability Research, 54*(3), 266–280.

Davidson, B., & Dosser Jr, D. A. (1982). A support system for families with developmentally disabled infants. *Family Relations*, 295–299.

Davis, N. O., & Carter, A. S. (2008). Parenting stress in mothers and fathers of toddlers with autism spectrum disorders: Associations with child characteristics. *Journal of Autism and Developmental Disorders, 38*(7), 1278–1291.

Deater-Deckard, K. (1998). Parenting stress and child adjustment: Some old hypotheses and new questions. *Clinical Psychology: Science and Practice, 5*(3), 314–332.

Deater-Deckard, K., & Scarr, S. (1996). Parenting stress among dual-earner mothers and fathers: Are there gender differences? *Journal of Family Psychology, 10*(1), 45–59.

Donenberg, G., & Baker, B. L. (1993). The impact of young children with externalizing behaviours on their families. *Journal of Abnormal Child Psychology, 21*(2), 179–198.

Dunn, M. E., Burbine, T., Bowers, C. A., & Tantleff-Dunn, S. (2001). Moderators of stress in parents of children with autism. *Community Mental Health Journal, 37*(1), 39–52.

DuPaul, G. J., Weyandt, L. L., O'Dell, S. M., & Varejao, M. (2009). College students with ADHD. *Journal of Attention Disorders, 13*(3), 234–250.

Dykens, E., Fisher, M., & Taylor, J. (2014). Reducing distress in mothers of children with autism and other disabilities: A randomized trial. *Pediatrics, 134*(2), 454–463.

Eisenhower, A., Baker, B., & Blacher, J. (2005). Preschool children with intellectual disability: Syndrome specificity, behaviour problems, and maternal well-being. *Journal of Intellectual Disability Research, 49*(9), 657–671.

Eisenhower, A. S., Baker, B. L., & Blacher, J. (2009). Children's delayed development and behavior problems: Impact on mothers' perceived physical health across early childhood. *Social Science and Medicine, 68*(1), 89–99.

Emerson, E., & Einfeld, S. (2010). Emotional and behavioural difficulties in young children with and without developmental delay: A bi-national perspective. *Journal of Child Psychology and Psychiatry and Allied Disciplines, 51*(5), 583–593.

Estes, A., Munson, J., Dawson, G., Koehler, E., Zhou, X.-H., & Abbott, R. (2009). Parenting stress and psychological functioning among mothers of preschool children with autism and developmental delay. *Autism: The International Journal of Research and Practice, 13*(4), 375–87.

Feldman, M. A., & Werner, S. E. (2002). Collateral effects of behavioral parent training on families of children with developmental disabilities and severe behavior disorders. *Behavioral Interventions, 17*(2), 75–83.

Gammon, E., & Rose, S. (1991). The coping skills training program for parents of children with developmental disabilities: An experimental evaluation. *Research on Social Work Practice, 1*(3), 244–256.

Gerstein, E. D., Crnic, K. A., Blacher, J., & Baker, B. L. (2009). Resilience and the course of daily parenting stress in families of young children with intellectual disabilities. *Journal of Intellectual Disability Research, 53*(12), 981–997.

Glidden, L. M., & Schoolcraft, S. A. (2003). Depression: Its trajectory and correlates in mothers rearing children with intellectual disability. *Journal of Intellectual Disability Research, 47*(4–5), 250–263.

Greaves, D. (1997). The effect of rational-emotive parent education on the stress of mothers of young children with Down syndrome. *Journal of Rational-Emotive and Cognitive-Behavior, 15*(4), 249–267.

Gupta, V. B. (2007). Comparison of parenting stress in different developmental disabilities. *Journal of Developmental and Physical Disabilities, 19*(4), 417–425.

Guralnick, M. J., Neville, B., Connor, R. T., & Hammond, M. A. (2003). Family factors associated with the peer social competence of young children with mild delays. *American Journal of Mental Retardation, 108*(4), 272–287.

Hastings, R. P., & Beck, A. (2004). Practitioner review: Stress intervention for parents of children with intellectual disabilities. *Journal of Child Psychology and Psychiatry and Allied Disciplines, 45*(8), 1338–1349.

Hastings, R. P., Daley, D., Burns, C., & Beck, A. (2006). Maternal distress and expressed emotion: Cross-sectional and longitudinal relationships with behavior problems of children with intellectual disabilities. *American Journal of Mental Retardation, 111*(1), 48–61.

Hauser-Cram, P., Warfield, M. E., Shonkoff, J. P., & Krauss, M. W. (2001). Children with disabilities: A longitudinal study of child development and parent well-being. *Monographs of the Society for Research in Child Development, 66*(3), 1–131. doi:10.1111/1540-5834.00151.

Herring, S., Gray, K. M., Taffe, J., Tonge, B., Sweeney, D., & Einfeld, S. (2006). Behaviour and emotional problems in toddlers with pervasive developmental disorders and developmental delay: Associations with parental mental health and family functioning. *Journal of Intellectual Disability Research, 50*(12), 874–882.

Hoare, P., Harris, M., Jackson, P., & Kerley, S. (1998). A community survey of children with severe intellectual disability and their families: Psychological adjustment, carer distress and the effect of respite care. *Journal of Intellectual Disability Research, 42*(3), 218–227.

Hodapp, R. M., Fidler, D. J., & Smith, A. C. M. (1998). Families of children with Prader-Willi syndrome: Stress-support and relations to child characteristics. *Journal of Intellectual Disability Research, 42*(5), 331–340.

Kabat-Zinn, J. (2003). Mindfulness-based interventions in context: Past, present, and future. *Clinical Psychology: Science and Practice, 10*(2), 144–156.

Kazdin, A., & Whitley, M. (2003). Treatment of parental stress to enhance therapeutic change among children referred for aggressive and antisocial behavior. *Journal of Consulting and Clinical Psychology, 71*(3), 504.

Kersh, J., Hedvat, T. T., Warfield, M. E., Hauser-Cram, P., & Warfield, M. E. (2006). The contribution of marital quality to the well-being of parents of children with developmental disabilities. *Journal of Intellectual Disability Research, 50*(Pt 12), 883–93.

Kirkham, M. (1993). Two-year follow-up of skills training with mothers of children with disabilities. *American Journal on Mental Retardation*.

Kirkham, M., & Schilling, R. (1990). Life skills training with mothers of handicapped children. *Journal of Social Service Research, 13*(2), 67–87.

Lecavalier, L., Leone, S., & Wiltz, J. (2006). The impact of behaviour problems on caregiver stress in young people with autism spectrum disorders. *Journal of Intellectual Disability Research, 50*(3), 172–183.

Lopez, V., Clifford, T., Minnes, P., & Ouellette-Kuntz, H. (2008). Parental stress and coping in families of children with and without developmental delays. *Journal on Developmental Disabilities, 14*(2), 99–104.

Lyons, A. M., Leon, S. C., Phelps, C. E. R., & Dunleavy, A. M. (2010). The impact of child symptom severity on stress among parents of children with ASD: The moderating role of coping styles. *Journal of Child and Family Studies, 19*(4), 516–524.

Mackler, J. S., Kelleher, R. T., Shanahan, L., Calkins, S. D., Keane, S. P., & O'Brien, M. (2015). Parenting stress, parental reactions, and externalizing behavior from ages 4 to 10. *Journal of Marriage and Family, 77*(2), 388–406.

Madan-Swain, A., Katz, E., & LaGory, J. (2004). School and social reintegration after a serious illness or injury. *Handbook of Pediatric Psychology in School Settings*, 637–655.

Mathis, E. T., & Bierman, K. L. (2015). Dimensions of parenting associated with child prekindergarten emotion regulation and attention control in low income families. *Social Development, 24*(3), 601–620.

McIntyre, L., & Abbeduto, L. (2008). Parent training for young children with developmental disabilities: Randomized controlled trial. *American Journal on Mental Retardation, 113*(5), 356–368.

Merrell, K. W., & Holland, M. L. (1997). Social-emotional behavior of preschool-age children with and without developmental delays. *Research in Developmental Disabilities, 18*(6), 393–405.

Minor, H., Carlson, L., Mackenzie, M., Zernicke, K., & Jones, L. (2006). Mindfulness based stress reduction (MBSR) for parents and caregivers of individuals with developmental disabilities: A community-based approach. *Social Work in Health Care, 43*(1), 91–109.

Moreira, H., Gouveia, M. J., Carona, C., Silva, N., & Canavarro, M. C. (2014). Maternal attachment and children's quality of life: The mediating role of self-compassion and parenting stress. *Journal of Child and Family Studies, 24*(8), 2332–2344.

Mullins, L. L., Aniol, K., Boyd, M. L., Page, M. C., & Chaney, J. M. (2002). The influence of respite care on psychological distress in parents of children with developmental disabilities: A longitudinal study. *Children's Services: Social Policy, Research, and Practice, 5*(2), 123–138.

Neece, C. L. (2013). Mindfulness-based stress reduction for parents of young children with developmental delays: Implications for parental mental health and child behavior problems. *Journal of Applied Research in Intellectual Disabilities, 27*(2), 174–186.

Neece, C. L., & Baker, B. L. (2008). Predicting maternal parenting stress in middle childhood: The roles of child intellectual status, behaviour problems and social skills. *Journal of Intellectual Disability Research, 52*(12), 1114–1128.

Neece, C. L., Green, S. A., & Baker, B. L. (2012). Parenting stress and child behavior problems: A transactional relationship across time. *American Journal on Intellectual and Developmental Disabilities, 117*(1), 48–66.

NICHD Early Child Care Research Network. (2004). Affect dysregulation in the mother-child relationship in the toddler years: Antecedents and consequences. *Development and Psychopathology, 16,* 43–68.

Nieter, L., Thornberry, T., & Brestan-Knight, E. (2013). The effectiveness of group parent–child interaction therapy with community families. *Journal of Child and Family Studies, 22*(4), 490–501.

Nixon, C., & Singer, G. (1993). Group cognitive behavioral treatment for excessive parental self-blame and guilt. *American Journal on Mental Retardation.*

Oelofsen, N., & Richardson, P. (2006). Sense of coherence and parenting stress in mothers and fathers of preschool children with developmental disability. *Journal of Intellectual and Developmental Disability, 31*(1), 1–12.

Orsmond, G. I., Seltzer, M. M., Krauss, M. W., & Hong, J. (2003). Behavior problems in adults with mental retardation and maternal well-being: Examination of the direction of effects. *American Journal of Mental Retardation, 108*(4), 257–271.

Osborne, L. A., McHugh, L., Saunders, J., & Reed, P. (2008). Parenting stress reduces the effectiveness of early teaching interventions for autistic spectrum disorders. *Journal of Autism and Developmental Disorders, 38*(6), 1092–1103.

Osborne, L., & Reed, P. (2009). The relationship between parenting stress and behavior problems of children with autistic spectrum disorders. *Exceptional Children, 76*(1), 54–73.

Pai, A. L., Greenley, R. N., Lewandowski, A., Drotar, D., Youngstrom, E., & Peterson, C. C. (2007). A meta-analytic review of the influence of pediatric cancer on parent and family functioning. *Journal of Family Psychology, 21*(3), 407.

Painter, L., Cook, J., & Silverman, P. (1999). The effects of therapeutic storytelling and behavioral parent training on noncompliant behavior in young boys. *Child & Family Behavior Therapy, 21*(2), 47–66.

Parish, S. L., Seltzer, M. M., Greenberg, J. S., & Floyd, F. (2004). Economic implications of caregiving at midlife: Comparing parents with and without children who have developmental disabilities. *Mental Retardation, 42*(6), 413–426.

Pisula, E. (2007). A comparative study of stress profiles in mothers of children with autism and those of children with Down's syndrome. *Journal of Applied Research in Intellectual Disabilities, 20*(3), 274–278.

Quine, L., & Pahl, J. (1991). Stress and coping in mothers caring for a child with severe learning difficulties: A test of Lazarus' transactional model of coping. *Journal of Community & Applied Social Psychology, 1*(1), 57–70.

Rimmerman, A., Kramer, R., Levy, J. M., & Levy, P. H. (1989). Who benefits most from respite care? *International Journal of Rehabilitation Research, 12*(1), 41–48.

Robbins, F. R., Dunlap, G., & Plienis, A. J. (1991). Family characteristics, family training, and the progress of young children with autism. *Journal of Early Intervention, 15*(2), 173–184.

Roberts, L. R., & Neece, C. L. (2015). Feasibility of mindfulness-based stress reduction intervention for parents of children with developmental delays. *Issues in Mental Health Nursing, 36*(8), 592–602.

Rodrigue, J., Morgan, S., & Geffken, G. (1990). Families of autistic children: Psychological functioning of mothers. *Journal of Clinical Child Psychology, 19*(4), 371–379.

Rothbaum, F., & Weisz, J. R. (1994). Parental caregiving and child externalizing behavior in nonclinical samples: A meta-analysis. *Psychological Bulletin, 116*(1), 55.

Sanders, J., & Morgan, S. (1997). Family stress and adjustment as perceived by parents of children with autism or down syndrome: Implications for intervention. *Child & Family Behavior Therapy, 19*(4), 15–32.

Singer, G. H., Ethridge, B. L., & Aldana, S. I. (2007). Primary and secondary effects of parenting and stress management interventions for parents of children with developmental disabilities: A meta-analysis. *Mental Retardation and Developmental Disabilities Research Reviews, 13*(4), 357–369.

Singer, G. H., Irvin, L., & Hawkins, N. (1988). Stress management training for parents of children with severe handicaps. *Mental Retardation, 26*(3), 269–277.

Singer, G. H., Marquis, J., Powers, L. K., Blanchard, L., DiVenere, N., Santelli, B., … Sharp, M. (1999). A multi-site evaluation of parent to parent programs for parents of children with disabilities. *Journal of Early Intervention, 22*(3), 217–229.

Singh, N. N., Lancioni, G. E., Winton, A. S., Fisher, B. C., Wahler, R. G., Mcaleavey, K., … & Sabaawi, M. (2006). Mindful parenting decreases aggression, noncompliance, and self-injury in children with autism. *Journal of Emotional and Behavioral Disorders, 14*(3), 169–177.

Singh, N. N., Lancioni, G. E., Winton, A. S. W., Karazsia, B. T., Myers, R. E., Latham, L. L., et al. (2014). Mindfulness-based positive behavior support (MBPBS) for mothers of adolescents with autism spectrum disorder: Effects on adolescents' behavior and parental stress. *Mindfulness, 5*(6), 646–657.

Singh, N. N., Lancioni, G. E., Winton, A. S., Singh, A. N., Adkins, A. D., & Singh, J. (2009). Mindful staff can reduce the use of physical restraints when providing care to individuals with intellectual disabilities. *Journal of Applied Research in Intellectual Disabilities, 22*(2), 194–202.

Singh, N. N., Lancioni, G. E., Winton, A. S., Singh, J., Curtis, W. J., Wahler, R. G., et al. (2007). Mindful parenting decreases aggression and increases social behavior in children with developmental disabilities. *Behavior Modification, 31*(6), 749–771.

Singh, N. N., Singh, A., & Lancioni, G. (2010). Mindfulness training for parents and their children with ADHD increases the children's compliance. *Journal of Child and Family Studies, 19*(2), 157–166.

Sloper, P., Knussen, C., Turner, S., & Cunningham, C. (1991). Factors related to stress and satisfaction with life in families of children with down's syndrome. *Journal of Child Psychology and Psychiatry, 32*(4), 655–676.

Smith, A. L., Romski, M., Sevcik, R. A., Adamson, L. B., & Barker, R. M. (2014). Parent stress and perceptions of language development: Comparing down syndrome and other developmental disabilities. *Family Relations, 63*(1), 71–84.

Strauss, K., Vicari, S., Valeri, G., D'Elia, L., Arima, S., & Fava, L. (2012). Parent inclusion in early intensive behavioral intervention: The influence of parental stress, parent treatment fidelity and parent-mediated generalization of behavior targets on child outcomes. *Research in Developmental Disabilities, 33*(2), 688–703.

Suárez, L. M., & Baker, B. L. (1997). Child externalizing behavior and parents' stress: The role of social support. *Family Relations, 46*(4), 373–381.

Theule, J., Wiener, J., Tannock, R., & Jenkins, J. M. (2013). Parenting stress in families of children with ADHD: A meta-analysis. *Journal of Emotional and Behavioral Disorders, 21*(1), 3–17.

Tomanik, S., Harris, G. E., & Hawkins, J. (2004). The relationship between behaviours exhibited by children with autism and maternal stress. *Journal of Intellectual and Developmental Disability, 29*(1), 16–26.

Wainberg, H. A. (1999). Parent training for attention-deficit hyperactivity disorder: Parental and child outcome. *Journal of Clinical Psychology, 55*(7), 907–913.

Warren, R., & Cohen, S. (1985). Respite care. *Rehabilitation Literature, 46,* 66–71.

Weiss, M. J. (2002). Hardiness and social support as predictors of stress in mothers of typical children, children with autism, and children with mental retardation. *Autism, 6*(1), 115–130.
Wong, F. K., & Poon, A. (2010). Cognitive behavioural group treatment for Chinese parents with children with developmental disabilities in Melbourne, Australia: An efficacy study. *The Australian and New Zealand Journal of Psychiatry, 44*(8), 742–9.
Woodman, A. C. (2014). Trajectories of stress among parents of children with disabilities: A dyadic analysis. *Family Relations, 63*(1), 39–54.
Woodman, A. C., & Hauser-Cram, P. (2013). The role of coping strategies in predicting change in parenting efficacy and depressive symptoms among mothers of adolescents with developmental disabilities. *Journal of Intellectual Disability Research, 57*(6), 513–530.
Woodman, A. C., Mawdsley, H. P., & Hauser-Cram, P. (2015). Parenting stress and child behavior problems within families of children with developmental disabilities: Transactional relations across 15 years. *Research in Developmental Disabilities, 36*, 246–276.

Part II
Consequences of Parenting Stress for Children

Chapter 6
Developmental Origins of Self-regulation: Prenatal Maternal Stress and Psychobiological Development During Childhood

Regula Neuenschwander and Timothy F. Oberlander

Introduction: Setting the Scene

Even before birth, a mother's psychological state is shaping her child's subsequent development of self-regulation. The premise that fetal development sets pathways for health and well-being as well as risk and challenge across the life span is generally referred to as *fetal programming* (cf. Developmental Origins of Health and Disease, Barker, 2003). The notion of fetal programming implies that fetal development is altered in a way that prepares the offspring for the particular environment in which it will find itself (cf. predictive adaptive response, Gluckman & Hanson, 2005). Thus, not all outcomes reflect conditions of risk or disease. Some fetal adaptations that increase vigilance to the environment or alter one's capacity to respond to stress could be maladaptive in one context but quite adaptive in another (Glover, 2011), thus shaping the developmental outcomes for better *and* worse (Belsky & Pluess, 2009).

The period of intrauterine life represents one of the most sensitive windows during which the effects of stress may be transmitted inter-generationally from a mother to her as-yet-unborn child. The fact that maternal mood disturbances (e.g., negative emotions and perceived stress) during pregnancy are linked with later child behavior, even after controlling for effects of postnatal maternal mood and other relevant prenatal and postnatal confounders, suggests that, as in animal models, some of the risk is conferred prenatally via changes in women's mood-based physiology affecting fetal neurobehavioral development (M. Weinstock, 2008). While multiple underlying mechanisms and systems are involved in fetal programming (Talge, Neal, & Glover, 2007), the

R. Neuenschwander (✉) · T.F. Oberlander
Department of Pediatrics, BC Children's Hospital Research Institute,
University of British Columbia, Vancouver, BC, Canada
e-mail: rneuenschwander@bcchr.ca

T.F. Oberlander
e-mail: toberlander@bcchr.ca

K. Deater-Deckard and R. Panneton (eds.), *Parental Stress and Early Child Development*, DOI 10.1007/978-3-319-55376-4_6

stress regulatory system in general and the hypothalamic pituitary adrenal (HPA) axis in particular may play a significant role in mediating the effects of maternal stress/anxiety and child outcomes (Glover, O'Connor, & O'Donnell, 2010). Despite the popularity of the fetal programming model, it is also important to acknowledge that such effects are not necessarily permanent as research has shown that young animals show remarkable neuronal resilience if the stress is discontinued (McEwen & Morrison, 2013). Thus, while in this chapter we will focus on prenatal maternal mood exposure and its associations with child self-regulatory abilities, it is important to bear in mind that postnatal factors (e.g., parenting, secure attachment, and socioeconomic status) matter as well and will be the main focus of the other chapters in this book (e.g., Chap. 8 by Finegood & Blair; Chap. 11 by Crnic & Ross in this volume).

A key assumption underlying the fetal programming hypothesis is that biological systems undergoing rapid developmental changes are especially vulnerable to organizing and disorganizing influences (Seckl & Meaney, 1993). Stress early in life, and specifically prenatal maternal stress, may have a particularly large effect on prefrontal cortex (PFC) structure and function because of its rapid growth during gestation and its high density of glucocorticoid receptors (Arnsten, 2009; Fuster, 2008; Sanchez, Young, Plotsky, & Insel, 2000). In particular, executive function (EF)—a set of higher order cognitive processes, such as working memory, inhibition, and attention shifting, associated with PFC and integral to emerging self-regulatory behavior (Blair, 2002)—is the first to suffer and suffer disproportionately, if we are stressed (Arnsten, 2009; Diamond & Ling, 2016). Here we will examine the possiblity that prenatal maternal stress may have a similarly strong impact on children's emerging EF.

Several independent prospective longitudinal studies using behavioral questionnaires and clinical scales administered at varying time points during development have established an association between prenatal maternal mood and child self-regulatory abilities. Specifically, children of mothers who were stressed during pregnancy (high anxiety/depression) had more difficulties than children not exposed to prenatal maternal stress with cognitive, behavioral, and emotional self-regulation as reflected in difficult temperament, attention regulation problems, hyperactivity, clinical diagnosis of ADHD, ADHD symptoms, conduct disorders, and emotional problems (after controlling for possible confounding factors such as prenatal maternal smoking or alcohol consumption, maternal education, birthweight, gestational age, and postnatal maternal mood; Huizink, Robles de Medina, Mulder, Visser, & Buitelaar, 2003; O'Connor, Heron, Golding, Beveridge, & Glover, 2002; O'Connor, Heron, Golding, Glover, & Team, 2003; Oberlander et al., 2007; Van den Bergh & Marcoen, 2004). More recently, human studies have begun to examine the neurodevelopmental consequences in children exposed to maternal stress during gestation in more depth and more specifically (e.g., Entringer, Buss, & Wadhwa, 2015; Van den Bergh, Mulder, Mennes, & Glover, 2005). In this chapter, we will specifically focus on current studies using laboratory-based measurement of child EF or neurophysiological measures indexing PFC activity to examine the long-term consequences of maternal stress during pregnancy on emerging regulatory mechanisms in children. These findings provide a unique opportunity to elucidate which specific aspects of children's self-regulation (including underlying structure–function relations) may be altered following exposure to prenatal maternal stress.

Increasingly, research has focused on how fetal programming models explain variations in psychiatric outcomes (Glover, 2011). A case in point is illustrated by the role the neurotransmitter serotonin (5-hydroxytryptamine, 5-HT) plays in shaping developmental risk and resiliency. Increased use of selective serotonin reuptake inhibitor (SSRI) antidepressants to manage mood disorders during pregnancy highlights the role psychotropic medication exposure during critical prenatal periods has in shaping children's development. We will review how exposure to prenatal antidepressants shape—possibly via altered central 5-HT levels—the development of systems that regulate attention, cognition, emotion, and stress responses (Hanley & Oberlander, 2012).

In this chapter, we focus on empirical evidence examining associations between prenatal maternal stress (i.e., pregnancy-specific anxiety, stress exposure, depression, and antidepressants) and child self-regulatory capacities reflected in neurobiological processes such as EF and stress regulation spanning fetal periods to early adulthood. We take the view that psychobiological processes comprising EF and stress regulation are shaped by early exposures related to maternal mood during gestation that influence the developing central nervous system (CNS) and autonomic nervous system (ANS). Furthermore, we will review current evidence within a conceptual perspective whereby prenatal maternal mood during sensitive periods of fetal development may act as a "plasticity factor" rather than "risk factor" associated with vulnerability that predicts disordered development and behavior. With this perspective in mind, we will critically review empirical studies examining the association of maternal mood during gestation on stress regulation and higher order cognitive abilities (behavioral measures of EF and neurophysiological measures indexing PFC) during childhood and adolescence, as well as the role of altered 5-HT signaling (i.e., antidepressant exposure). Understanding the role of maternal stress during gestation for child development offers critical insights that may explain why variations in early typical environment are associated with shaping both developmental risk *and* resilience.

Developmental Origins of Self-regulation

The development of self-regulation is central to a child's emerging ability to adaptively respond to environmental demands and to engage in goal-directed behavior (Baumeister & Vohs, 2004; Calkins & Howse, 2004). It is marked by the acquisition of an integrated set of domain specific (biological, attentional, emotional, behavioral, and cognitive) self-regulatory mechanisms that are hierarchical in nature and that build upon each other (Calkins & Williford, 2009). Biological components of self-regulation include serotonin and dopamine neurotransmitter system genes and central and peripheral nervous system connectivity (Bell & Deater-Deckard, 2007). Cognitive components are generally referred to as EF representing a complex and interrelated set of higher order cognitive processes associated with the PFC, including the maintenance and manipulation of relevant information (working memory), inhibition of predominant responses (inhibition), and mental set shifting (shifting, Miyake, Friedman, Emerson, Witzki, & Howerter, 2000). EF serves a critical higher level or top-down role in behavior regulation, such as directing attention and organizing cognitive resources (Miller & Cohen, 2001) and/or regulating emotions (Ochsner & Gross, 2005). Over the past two decades, a strong body of developmental research has established that EFs are crucial for social, emotional, and academic success during childhood (e.g., Blair & Razza, 2007; Hughes & Ensor, 2011; Neuenschwander, Röthlisberger, Cimeli, & Roebers, 2012) and self-regulation has been shown to shape physical and mental health risk trajectories across the life span (Moffitt et al., 2011). Importantly, EFs are malleable based on context-specific experiences both at home and at school (for reviews see Diamond & Lee, 2011; Hughes, 2011; see also Chap. 8 by Finegood & Blair).

Various aspects of parenting, including parenting stress, have been shown to be associated with child EF. For instance, sensitive parents that engage in age-appropriate scaffolding act as external regulators of child behavior and in these terms gradually facilitate children's ability to regulate their own emotions and behaviors (e.g., Bernier, Carlson, & Whipple, 2010). These parenting aspects also reflect the parent's ability to regulate their own emotions and behaviors, and suggest that parental EF is an important part of sensitive parenting (Barrett & Fleming, 2011) (see also Chap. 10 by Mileva-Seitz & Fleming in this volume). Specifically, parental EF may moderate the association between parental risk and child outcomes, such that the negative effects of parental risk are mostly evident when, for instance, mothers show low EF (Deater-Deckard, Wang, Chen, & Bell, 2012). In general, parenting stress may be one crucial mechanism through which stressors in a family's environment affect parent–child interactions and ultimately children and their neurocognitive development (see Chap. 8 by Finegood & Blair).

The PFC is the brain region that is most sensitive to the detrimental effects of stress exposure (Arnsten, 2009; McEwen & Morrison, 2013). Phylogenetically, the PFC is among the brain regions that evolved most recently or were most recently altered in the course of human evolution. In line with this, the PFC shows a protracted ontogenetic development into early adulthood and displays remarkable structural and functional plasticity over the life course (Fuster, 2008). Chief external landmarks of the PFC (i.e., its primary sulci) develop during gestational weeks 25–26 (Stiles & Jernigan, 2010). Importantly, the PFC intelligently regulates our thoughts, actions, and emotions through extensive connections with other more posterior and subcortical areas of the brain. Therefore, it is likely that a dysfunction of the PFC can be associated with a dysfunction in one or more of the related systems.

Chronic stress early in life may have a particularly large effect on PFC structure and function in adulthood because of its rapid growth during fetal life. This rapid growth rate and the high density of glucocorticoid receptors (Fuster, 2008; Sanchez et al., 2000) make the fetal PFC especially vulnerable to stress hormones that reach it in excess amounts as a result of *maternal* stress. Such hormones may impede the formation of correct neural connections and reduce plasticity and neurotransmitter activity, which in turn can induce subtle changes in subsequent cognitive function and behavior (Weinstock, 2008). For instance, in animal models, dendritic changes in fetuses have been documented in utero when the rat mother was exposed to stress (Murmu et al., 2006). In humans, growing up under social or economic disadvantage has been shown to increase young toddlers' cortisol levels which in turn mediated the effects of poverty and parenting on EF at the age of three (Blair et al., 2011). In adults, acute psychosocial stress exposure has been found to impair EF (e.g., Alexander, Hillier, Smith, Tivarus, & Beversdorf, 2007; Lupien, Gillin, & Hauger, 1999). To some extent, these effects are believed to reflect the fact that glucocorticoid levels (i.e., cortisol) modulate synaptic activity in the neural circuitry of the PFC. Importantly, the functional relation between cortisol levels and PFC activity or EF performance is curvilinear (Arnsten, 2009; de Kloet, Oitzl, & Joëls, 1999; Lupien, Maheu, Tu, Fiocco, & Schramek, 2007), such that very high or very low levels of stress impair EF performance, whereas moderate stress/cortisol levels lead to optimal EF performance. This inverted U-shape relation may have important implications for beneficial effects of prenatal exposure to mild and moderate levels of maternal stress on certain child outcomes (cf. DiPietro, Novak, Costigan, Atella, & Reusing, 2006). Taken together, it can be concluded that prenatal stress may have a particularly strong effect on EF; however, the relationship between EF and stress is complex and appears to be context dependent.

Prenatal Maternal Mood and Stress

Pregnancy is a dramatic biological and psychological period in a woman's life. The woman's transition to motherhood not only does transform her physical landscape including the internal hormonal milieu but also has significant implications for her relationships and her societal role. Furthermore, for many women, the stereotypical image of pregnancy as a happy and joyful time in life when a mother and her partner are expecting a child they planned to have and that they are well prepared to love and care for does not apply. For many women, pregnancy is an experience characterized by a lack of adequate resources, both socioeconomic and psychosocial, and the presence of many stressors such as work responsibilities and conflict with the partner makes pregnancy a distant reflection of the ideal prototype (Dunkel Schetter, 2011). It is thus not surprising that pregnancy and the postpartum period tend to heighten risk for development or recurrence of mood disorders (Leight, Fitelson, Weston, & Wisner, 2010).

Prevalence estimates of antenatal depression vary greatly depending on the criteria used and may usually represent rather conservative estimates, because cases of maternal depression are underreported and underdiagnosed (Howard et al., 2014). A systematic review (Bennett, Einarson, Taddio, Koren, & Einarson, 2004) of studies conducted mostly in Europe and Northern America examining the prevalence of depression during pregnancy found the following estimates by trimester: 7.4% in the first, 12.8% in the second, and 12% in the third. For women of low socioeconomic status, in contrast, meta-analytic estimates, although based on few studies, were much higher: for the second and third trimesters 47% and 39%, respectively, when obtained by self-report, and 28% and 25% when determined by structured clinical interviews. Estimates for prenatal anxiety, in contrast, are scarce, probably because the interplay between the perinatal period and anxiety disorders remains poorly studied (Leight et al., 2010). Some of the stressors that commonly affect women in pregnancy around the globe are low material resources, unfavorable employment conditions, heavy family and household responsibilities, strain in intimate relationships, and pregnancy complications (Dunkel Schetter & Tanner, 2012).

Antenatal maternal mood disturbances have been characterized on multiple dimensions, including measures reflecting stress-related disorders such as anxiety and/or depression. These outcomes are often used interchangeably, often implying similar constructs. Indeed, differentiating symptoms reflecting anxiety from depression remains challenging, and many of these symptoms may lie along a continuum of a maternal stress regulatory disorder. Stress is typically regarded as a physiological and psychological condition that is beyond the capacity of an individual's ability to cope, often leading to symptoms such as anxiety or depression. If severe enough, these symptoms may meet a clinical threshold and constitute a major affective disorder. Notwithstanding this perspective, while maternal symptoms of anxiety and depression often imply a common metric for stress, a distinction between these two dimensions can be drawn (DiPietro, 2012) and the differential impact of distinct types of maternal stress on developmental outcomes has been established in some studies.

Definitions and measurements of prenatal maternal stress have evolved over time. Whereas older studies often relied solely on a checklist of retrospectively assessed stressful life events (e.g., death of a family member or catastrophic community-wide disasters such as earthquakes), more recent studies have shifted toward considering prenatal maternal stress as a multi-dimensional concept. Given that an event or situation can be perceived differently by various individuals, it is really that subjective perception or interpretation of an external stressor rather than its objective nature that has the power to trigger an emotional response (Lazarus, 1991) and hence possibly influence health outcomes. Thus, more recent studies combine measures of acute (life events) and chronic (daily hassles) stress stimuli with more subjective measures including resources (personality and social support), stress perception, and mood outcomes (anxiety and depression) that reflect emotional responses to stressful stimuli (Dunkel Schetter, 2011). It is still unclear which types of prenatal emotional disturbances or stress are most harmful for fetal and child development. Interestingly, there is some evidence that levels of maternal self-reported pregnancy-specific anxiety are superior to general measures of distress (such as state anxiety or symptoms of depression) for predicting the developmental outcomes (e.g., Buss, Davis, Hobel, & Sandman, 2011; DiPietro et al., 2006). We will emphasize which types of maternal stress were assessed and most predictive for developmental outcomes in the studies that we review below.

Prenatal Maternal Stress Shaping Child Self-regulation

Accumulating research indicates that a mother's stress and related affective states experienced in pregnancy can have significant negative consequences for her child's long-term learning, stress physiology, motor, cognitive, and emotional development, behavior, and health (reviewed in, Beydoun & Saftlas, 2008; Dunkel Schetter & Tanner, 2012; Entringer et al., 2015; Glover, 2011; Kinsella & Monk, 2009; Mennes, Stiers, Lagae, & Van den Bergh, 2006; Talge et al., 2007; Van den Bergh, Mulder, et al., 2005; M. Weinstock, 2008)—even when accounting for postnatal maternal psychological state. Specifically, with regard to developmental origins of self-regulation, antenatal maternal stress disrupts fetal neurobehavioral development (DiPietro et al., 1996; Tronick & Weinberg, 1997), alters behavioral reactivity in utero (Allister et al., 2001; Monk et al., 2000), and in the newborn period is reflected in reduced birthweight and increased risk of prematurity (Glover, 2011; Talge et al., 2007). The exact mechanisms by which antenatal anxiety and stress influence fetal brain development remain unclear, yet the magnitude of their effects is clinically significant, with approximately 15% of emotional and behavioral problems in childhood attributable to antenatal stress/anxiety (Talge et al., 2007). Furthermore, emerging evidence suggests that the combination of early life stress, genetics, and ongoing stress may ultimately determine individual responsiveness to stress and the vulnerability to psychiatric disorders, such as depression (Charney & Manji, 2004). Importantly, not all outcomes following stressful early life events reflect adversity. Antenatal exposure to mild-to-moderate levels of psychological distress may actually advance motor and mental development in a healthy population (DiPietro et al., 2006), suggesting that early stress exposure shapes developmental outcomes for better *and* worse.

Laboratory-based measures of child neurocognitive development (behavioral measures of EF and neurophysiological measures indexing PFC structure and activity) offer a key insight into the neural correlates (i.e., specific aspects of children's EF including underlying structure–function relations) that may be affected by prenatal maternal stress. The first study that measured cognitive functioning (or cognitive regulation problems) with computerized and standardized tasks placing a load on PFC functions comes from the prospective study of the Van den Bergh and Marcoen group in the Netherlands (e.g., Van den Bergh & Marcoen, 2004). Van den Bergh and colleagues (Van den Bergh, Mennes, et al., 2005) reported that adolescents of mothers who experienced high levels of anxiety (state subscale of the State-Trait Anxiety Inventory, Spielberger, Gorsuch, & Lushene, 1970) during the second trimester of their pregnancy were reported to be more impulsive on visual attention control tasks compared to adolescents exposed to low to average levels of prenatal maternal anxiety. Specifically, adolescents of mothers who were highly anxious during the 12–22 weeks of pregnancy, but not later, responded faster and made more errors in the target present condition of the "endcoding" task compared to the low-average group, reflecting an impulsive response pattern. Importantly, this impulsive response pattern did not disappear when controlling for performance on two subtests of the Wechsler Intelligence Scale for Children (WISC-R), suggesting a specific cognitive regulation impairment. Furthermore, as anxiety did not interact with memory load, this specific pattern of cognitive regulation impairment did not appear to be related to a working memory problem, nor to an impairment in a stop signal task tapping exogenous response control processes. Therefore, the authors concluded that the cognitive regulation problem of adolescents of mothers who were highly anxious at 12–22 weeks of pregnancy was related to altered endogenous response control processes. This control deficit, for instance, is expressed when individuals are required to continue the inhibition of a response for a longer time without external signals encouraging the inhibition.

Support for this interpretation was provided by a second study with the same group of adolescents (Van den Bergh et al., 2006). Performance on a computerized continuous performance task measuring sustained attention declined as the task progressed in 15-year-old boys of mothers with high levels of state anxiety during 12–22 weeks of their pregnancy, but not at later points in gestation. Specifically, these adolescent boys' processing speeds became slower and their reaction times became more variable as the task progressed compared to a group of adolescents of mothers with low to moderate levels of prenatal anxiety. These results indicated that boys, but not girls, of highly anxious mothers were less able than boys of low to moderate anxious mothers to sustain their attention and stay focused on the task at hand, thus showing impaired endogenous attention control (e.g., resisting thinking about other things; resisting looking away). Of note, no significant associations with antenatal maternal anxiety were found in the number of errors (neither commission nor omission errors) made. The fact, however, that these results held when controlling for two subtests of the WISC-R indicates that maternal anxiety was uniquely associated with sustained attention/endogenous response inhibition.

To further delineate the cognitive sequelae associated with antenatal maternal anxiety, Van den Bergh and colleagues (Mennes et al., 2006) reviewed recent neuroimaging studies to create a cortical map of regions commonly and selectively activated by well-known EF tasks. The pragmatic value of this cortical map was tested in a subsample of the previous reported adolescents who were now 17-years-old. Adolescents of mothers with high levels of anxiety during 12–22 weeks of their pregnancy performed significantly lower in tasks that required integration and control of different task parameters compared to adolescents of mothers with normal levels of antenatal anxiety. Specifically, the percentage of correct answers in a response-shifting task was lower overall—and especially during the incompatible trials—in the high maternal anxiety group as compared to the normal maternal anxiety group. Moreover, a decrease in performance when the cognitive load of dual tasks increased was observed in adolescents in the high maternal anxiety group. Together these results suggest that the adolescents in the high anxiety group experienced difficulties organizing their cognitive resources in order to handle two tasks at the same time. In contrast, working memory (N-back task), inhibition of a prepotent response (Go/NoGo task), and visual orienting of attention (visual cued-attention orientation task) were not impaired, suggesting that adolescents of mothers experiencing high levels of anxiety during the second trimester performed selectively poorer in tasks that require subjects to perform two tasks simultaneously and switch between different task rules. This conclusion was based on the established cortical map found to be linked to a part of, or in cortical and subcortical regions linked to, the orbitofrontal cortex. Importantly, although several other areas were activated by dual- and response-shifting tasks, this part of the orbitofrontal cortex was found to respond exclusively during performance on these two tasks (and not during performance on the other EF tasks).

Further evidence of neurodevelopmental consequences in the offspring of maternal stress during pregnancy comes from the prospective study of the multi-investigator research program at the University of California, Irvine. The first study examined links between pregnancy-specific anxiety (a self-developed measure by Glynn, Schetter, Hobel, & Sandman, 2008) and prefrontal cortical volumes in 6- to 9-year-old children (Buss, Davis, Muftuler, Head, & Sandman, 2010). Pregnancy-specific anxiety at 19 weeks' gestation, but not at 25 and 31 weeks' gestation, was associated with diffuse cortical volume reductions (in gray matter) in the PFC, the premotor and temporal cortices, as well as the postcentral gyrus and the cerebellum extending to the middle occipital gyrus and the fusiform gyrus. Interestingly, the prefrontal regions that were found to be associated with high anxiety during pregnancy have been shown to be involved in the regulation of stress hormone secretion (Pruessner et al., 2008). These same brain regions appear to be particularly vulnerable to conditions of chronic stress due to their high density of glucocorticoid receptors (Sapolsky, Uno, Rebert, & Finch, 1990). Thus, high prenatal anxiety in mothers may increase the risk of higher stress susceptibility and reactivity in their developing children, rendering the children more vulnerable to neurodevelopmental and psychiatric disorders as well as cognitive and intellectual impairment.

In a second study, Buss and colleagues (2011) examined the association of pregnancy-specific anxiety with EF in a larger subset of the same cohort of 6–9 year-old children. High levels of maternal pregnancy-specific anxiety over the course of gestation were associated with lower inhibitory control (Flanker task), in girls only, and lower visuospatial working memory performance (Corsi block-tapping test), both in boys and girls. Specifically, girls showed slower reaction times as a function of maternal anxiety, and this difference was most pronounced in the incongruent trials. Of note, higher state anxiety and depression were also associated with lower visuospatial working memory performance. However, neither state anxiety nor depression explained any additional variance after accounting for pregnancy-specific anxiety. These results are especially interesting in light of the gray matter reductions in PFC regions in association with pregnancy-specific anxiety reported above (cf. Buss et al., 2010). A lack of power, though, prevented the authors from testing if PFC volume reductions mediated the association between pregnancy-specific anxiety and EF. Nevertheless, the fact that these associations between pregnancy-specific anxiety and child EF were observed among a group of low-risk women that did not smoke or consume alcohol during pregnancy and had a slightly higher than average socioeconomic status strengthens the results of the study.

A third study from the same cohort examined the associations of cortical changes and child externalizing behavior in 7-year-olds exposed to maternal depressive symptoms during pregnancy (Sandman, Buss, Head, & Davis, 2015). Using MRI, changes in cortical thickness were analyzed by measuring the width of the cortical gray matter layer that covers the surface of the brain. Significant cortical thinning (i.e., selective diminishment of gray matter brain regions which implies reduced synaptic density) primarily in children's right frontal lobes (right superior, medial orbital, and frontal pole regions of the PFC) was associated with exposure to prenatal maternal depression across gestation, with the strongest associations found at 25 weeks' gestation (compared to 19 and 31 weeks). This pattern of cortical thinning seems to be similar to patterns in depressed patients and individuals with risk of depression (Lagopoulos, Hermens, Naismith, Scott, & Hickie, 2012). Interestingly, the significant association between prenatal maternal depression and child externalizing behavior (assessed with the Child Behavior Checklist) was mediated by cortical thinning in prefrontal areas of the right hemisphere.

Further evidence of differential prenatal stress-dependent effects on neurodevelopmental consequences in the offspring comes from a retrospective study in Germany (Entringer, Buss et al., 2009). These authors hypothesized that if there is only a subtle vulnerability in subjects exposed to prenatal psychosocial stress, small differences between groups may not emerge under basal conditions but will emerge when a substantial challenge is imposed on the system. Indeed, young women whose mothers experienced a major negative life event during their pregnancy did not differ from a matched non-exposed comparison group in their working memory performance (item-recognition task). However, after hydrocortisone (cortisol) administration, women in the prenatal stress group showed significantly longer reaction times compared to women in the control group. These findings provide support for the potential modulatory effect of acute stress exposure (cortisol) on the association between prenatal stress exposure and subsequent working memory performance in young adults.

Finally, Pearson and colleagues (Pearson et al., 2016) examined prospective observational data from a large UK population cohort (Avon Longitudinal Study of Parents and Children, ALSPAC) looking at associations between prenatal maternal anxiety (anxiety items from the Crown-Crisp Index, Birtchnell, Evans, & Kennard, 1988), several EF measures at age 8, and academic achievement at the end of compulsory school at age 16. Prenatal anxiety (not specified at what time point) was neither associated with attentional control (basic form of a Stroop task), selective attention (baseline of Sky search task), nor attentional switching (Sky search task) after controlling for postnatal depression. However, there was evidence that prenatal anxiety was associated with impaired working memory (digit span and non-word memory). Interestingly, impaired working memory mediated the effect of prenatal anxiety to math grades at age 16, with 17% of the total association between prenatal anxiety and math being explained by indirect paths through working memory. A similar pattern was seen for language grades, but associations were confounded by maternal education. This is the first study to demonstrate that EF mediates the association between prenatal stress and later academic outcomes.

Taken together, these studies indicate that prenatal maternal stress (mostly anxiety in the second trimester) is associated with subtle changes in EF and the PFC in middle childhood, adolescence, and early adulthood. The specific findings, however, are not always consistent, and in some cases, they are sex-specific. For example, Buss and colleagues (2011) only found an association between maternal pregnancy-specific anxiety and inhibitory control in girls but not in boys, whereas Van den Bergh and colleagues (2006) detected impaired endogenous response inhibition in adolescent boys but not in girls. To date, few human studies have addressed sex-specific differences in child outcomes following prenatal stress exposure. Future research needs to further explore the possibility that differences in the effects of timing in boys and girls may be based on the differences in the amount of sex hormones in the developing fetus (de Bruijn, van Bakel, & van Baar, 2009).

With regard to which specific types of prenatal maternal emotional disturbances or stress have the strongest impact on child development, the reviewed studies indicate that maternal anxiety may be especially predictive for developmental outcomes. Whereas the Van den Bergh and Marcoen group as well as the Pearson study only included or analyzed anxiety measures during pregnancy, the multi-investigator research group from California assessed multiple measures of maternal stress during pregnancy, possibly allowing to draw conclusions about the most sensitive measure for developmental outcomes. This, however, was only possible in one of their studies (Buss et al., 2011), since selection of prenatal stress measures was reduced to only include one of the available measures in the two other studies reviewed above.

An important question with regard to fetal programming is the time period of pregnancy during which the fetus is most vulnerable to maternal stress. The finding of a specific time window makes it unlikely that the associations found can be explained by shared genetic variance only, as this does not explain why effects only involve prenatal maternal anxiety at a specific time period (here mostly in the second trimester) and not earlier in pregnancy or after birth. In most of the reviewed studies, the relationship seems to be more evident when stress by mothers is experienced in the second trimester (12–27 weeks)—although some studies did only find specific associations with some time points in the second trimester and not others (Buss et al., 2010; Sandman et al., 2015). In humans, key external markers of the PFC develop during gestational weeks 25–26 (Stiles & Jernigan, 2010) and key brain developmental processes such as neuron proliferation, migration, and differentiation take place between gestational weeks 8 and 24 in brain areas connected to the PFC (e.g., amygdala, ACC, brain stem, and basal ganglia) (Levitt, 2003). Therefore, it is plausible that in the reviewed studies, physiological factors related to maternal anxiety interfered with some of the complex neurodevelopmental processes taking place at that gestation period. However, the level of antenatal maternal anxiety before 12 weeks of gestation and its association with child EF remains unknown. Moreover, the effect of timing may be due to the fact that pregnancy anxiety is highest at 19 weeks' gestation and decreases over the course of gestation, which is in line with previous observations of reduced physiological and psychological stress reactivity as pregnancy advances (de Weerth & Buitelaar, 2005; Glynn et al., 2008). In general, there is currently little agreement about the gestational age most sensitive to maternal prenatal stress, and the fact that several gestational ages have been reported to be critical for the long-term effects of antenatal anxiety/stress may indicate that different mechanisms are operating at different stages (Van den Bergh, Mulder, et al., 2005).

There is now ample evidence suggesting that prenatal maternal stress is associated with long-term neurodevelopmental alterations in the offspring: Across all studies, prenatal stress was associated with each one of the EF components—inhibition, shifting, and working memory. These findings, however, lack robustness as in several studies multiple EF tasks tapping various EF components have been administered, but associations with prenatal maternal stress were only found for selected EF tasks (Mennes et al., 2006; Pearson et al., 2016; Van den Bergh, Mennes, et al., 2005). Therefore, it is too early to draw firm conclusions as to which specific aspects of children's EF including underlying PFC structures and functions may be altered following exposure to prenatal maternal stress. For instance, some authors report impaired performance on working memory tasks (Buss et al., 2011; Pearson et al., 2016), others do not (Mennes et al., 2006; Van den Bergh, Mennes, et al., 2005), and still others only find a difference between prenatally stress exposed individuals and non-exposed individuals after hydrocortisone administration (Entringer, Kumsta, et al. 2009). A way to reconcile these seeming inconsistencies rests in the idea that earlier in development (early-to-middle childhood), prenatal stress effects on working memory are more pervasive, whereas later in development (adolescence and early adulthood), the subtle vulnerability in these subjects can only be detected when a challenge is imposed on the system. This interpretation, however, is speculative at best and requires further investigation in future studies. Nevertheless, of particular interest are the studies (Buss et al., 2010; Entringer, Buss, et al., 2009) that provide indirect evidence that prenatal maternal stress affects brain development in a way that may also affect the regulation of stress (HPA axis) in subsequent offspring.

Prenatal Maternal Stress Shaping Child Stress Regulation

The HPA axis may play a significant role in mediating the effects of maternal stress/anxiety on child EF. Animal models have helped illustrate a central role for the HPA axis in mediating prenatal stress effects on behavioral or cognitive alterations in the offspring (M. Weinstock, 2008). Emerging evidence shows that prenatal maternal stress also affects the HPA axis in humans (Glover et al., 2010). Thus, evaluating how children's stress regulation is affected by prenatal stress exposure should help elucidate our understanding of potential pathways through which the development of EF may be affected by prenatal maternal stress.

Two main systems comprise the psychobiology of stress: the HPA axis with its end product cortisol and the adrenal medullary system (SAM, which is part of the autonomic nervous system or ANS) with its end products epinephrine and norepinephrine. The acute secretion of glucocorticoids (called corticosterone in animals and cortisol in humans) and catecholamines (epinephrine and norepinephrine, also known as adrenaline) constitutes the primary agents in the chain of hormonal events triggered in response to stress. In response to stress, these neurochemicals act to give rise to the "fight-or-flight response" reflected in increased heart rate and blood pressure. In this way, stress responses serve an adaptive survival mechanism consisting of a carefully orchestrated yet near-instantaneous sequence of hormonal changes and physiological responses enabling an individual to react quickly to threat. However, frequent activation can result in a permanent dysregulation of the HPA axis, particularly when experienced during phases of rapid brain development such as the prenatal period and infancy (Gunnar & Quevedo, 2007). Moreover, chronic stress exposure has long-term effects on physical and psychological health such as high blood pressure, increased risk of infection, arterial disease, and brain changes that may contribute to anxiety, depression, and addiction (for a general review, see McEwen, 2000).

A series of developmental studies in animals, both rodent and non-human primate, established the central role of the HPA axis in mediating prenatal stress effects in both mother and offspring (M. Weinstock, 2008), although other neurocircuits, such as the dopaminergic and serotonergic systems, are also likely to be involved. In rodents, many studies have found that prenatal stress causes both an increase in basal levels and an increase in corticosterone response in the offspring (although variability of the findings is high). In humans, equivalent work is only just starting, but there is suggestive evidence that there may be similar reprogramming effects (Glover et al., 2010). Whereas maternal stress could affect fetal development by exposure to stress hormones that are transported through the placenta, noradrenaline does not appear to cross from mother to fetus (Giannakoulopoulos, Teixeira, Fisk, & Glover, 1999) but may have an indirect effect via changes in the maternal muscular or vascular tone which in turn may cause stress to the fetus and raise cortisol levels (Van den Bergh, Mulder, et al., 2005). We will now review recent studies examining long-term effects of prenatal maternal stress on basal cortisol levels and cortisol responses to stress in the offspring.

Glover and colleagues' (2010) review of the literature revealed 11 studies in the last 10 years that have examined the association between prenatal maternal mood or stress and the function of the HPA axis in human offspring. The method of measuring the outcome varied from diurnal saliva cortisol to single basal samples, or saliva or plasma cortisol and ACTH response to a stressor. The age of the subjects ranged from 1 week up to young adulthood. All studies found that there were associations between prenatal maternal stress and some aspect of HPA axis function in the child. However, perhaps unsurprisingly, the nature of this association varied and solid replications seem to be missing. Nevertheless, the authors concluded that the reviewed studies mostly suggested that prenatal stress or anxiety is associated with raised basal cortisol or raised cortisol reactivity in the offspring. Furthermore, the effect was particularly apparent in the children of mothers exposed in their third, rather than earlier trimesters. Note that for the relationship between prenatal maternal stress and EF/PFC, the second trimester seems to be the most sensitive period, indicating that a different—yet to be established—mechanism may underlie the association between prenatal maternal stress and child stress regulation as opposed to prenatal maternal stress and EF. Most importantly, though, as mentioned before, the finding of a specific time window supports the possibility of fetal programming, rather than a shared genetic vulnerability. Finally, in their review, there was only one study (Van den Bergh, Van Calster, Smits, Van Huffel, & Lagae, 2008) that provided evidence that an altered diurnal cortisol profile associated with prenatal anxiety was mediating an altered behavioral phenotype (i.e., depressive symptoms) in adolescent girls (but not in boys).

Recently published studies that were not part of Glover and colleague's review expand on their conclusions and provide some interesting new insights. O'Donnell and colleagues (2013), for instance, followed 889 mother–child dyads and found that high levels of mother's anxiety in the third trimester predicted both a reduced cortisol awakening response (CAR) and a reduced diurnal cortisol decline (DCD) among 15-year-old males and females. Interestingly and in contrast, an earlier study (that was part of Glover's review) based on a smaller selection ($n = 74$) of this sample showed that higher maternal prenatal anxiety in the third trimester predicted higher morning cortisol levels (single assessment after awakening) among 10-year-olds (O'Connor et al., 2005). The reduced CAR and DCD in adolescents, however, are in line with Van den Bergh and colleagues' (2008) findings, indicating that maternal anxiety during the second trimester predicted a combination of a low morning cortisol level (single assessment after awakening) and a reduced DCD among 14- to 15-year-olds. These findings provide preliminary evidence that early stress exposure may be associated with elevated or hyperactivation of the HPA axis that, over time, leads to adrenocortical counter-regulation and hypo-activation (Miller, Chen, & Zhou, 2007). More research, however, is needed to confirm this longitudinal pattern of the HPA axis following prenatal stress exposure, possibly getting exhausted over time, resulting in long-term dampened stress responses. To date, very few studies have assessed diurnal cortisol patterns in middle childhood and adolescence in the offspring of maternal stress during pregnancy, and findings are not always consistent (see Vänskä et al., 2015 for an intensified CAR but non-affected DCD in 10- to 12-year-olds) or applied analytical approaches prevent to compare specific findings with regard to CAR and DCD (Simons, Beijers, Cillessen, & de Weerth, 2015).

Furthermore, dysregulation of the HPA axis following prenatal stress exposure may not be detectable in diurnal cortisol patterns, but in stress reactivity. For instance, Entringer and colleagues (2009) did not find differences in the diurnal patterns of young adults whose mothers experienced severe stress during their pregnancy compared to an age-matched comparison group, but in stress responses to the Trier Social Stress Test (TSST). In particular, pre-TSST cortisol levels were lower (possibly reflecting hypo-activation), whereas the increase in cortisol in response to the TSST was higher in exposed subjects compared to subjects from the comparison group. This pattern of raised cortisol reactivity to a stressor as noted in Glover's review has also been confirmed by recent studies in infants (Davis, Glynn, Waffarn, & Sandman, 2011) although some found that the direction of the effect depends on infant age and/or the nature of the stressor (Tollenaar, Beijers, Jansen, Riksen-Walraven, & de Weerth, 2011).

Additionally, not all children or adolescents are equally affected by prenatal maternal stress. A recent study (Buchmann et al., 2014) shows that in 19 year-old adolescents exposed to prenatal maternal stress, only carriers of the DRD4 seven-repeat allele were found to have an altered (i.e., attenuated) cortisol secretion during the TSST. These results suggest that prenatal maternal stress may only affect the HPA axis of carriers of certain "risk alleles" (the DRD4 7r allele has been shown to be a "risk allele" for externalizing problems, particularly in the presence of environmental adversity; Bakermans-Kranenburg & van IJzendoorn, 2006). Importantly, the notion of a "biological sensitivity to context" (Ellis, Boyce, Belsky, Bakermans-Kranenburg, & van IJzendoorn, 2011) illustrates how an allelic variation in the context of both early (i.e., fetal) and ongoing (i.e., postnatal/childhood) life experience shapes adaptation and diversity of child developmental outcomes. In this context, allelic variations may confer advantages for some children in supportive environments, but disadvantages when facing social adversity in the context of maternal depression (Boyce & Ellis, 2005). Intriguingly, the biological sensitivity to context concept offers a critical perspective that allows us to move our thinking about fetal programming from "invariant" developmental outcomes associated with early adverse exposure to a perspective that outcomes in childhood represent interactions between biological (a child's genotype) and contextual (maternal mood) variables enabling both positive and negative outcomes. Further, DNA methylation—an epigenetic mechanism—may be a crucial component of genetic differential susceptibility/biological sensitivity to context (see Chap. 7 by Mulder, Rijlaarsdam & Van IJzendoorn).

Taken together, emerging evidence suggests that prenatal maternal stress affects both diurnal profiles and reactivity patterns of the HPA axis in the offspring. Studies providing evidence that an altered HPA axis mediates the association of prenatal maternal stress and neurodevelopmental outcomes, however, are still missing and needed (Glover et al., 2010). Detecting these relationships, though, may be quite challenging as studies have shown that the relation between HPA axis reactivity and measures of EF is of a complex nature (e.g., Blair, Granger, & Peters Razza, 2005; see also Chap. 8 by Finegood & Blair).

Whether or not prenatal maternal stress is initially associated with a hyperactivation of the HPA axis and later in development with a hypo-activation needs to be determined. Hyperactivation is in general suggested to be indicative of a currently stressed, hyperactive HPA axis (e.g., McEwen & Wingfield, 2003), whereas hypo-activation reflects reduced cortisol production, possibly due to more chronic stress that has caused "exhaustment" of the mechanisms underlying the HPA axis (e.g., Doom, Cicchetti, & Rogosch, 2014). In line with this, a recent meta-analysis on chronic stress in adults (G. E. Miller et al., 2007) found that the more months that had elapsed since the stress first emerged, the lower a person's morning cortisol, daily cortisol volume, and ACTH levels. In contrast, when chronic stressors were still present in a person's life (e.g., unemployment), morning, afternoon, evening, and daily cortisol outputs were significantly higher. Importantly though, exposure to chronic stress in the early years of life, when the nervous system is still developing, may result in a distinct pattern of dysregulation.

Molecules Matter Too: In Utero Exposure to Antidepressants

With increased understanding that prenatal maternal stress and related mood disturbances have consequences for child behavior and development, antenatal mood disorders are treated with selective serotonin reuptake inhibitor (SSRI) antidepressants. This is raising critical and unanswered questions about the long-term impact of serotonin exposure in combination with maternal mood disturbances on the developing brain. Importantly, both exposures (i.e., maternal mood and SSRIs) are increasingly common and the developmental impact of SSRIs is often indistinguishable from the impact of antenatal maternal mood disturbances (Oberlander, Gingrich, & Ansorge, 2009). Maternal mood disturbances during gestation occur in 10–20% of pregnancies, and up to a third of all depressed mothers have been reported to be treated with an SSRI during pregnancy (Oberlander, Warburton, Misri, Aghajanian, & Hertzman, 2006). SSRIs primarily act by blocking the serotonin transporter (5-HTT) leading to increased intrasynaptic 5-HT levels, thereby potentiating 5-HT neural transmission. SSRIs readily cross the placenta and the blood–brain barrier (Laine, Heikkinen, Ekblad, & Kero, 2003), thereby altering fetal central 5-HT signaling. Such exposure adds a new dimension to how maternal mood disturbances including their treatment by antidepressants during pregnancy potentially shape early human development, possibly via changes in levels of the central neurotransmitter 5-HT during critical periods of neurodevelopment. Maternal mood symptoms, however, do not have to reach clinical levels to have an impact on development (Dunkel Schetter & Tanner, 2012). Our current understanding of negative affective states in pregnancy is based largely on studies—such as reviewed above—of symptomatology (i.e., symptoms of anxiety and depression during pregnancy, as measured with screening tools such as the Edinburgh Postpartum Depression Scale (EPDS)) as opposed to confirmed diagnoses of mental disorders. Further, even in the presence of prenatal SSRI antidepressant treatment, maternal mood disturbances can still have an impact on infant development (Weikum, Oberlander, Hensch, & Werker, 2012). Clearly, regardless of SSRI treatment, maternal mood during pregnancy can affect infant and child development for better *and* worse.

Because prenatal SSRI exposure has not been associated with gross structural teratogenic effects, they are often considered for antenatal therapy (Misri et al., 2006), with the expectation that they confer benefit to mothers (improved prenatal mood) and by extension to her offspring (i.e., via improved prenatal and possibly postnatal maternal mood). However, a substantial number of pregnant women with depression and anxiety remain partially or fully symptomatic even after treatment (Cohen et al., 2006). Failure to achieve remission leaves mothers' mood disturbances (and inherent confounding factors, such as smoking, alcohol, and socioeconomic status) and antenatal SSRI exposure to continue incurring consequences for mothers, and cognitive and emotional child development. Thus, mothers and clinicians must balance the potential consequences of untreated or poorly treated mental illness against risks of antenatal psychopharmacotherapy.

Central to our understanding of how in utero SSRI exposure influences early brain development is the diverse role played by the neurotransmitter 5-HT and its role as a mediator between early life experience and subsequent development. Serotonin is a phylogenetically ancient neurotransmitter widely distributed throughout the entire brain. As early as 5 weeks of gestation, serotonergic neurons are already evident in the human brain (Sundstrom et al., 1993), and by 15 weeks, the raphe nuclei already contain 5-HT neurons (Takahashi, Nakashima, Ohama, Takeda, & Ikuta, 1986). Serotonin plays two critical roles: First, during early developmental periods, 5-HT acts as a growth factor, regulating the development of its own and related neural systems (Whitaker-Azmitia, Druse, Walker, & Lauder, 1996). As a trophic factor, 5-HT also regulates cell division, differentiation, migration, myelination, synaptogenesis, and dendritic pruning (Gaspar, Cases, & Maroteaux, 2003). Then in the mature brain, 5-HT acts as a modulatory neurotransmitter regulating cognition, attention, emotion, learning, sleep, arousal, and stress responsivity. Given these dual roles (i.e., growth and nurturance), it is conceivable that altering 5-HT levels during early sensitive periods might have developmentally lasting consequences for stress and self-regulation.

Effects are evident even before SSRI exposure ends during gestation. Changes in fetal neurobehavioral disturbances include disrupted non-rapid eye movement sleep (Mulder, Ververs, de Heus, & Visser, 2011), reduced brain flow indices (Rurak et al., 2011), and reduced fetal heart rate variability (Rurak et al., 2011). Importantly, such effects are apparent before and following a typical daily maternal SSRI dose, possibly reflecting an early and sustained effect on brain function beyond an acute medication-related effect. Soon after the introduction of SSRI antidepressants in 1988 to manage mood disorders during pregnancy, reports emerged of newborn neurobehavioral disturbances (irritability, weak or absent cry, increased motor activity) or "withdrawal" symptoms, shorter mean gestational age, and lower birthweight (Moses-Kolko et al., 2005). SSRI-exposed neonates have been reported to be more motorically active and tremulous, and had lower heart rate variability and state regulation (Zeskind & Stephens, 2004). Some of these behaviors may be predictors of altered behavior in childhood (Oberlander et al., 2007), and these effects may be mediated through the pharmacological variables (Laine et al., 2003; Oberlander et al., 2004).

Prenatal SSRI Exposure Shaping Child Stress Regulation

Serotonin plays central roles in the early development and function of the two key stress response systems—the HPA axis and the ANS system. Both systems are highly interrelated, and possibly via 5-HT, they are exquisitely sensitive to the effects of early adverse experience (Laplante, Diorio, & Meaney, 2002). Alterations in HPA function that frequently characterize anxiety and depressive disorders (Lowry, 2002) may link altered serotonin levels to neuroendocrine stress regulation and psychopathology (Chrousos, 2000; Homberg & Contet, 2009; McEwen, 2005). In animal models, changing prenatal serotonergic tone affects neurodevelopmental processes associated with stress regulation (Ansorge, Hen, & Gingrich, 2007). Importantly, the relationship between 5-HT and stress reactivity is bidirectional. That is, stressors may alter 5-HT metabolism as well as bias how an individual copes with subsequent stressful challenges (L. Weinstock, Cohen, Bailey, Blatman, & Rosenbaum, 2001; M. Weinstock, 2001). Chronic unpredictable stress during pregnancy alters 5-HT levels that have lasting effects on monoaminergic system function and behavior in rodent offspring (Schneider, Roughton, Koehler, & Lubach, 1999; Weinberg & Tronick, 1998). Prenatal stress lowers plasma and hippocampal serotonergic activity (Peters, 1990) leading to reduced HPA adaptation to stressors reflecting 5-HT's role in HPA function (Firk & Markus, 2007). Serotonin and cardiovascular/autonomic stress regulation are also highly interrelated via links between reflex control of parasympathetic outflow to the heart that involve regulation of central sympathetic and parasympathetic autonomic tone (Ramage, 2001). Given these relationships, it is conceivable that early manipulation of 5-HT levels (i.e., in utero or early life in animal models) alters subsequent stress regulation (Ishiwata, Shiga, & Okado, 2005).

In human newborns, prenatal SSRI exposure is associated with altered stress regulation. A case in point is the duration of facial action and cardiac responses in response to an acute painful event—particularly, parasympathetic cardiac activity is shorter and less intense in SSRI-exposed compared to non-exposed neonates (Oberlander et al., 2002). Altered pain reactivity persists at 2 months of age, after controlling for postnatal drug level and maternal mood (Oberlander et al., 2005). Neurobehavioral changes have been associated with measures of central serotonergic levels in utero and levels of the serotonin metabolite 5-HIAA specifically (Laine et al., 2003). Further, SSRI-exposed neonates exhibit lower cord blood levels of a biomarker of early brain maturation and central serotonergic function (i.e., the astroglial-specific calcium-binding protein, S100B, Hilli et al., 2009; Pawluski, Galea, Brain, Papsdorf, & Oberlander, 2009) and increased norepinephrine metabolite levels (Davidson et al., 2009).

SSRIs are thought to act via increased central 5-HT activity to "normalize" the hypercortisolism and stress dysregulation (Barden, Reul, & Holsboer, 1995) that characterizes depression (Gillespie & Nemeroff, 2005). In an animal model, Ishiwata and colleagues (2005) observed that early SSRI treatment of prenatally stressed mice "normalized" corticosterone responses to a subsequent stressor, increased 5-HT turnover in the hippocampus, and restored the ability to learn spatial information compared with the effects of exposure to prenatal stress alone. In human infants, effects of SSRI exposure on stress regulation may only became evident in the presence of a specific postnatal environment (Oberlander et al., 2008). That is, in response to a non-noxious challenge, SSRI-exposed and non-exposed infants exhibited similar salivary cortisol levels. However, when infant feeding status was considered, differences associated with SSRI exposure emerged. Specifically, compared with breastfed SSRI-exposed and breastfed non-exposed infants, the latter showed a blunted post-stress cortisol response. These findings suggest an SSRI-related effect on the HPA stress system that only becomes apparent in a particular postnatal maternal caregiving context.

Importantly, altered HPA function is characteristic of mood disorders such as anxiety and depression (Fuller, 1996; Lowry, 2002) and links stress regulation with altered serotonergic tone as a key related risk factor for psychopathology (Chrousos, 2000; Homberg & Contet, 2009; McEwen, 2005). Moreover, disruption of 5-HT signaling is considered a key developmental component underlying a number of neuropsychiatric disorders, such as schizophrenia, affective disorders, anxiety, and autism (Bonnin & Levitt, 2011; Chugani et al., 1999; Sodhi & Sanders-Bush, 2004; Whitaker-Azmitia, 2001). With this perspective, the importance of understanding the implications of changing 5-HT signaling during critical periods and altered stress regulation in the emergence of neurodevelopment disorders becomes particularly evident. These concerns have been further raised by recent studies linking in utero SSRI exposure to an increased risk of complex development disorders such as autism spectrum disorders (Boukhris, Sheehy, Mottron, & Berard, 2016; Croen, Grether, Yoshida, Odouli, & Hendrick, 2011; Man et al., 2015; Rai et al., 2013), anxiety (Hanley, Brain, & Oberlander, 2015), depression (Malm et al., 2016), and ADHD (Clements et al., 2015) during childhood. Whether these developmental outcomes reflect a long-term impact of increased serotonin signaling associated with prenatal SSRI exposure, maternal mood disturbances, or a genetic predisposition for these developmental disorders remains a focus for future research.

In summarizing our current knowledge about whether SSRI treatment can potentially have advantages or disadvantages for development, three key themes emerge: First, while prenatal SSRIs alter central 5-HT levels, developmental outcomes do not necessarily reflect a "main effects" story that can be easily attributed to one causal factor (i.e., maternal mood, genetics, or the drug itself). Rather, outcomes in this setting represent an interplay between maternal mood, pharmacological, genetic, and contextual factors related to both mother and her developing child. Second, while SSRIs are typically prescribed during pregnancy with the expectation of optimizing maternal mood and by extension infant developmental health, children may continue to be at risk as maternal pharmacotherapy might not "buffer" or protect them from antenatal maternal mood disturbances (i.e., a lack of drug efficacy). Finally, this is a context of developmental vulnerability *and* plasticity. Therefore, identifying settings whereby individuals might benefit from prenatal maternal pharmacotherapy remains a key and pressing question. Longitudinal study designs that integrate a maternal and infant/child developmental perspective should help us move away from characterizing prenatal SSRI exposure, maternal mood, or even genetic variations as "bad" or "harmful" and rather look at these as adversity- or risk-related factors that heighten or lessen vulnerability associated with early development.

Putting It All Together

The notion that a mother's mood during pregnancy shapes the developing fetal brain and influences risks of mental and physical health across the life span has been a part of popular beliefs for millennia (Murphy, 2010). More than six decades of empirical research has shed light onto the role a mother's psychological state in pregnancy plays for her offspring, although the underlying specific mechanisms remain unclear. In this chapter, we have provided an overview of more recent studies examining the role of prenatal maternal stress (stress exposure, anxiety, depression, and antidepressants) on developmental origins of self-regulation reflected by neurobiological processes such as EF and HPA axis functioning in the offspring spanning from early childhood to early adulthood. These findings highlight the importance of incorporating the prenatal period into our models of parent–child interactions. Some of the stressors that commonly affect women in pregnancy (e.g., low material resources, employment conditions, and strain in intimate relationships) are the same that underlie parenting stress, as discussed in several other chapters of this book.

Understanding the role of maternal stress during gestation in shaping child development offers important insights that may explain why variations in early typical environment are associated with shaping both developmental risk *and* resilience. Importantly, not all gestational stress associated with maternal mood disorders results in negative developmental outcomes; ultimately, understanding the complex relation between maternal stress during pregnancy and effects on children after birth requires the systematic unpacking of interrelations between micro-level factors (e.g., genes), macro-level factors (e.g., medications), and niche (e.g., where the child lives), all couched within time and timing.

Given the central role of EF for child developmental health and the fact that stress early in life may have a particularly large impact on PFC structure and function, this chapter reviewed evidence linking prenatal maternal stress to long-term neurocognitive alterations in the offspring. Across all studies, evidence was found that prenatal stress is associated with each one of the EF components: inhibition (Buss et al., 2011; Van den Bergh, Mennes, et al., 2005), shifting (Mennes et al., 2006), and working memory (Buss et al., 2011; Entringer, Buss, et al., 2009; Pearson et al., 2016), as well as with cortical reductions in the PFC (Buss et al., 2010) and cortical thinning in the right frontal lobes (Sandman et al., 2015). However, no conclusions can be firmly drawn as to which specific aspects of children's EF including underlying PFC structures and functions may be most strongly or consistently altered following exposure to prenatal maternal stress. Future research is needed to examine how prenatal stress shapes EF during childhood and determine whether the functional relation between early stress exposure and EF performance is curvilinear (Arnsten, 2009; de Kloet et al., 1999; Lupien et al., 2007), such that moderate levels of stress exposure may actually enhance EF performance. Evidence that the relationship between prenatal stress exposure and child outcomes may not be necessarily linear is supported by DiPietro and colleagues' (2006) findings, showing that exposure to moderate levels of prenatal stress may actually advance motor and mental development. Critical insight may also be gained by investigating whether child EF mediates the association between prenatal stress exposure and later emotional and behavioral outcomes. Such findings may allow us to understand how exposure to prenatal stress affects children's functioning *across* different developmental domains.

One of the most studied mechanisms involved in fetal programming is the HPA axis, which may play a significant role in mediating the effects of prenatal maternal stress on child EF. We reviewed emerging evidence linking prenatal stress to diurnal and reactivity patterns of the HPA axis in the offspring. Whereas variability in the findings is high, many studies have found that prenatal stress is associated with raised basal and reactivity cortisol levels in infancy (Davis et al., 2011; Glover et al., 2010; Tollenaar et al., 2011), and early-to-middle childhood (Glover et al., 2010; O'Connor et al., 2005; Simons et al., 2015). Later in development, some studies have found either reduced CAR and DCD in adolescents (O'Donnell et al., 2013; Van den Bergh et al., 2008) or no detectable differences in diurnal patterns among young adults exposed to early stress vs. an age-matched comparison group (Entringer, Kumsta, et al., 2009). In this later sample, however, differences between the two groups were found in stress reactivity with raised cortisol reactivity during the TSST for the early stress group. Another study (Buchmann et al., 2014), however, only found attenuated cortisol secretion during the TSST for a subgroup of adolescents (DRD4 7r allele carriers) following prenatal stress exposure. Future research may clarify for whom, in which domain/situation, and during which developmental stage prenatal stress exposure is associated with dysregulation of the HPA axis.

Whether alterations in HPA axis function mediate the association between early stress exposure and altered behavioral outcomes (Van den Bergh et al., 2008) remains a critical question. Alternatively, a child's stress regulation may moderate the association between prenatal stress exposure and later child outcomes. As Entringer and colleagues (2009) have shown, acute stress exposure can have a modulatory effect on the association between prenatal stress exposure and subsequent working memory performance in young adults. Thus, subtle vulnerabilities in the offspring of prenatal stress may be found in the intricate interplay between stress regulation and EF.

Importantly, not all children are affected in the same fashion by prenatal maternal stress and some may even be positively affected, raising questions about the role of genetic and epigenetic influences that shape interactions between early experience and developmental outcomes. As brain development is a product of the dynamic, bidirectional interplay between the individual's genotype and the nature of the early environment, a number of genetic factors (DRD4r, SERT, and COMT) have been identified that determine how children respond to various exposures. While this chapter did not specifically review studies examining the idea of "biological sensitivity to context" (Ellis et al., 2011), there is supporting evidence for it (Buchmann et al., 2014; Weikum et al., 2013). For instance, Pluess and colleagues (2011) have shown that the association between maternal anxiety during pregnancy and negative emotionality in early infancy was only significant in infants carrying one or more copies of the 5-HTTLPR short allele but not in those homozygous for the long allele. In this way, the 5-HTTLPR allelic variations might increase vulnerability to adverse environmental influences as early as the fetal period for some, while in other settings, 5-HTTLPR allelic variations may be associated with resiliency for other infants (Weikum et al., 2013).

The combination of early life stress, genetics, and ongoing challenge may ultimately shape or calibrate individual responsiveness to subsequent stress and vulnerability for behavioral or psychiatric disorders (Charney & Manji, 2004). Recent work with rodents suggests that long-term behavioral outcomes are determined by characteristics of both the pre- and postnatal environment (Francis, Szegda, Campbell, Martin, & Insel, 2003). The interactive effects of pre- and postnatal environmental influences represent an important area for future investigation. In fact, the congruence between prenatal and postnatal environments may be crucial. For instance, Sandman and colleagues (2012) found increased motor and mental development during the first year of life among infants whose mothers experienced congruent levels of depressive symptoms during and after pregnancy, even when the levels of symptoms were relatively high and the prenatal and postnatal environments were unfavorable. In this sense, prenatal environments prepare the fetus for postnatal life and confer an adaptive advantage for critical survival functions during early development. Furthermore, maternal prenatal and postnatal mental health problems may be differentially associated with later outcomes in the offspring. For instance, Vänskä et al., (2015) showed that both maternal prenatal and postnatal mental health problems predicted children's later stress regulation, but in unique ways.

In conclusion, we presented evidence that perinatal maternal stress shapes key elements of self-regulatory abilities during childhood. Conceptualization of these associations has drawn on the concept of fetal programming (Barker, 2003) which implies that changes in the fetal environment may shape a "predictive adaptive response" in which fetal development sets a forecast for a place in the world ahead (Gluckman & Hanson, 2005). Altered PFC function and stress regulation are not inevitably associated with dysfunctional outcomes. Increasingly, research is pointing to the possibility that early stress exposure works to "calibrate" developmental systems that only become "vulnerable" or "resilent" in particular childhood contexts (Glover, 2011). In this way, whether via developmental alterations in serotonin signaling or altered levels of cortisol, maternal mood during gestation may shape a sensitivity to negative and positive life experiences that predicts variations in long-term behavioral and psychiatric health and illness (Homberg, Schubert, & Gaspar, 2010).

Acknowledgements This work was supported by a postdoctoral fellowship from Kids Brain Health Network (formerly NeuroDevNet)/Brain Canada/Health Canada to R.N. T.F.O is the R. Howard Webster Professor in Brain Imaging and Early Child Development at the University of British Columbia, and his work is supported by the BC Children's Hospital Research Institute and the Canadian Institutes for Health Research.

References

Alexander, J. K., Hillier, A., Smith, R. M., Tivarus, M. E., & Beversdorf, D. Q. (2007). Beta-adrenergic modulation of cognitive flexibility during stress. *Journal of Cognitive Neuroscience, 19,* 468–478.

Allister, L., Lester, B. M., Carr, S., & Liu, J. (2001). The effects of maternal depression on fetal heart rate response to vibroacoustic stimulation. *Developmental Neuropsychology, 20,* 639–651.

Ansorge, M. S., Hen, R., & Gingrich, J. A. (2007). Neurodevelopmental origins of depressive disorders. *Current Opinion in Pharmacology, 7,* 8–17.

Arnsten, A. F. T. (2009). Stress signalling pathways that impair prefrontal cortex structure and function. *Nature Review Neuroscience, 10,* 410–422.

Bakermans-Kranenburg, M. J., & van IJzendoorn, M. H. (2006). Gene-environment interaction of the dopamine D4 receptor (DRD4) and observed maternal insensitivity predicting externalizing behavior in preschoolers. *Developmental Psychobiology, 48,* 406–409.

Barden, N., Reul, J. M., & Holsboer, F. (1995). Do antidepressants stabilize mood through actions on the hypothalamic-pituitary-adrenocortical system? *Trends in Neuroscience, 18,* 6–11.

Barker, D. J. (2003). The developmental origins of adult disease. *European Journal of Epidemiology, 18,* 733–736.

Barrett, J., & Fleming, A. (2011). Annual research review: All mothers are not created equal: Neural and psychobiological perspectives on mothering and the importance of individual differences. *Journal of Child Psychology and Psychiatry, 52,* 368–397.

Baumeister, R. F., & Vohs, K. D. (Eds.). (2004). *Handbook of self-regulation: Research, theory, and applications*. New York: Guilford Press.

Bell, M. A., & Deater-Deckard, K. (2007). Biological systems and the development of self-regulation: Integrating behavior, genetics, and psychophysiology. *Journal of Developmental and Behavioral Pediatrics, 28,* 409–420.

Belsky, J., & Pluess, M. (2009). Beyond diathesis stress: Differential susceptibility to environmental influences. *Psychological Bulletin, 135,* 885–908.

Bennett, H. A., Einarson, A., Taddio, A., Koren, G., & Einarson, T. R. (2004). Prevalence of depression during pregnancy: Systematic review. *Obstetrics and Gynecology, 103,* 698–709.

Bernier, A., Carlson, S. M., & Whipple, N. (2010). From external regulation to self-regulation: Early parenting precursors of young children's executive functioning. *Child Development, 81,* 326–339.

Beydoun, H., & Saftlas, A. F. (2008). Physical and mental health outcomes of prenatal maternal stress in human and animal studies: A review of recent evidence. *Paediatric and Perinatal Epidemiology, 290,* 595–596.

Birtchnell, J., Evans, C., & Kennard, J. (1988). The total score of the crown-crisp experiential index: A useful and valid measure of psychoneurotic pathology. *British Journal of Medical Psychology, 61,* 255–266.

Blair, C. (2002). School readiness: Integrating cognition and emotion in a neurobiological conceptualization of children's functioning at school entry. *American Psychologist, 57,* 111–127.

Blair, C., Granger, D., & Peters Razza, R. (2005). Cortisol reactivity is positively related to executive function in preschool children attending head start. *Child Development, 76,* 554–567.

Blair, C., Granger, D. A., Willoughby, M., Mills-Koonce, R., Cox, M., Greenberg, M. T., … & F. L. P. I. (2011). Salivary cortisol mediates effects of poverty and parenting on executive functions in early childhood. *Child Development, 82*, 1970–1984.

Blair, C., & Razza, R. P. (2007). Relating effortful control, executive function, and false belief understanding to emerging math and literacy ability in Kindergarten. *Child Development, 78,* 647–663.

Bonnin, A., & Levitt, P. (2011). Fetal, maternal, and placental sources of serotonin and new implications for developmental programming of the brain. *Neuroscience, 197,* 1–7.

Boukhris, T., Sheehy, O., Mottron, L., & Berard, A. (2016). Antidepressant use during pregnancy and the risk of autism spectrum disorder in children. *JAMA Pediatrics, 170,* 117–124.

Boyce, W. T., & Ellis, B. J. (2005). Biological sensitivity to context: An evolutionary-developmental theory of the origins and functions of stress reactivity. *Developmental Psychopathology, 17,* 271–301.

Buchmann, A. F., Zohsel, K., Blomeyer, D., Hohm, E., Hohmann, S., Jennen-Steinmetz, C., et al. (2014). Interaction between prenatal stress and dopamine D4 receptor genotype in predicting aggression and cortisol levels in young adults. *Psychopharmacology (Berl), 231,* 3089–3097.

Buss, C., Davis, E. P., Hobel, C. J., & Sandman, C. A. (2011). Maternal pregnancy-specific anxiety is associated with child executive function at 6–9 years age. *Stress, 14,* 665–676.

Buss, C., Davis, E. P., Muftuler, L. T., Head, K., & Sandman, C. A. (2010). High pregnancy anxiety during mid-gestation is associated with decreased gray matter density in 6–9-year-old children. *Psychoneuroendocrinology, 35,* 141–153.

Calkins, S. D., & Howse, R. B. (2004). Individual differences in self-regulation: Implications for childhood adjustment. In P. Philippot & R. S. Feldman (Eds.), *The regulation of emotion* (pp. 307–332). Mahwah, NJ: Lawrence Erlbaum.

Calkins, S. D., & Williford, A. P. (2009). Taming the terrible twos: Self-regulation and school readiness. In O. A. Barbarin & B. H. Wasik (Eds.), *Handbook of child development and early education: Research to practice* (pp. 172–198). New York: Guilford Press.

Charney, D. S., & Manji, H. K. (2004). Life stress, genes, and depression: Multiple pathways lead to increased risk and new opportunities for intervention. *Science Signaling, 2004,* 5.

Chrousos, G. P. (2000). The role of stress and the hypothalamic-pituitary-adrenal axis in the pathogenesis of the metabolic syndrome: Neuro-endocrine and target tissue-related causes. *International Journal of Obesity Related Metabolic Disorders, 24*(Suppl 2), S50–S55.

Chugani, D. C., Niimura, K., Chaturvedi, S., Muzik, O., Fakhouri, M., Lee, M. L., et al. (1999). Increased brain serotonin synthesis in migraine. *Neurology, 53,* 1473–1479.

Clements, C. C., Castro, V. M., Blumenthal, S. R., Rosenfield, H. R., Murphy, S. N., Fava, M., et al. (2015). Prenatal antidepressant exposure is associated with risk for attention-deficit hyperactivity disorder but not autism spectrum disorder in a large health system. *Molecular Psychiatry, 20,* 727–734.

Cohen, L. S., Altshuler, L. L., Harlow, B. L., Nonacs, R., Newport, D. J., Viguera, A. C., et al. (2006). Relapse of major depression during pregnancy in women who maintain or discontinue antidepressant treatment. *JAMA, 295,* 499–507.

Croen, L. A., Grether, J. K., Yoshida, C. K., Odouli, R., & Hendrick, V. (2011). Antidepressant use during pregnancy and childhood autism spectrum disorders. *Archives of General Psychiatry, 68,* 1104–1112.

Davidson, S., Prokonov, D., Taler, M., Maayan, R., Harell, D., Gil-Ad, I., et al. (2009). Effect of exposure to selective serotonin reuptake inhibitors in utero on fetal growth: Potential role for the IGF-I and HPA axes. *Pediatric Research, 65,* 236–241.

Davis, E. P., Glynn, L. M., Waffarn, F., & Sandman, C. A. (2011). Prenatal maternal stress programs infant stress regulation. *Journal of Child Psychology and Psychiatry, 52,* 119–129.

de Bruijn, A. T., van Bakel, H. J., & van Baar, A. L. (2009). Sex differences in the relation between prenatal maternal emotional complaints and child outcome. *Early Human Development, 85,* 319–324.

de Kloet, E. R., Oitzl, M. S., & Joëls, M. (1999). Stress and cognition: Are corticosteroids good or bad guys? *Trends in Neurosciences, 22,* 422–426.

de Weerth, C., & Buitelaar, J. K. (2005). Physiological stress reactivity in human pregnancy: A review. *Neuroscience and Biobehavioral Reviews, 29,* 295–312.

Deater-Deckard, K., Wang, Z., Chen, N., & Bell, M. A. (2012). Maternal executive function, harsh parenting, and child conduct problems. *Journal of Child Psychology and Psychiatry, 53,* 1084–1091.

Diamond, A., & Lee, K. (2011). Interventions shown to aid executive function development in children 4 to 12 years old. *Science, 333,* 959–964.

Diamond, A., & Ling, D. S. (2016). Conclusions about interventions, programs, and approaches for improving executive functions that appear justified and those that, despite much hype, do not. *Developmental Cognitive Neuroscience, xx,* xx.

DiPietro, J. A. (2012). Maternal stress in pregnancy: Considerations for fetal development. *Journal of Adolescent Health, 51,* S3–8.

DiPietro, J. A., Hodgson, D. M., Costigan, K. A., & Johnson, T. R. (1996). Fetal antecedents of infant temperament. *Child Development, 67,* 2568–2583.

DiPietro, J. A., Novak, M. F., Costigan, K. A., Atella, L. D., & Reusing, S. P. (2006). Maternal psychological distress during pregnancy in relation to child development at age two. *Child Development, 77,* 573–587.

Doom, J. R., Cicchetti, D., & Rogosch, F. A. (2014). Longitudinal patterns of cortisol regulation differ in maltreated and nonmaltreated children. *Journal of the American Academy of Child and Adolescent Psychiatry, 53,* 1206–1215.

Dunkel Schetter, C. (2011). Psychological science on pregnancy: Stress processes, biopsychosocial models, and emerging research issues. *Annual Review of Psychology, 62,* 531–558.

Dunkel Schetter, C., & Tanner, L. (2012). Anxiety, depression and stress in pregnancy: Implications for mothers, children, research, and practice. *Current Opinion in Psychiatry, 25,* 141–148.

Ellis, B. J., Boyce, W. T., Belsky, J., Bakermans-Kranenburg, M. J., & van IJzendoorn, M. H. (2011). Differential susceptibility to the environment: An evolutionary–neurodevelopmental theory. *Development and Psychopathology, 23,* 7–28.

Entringer, S., Buss, C., Kumsta, R., Hellhammer, D. H., Wadhwa, P. D., & Wuest, S. (2009a). Prenatal psychosocial stress exposure is associated with subsequent working memory performance in young women. *Behavioral Neuroscience, 123,* 886–893.

Entringer, S., Buss, C., & Wadhwa, P. D. (2015). Prenatal stress, development, health and disease risk: A psychobiological perspective—2015 Curt Richter Award Paper. *Psychoneuroendocrinology, 62,* 366–375.

Entringer, S., Kumsta, R., Hellhammer, D. H., Wadhwa, P. D., & Wust, S. (2009b). Prenatal exposure to maternal psychosocial stress and HPA axis regulation in young adults. *Hormones and Behavior, 55,* 292–298.

Firk, C., & Markus, C. R. (2007). Serotonin by stress interaction: A susceptibility factor for the development of depression? *Journal of Psychopharmacology, 21,* 538–544.

Francis, D. D., Szegda, K., Campbell, G., Martin, W. D., & Insel, T. R. (2003). Epigenetic sources of behavioral differences in mice. *Nature Neuroscience, 6,* 445–446.

Fuller, R. W. (1996). Mechanisms and functions of serotonin neuronal systems: Opportunities for neuropeptide interactions. *Annals of the New York Academy of Sciences, 780,* 176–184.

Fuster, J. M. (2008). *The prefrontal cortex* (4th ed.). London: Academic Press.

Gaspar, P., Cases, O., & Maroteaux, L. (2003). The developmental role of serotonin: News from mouse molecular genetics. *Nature Review Neuroscience, 4,* 1002–1012.

Giannakoulopoulos, X., Teixeira, J., Fisk, N., & Glover, V. (1999). Human fetal and maternal noradrenaline responses to invasive procedures. *Pediatric Research, 45,* 494–499.

Gillespie, C. F., & Nemeroff, C. B. (2005). Hypercortisolemia and depression. *Psychosomatic Medicine, 67*(Suppl 1), S26–28.

Glover, V. (2011). Annual research review: Prenatal stress and the origins of psychopathology: An evolutionary perspectiv. *Journal of Child Psychology and Psychiatry, 52,* 356–367.

Glover, V., O'Connor, T. G., & O'Donnell, K. (2010). Prenatal stress and the programming of the HPA axis. *Neuroscience and Biobehavioral Reviews, 35,* 17–22.

Gluckman, P., & Hanson, M. (2005). *The fetal matrix: Evolution, development and disease*. New York: Cambridge University Press.

Glynn, L. M., Schetter, C. D., Hobel, C. J., & Sandman, C. A. (2008). Pattern of perceived stress and anxiety in pregnancy predicts preterm birth. *Health Psychology, 27,* 43–51.

Gunnar, M. R., & Quevedo, L. (2007). The neurobiology of stress and development. *Annual Review of Psychology, 58,* 145–173.

Hanley, G. E., Brain, U., & Oberlander, T. F. (2015). Prenatal exposure to serotonin reuptake inhibitor antidepressants and childhood behavior. *Pediatric Research, 78,* 174–180.

Hanley, G. E., & Oberlander, T. F. (2012). Neurodevelopmental outcomes following prenatal exposure to serotonin reuptake inhibitor antidepressants: A "social teratogen" or moderator of developmental risk? *Birth Defects Research (Part A), 94,* 651–659.

Hilli, J., Heikkinen, T., Rontu, R., Lehtimaki, T., Kishida, I., Aklillu, E., et al. (2009). MAO-A and COMT genotypes as possible regulators of perinatal serotonergic symptoms after in utero exposure to SSRIs. *European Neuropsychopharmacology, 19,* 363–370.

Homberg, J. R., & Contet, C. (2009). Deciphering the interaction of the corticotropin-releasing factor and serotonin brain systems in anxiety-related disorders. *Journal of Neuroscience, 29,* 13743–13745.

Homberg, J. R., Schubert, D., & Gaspar, P. (2010). New perspectives on the neurodevelopmental effects of SSRIs. *Trends in Pharmacological Sciencies, 31,* 60–65.

Howard, L. M., Molyneaux, E., Dennis, C.-L., Rochat, T., Stein, A., & Milgrom, J. (2014). Non-psychotic mental disorders in the perinatal period. *The Lancet, 384,* 1775–1788.

Hughes, C. (2011). Changes and challenges in 20 years of research into the development of executive functions. *Infant and Child Development, 20,* 251–271.

Hughes, C., & Ensor, R. (2011). Individual differences in growth in executive function across the transition to school predict externalizing and internalizing behaviors and self-perceived academic success at 6 years of age. *Journal of Experimental Child Psychology, 108,* 663–676.

Huizink, A. C., Robles de Medina, P. G., Mulder, E. J., Visser, G. H., & Buitelaar, J. K. (2003). Stress during pregnancy is associated with developmental outcome in infancy. *Journal of Child Psychology and Psychiatry, 44,* 810–818.

Ishiwata, H., Shiga, T., & Okado, N. (2005). Selective serotonin reuptake inhibitor treatment of early postnatal mice reverses their prenatal stress-induced brain dysfunction. *Neuroscience, 133,* 893–901.

Kinsella, M. T., & Monk, C. (2009). Impact of maternal stress, depression & anxiety on fetal neurobehavioral development. *Clinical Obstetrics and Gynecology, 52,* 425–440.

Lagopoulos, J., Hermens, D. F., Naismith, S. L., Scott, E. M., & Hickie, I. B. (2012). Frontal lobe changes occur early in the course of affective disorders in young people. *BMC Psychiatry, 12,* 1–7.

Laine, K., Heikkinen, T., Ekblad, U., & Kero, P. (2003). Effects of exposure to selective serotonin reuptake inhibitors during pregnancy on serotonergic symptoms in newborns and cord blood monoamine and prolactin concentrations. *Archives of General Psychiatry, 60,* 720–726.

Laplante, P., Diorio, J., & Meaney, M. J. (2002). Serotonin regulates hippocampal glucocorticoid receptor expression via a 5-HT7 receptor. *Brain Research. Developmental Brain Research, 139,* 199–203.

Lazarus, R. S. (1991). Progress on a cognitive-motivational-relational theory of emotion. *American Psychologist, 46,* 819–834.

Leight, K. L., Fitelson, E. M., Weston, C. A., & Wisner, K. L. (2010). Childbirth and mental disorders. *International Review of Psychiatry, 22,* 453–471.

Levitt, P. (2003). Structural and functional maturation of the developing primate brain. *Journal of Pediatrics, 143,* 35–45.

Lowry, C. A. (2002). Functional subsets of serotonergic neurones: Implications for control of the hypothalamic-pituitary-adrenal axis. *Journal of Neuroendocrinology, 14,* 911–923.

Lupien, S. J., Gillin, C. J., & Hauger, R. L. (1999). Working memory is more sensitive than declarative memory to the acute effects of corticosteroids: A dose-response study in humans. *Behavioral Neuroscience, 113,* 420–430.

Lupien, S. J., Maheu, F., Tu, M., Fiocco, A., & Schramek, T. E. (2007). The effects of stress and stress hormones on human cognition: Implications for the field of brain and cognition. *Brain and Cognition, 65,* 209–237.

Malm, H., Brown, A. S., Gissler, M., Gyllenberg, D., Hinkka-Yli-Salomäki, S., McKeague, I. W., et al. (2016). Gestational exposure to selective serotonin reuptake inhibitors and offspring psychiatric disorders: A national register-based study. *Journal of the American Academy of Child and Adolescent Psychiatry, 55,* 359–366.

Man, K. K., Tong, H. H., Wong, L. Y., Chan, E. W., Simonoff, E., & Wong, I. C. (2015). Exposure to selective serotonin reuptake inhibitors during pregnancy and risk of autism spectrum disorder in children: A systematic review and meta-analysis of observational studies. *Neuroscience and Biobehavioral Reviews, 49,* 82–89.

McEwen, B. S. (2000). Allostasis and allostatic load: Implications for neuropsychopharmacology. *Neuropsychopharmacology, 22,* 108–124.

McEwen, B. S. (2005). Glucocorticoids, depression, and mood disorders: Structural remodeling in the brain. *Metabolism, 54*(5 Suppl 1), 20–23.

McEwen, B. S., & Morrison, J. H. (2013). The brain on stress: Vulnerability and plasticity of the prefrontal cortex over the life course. *Neuron, 79,* 16–29.

McEwen, B. S., & Wingfield, J. C. (2003). The concept of allostasis in biology and biomedicine. *Hormones and Behavior, 43,* 2–16.

Mennes, M., Stiers, P., Lagae, L., & Van den Bergh, B. R. H. (2006). Long-term cognitive sequelae of antenatal maternal anxiety: Involvement of the orbitofrontal cortex. *Neuroscience and Biobehavioral Reviews, 30,* 1078–1086.

Miller, E. K., & Cohen, J. D. (2001). An integrative theory of prefrontal cortex function. *Annual Review of Neuroscience, 24,* 167–202.

Miller, G. E., Chen, E., & Zhou, E. S. (2007). If it goes up, must it come down? Chronic stress and the hypothalamic-pituitary-adrenocortical axis in humans. *Psychological Bulletin, 133,* 25–45.

Misri, S., Reebye, P., Kendrick, K., Carter, D., Ryan, D., Grunau, R. E., et al. (2006). Internalizing behaviors in 4-year-old children exposed in utero to psychotropic medications. *American Journal of Psychiatry, 163,* 1026–1032.

Miyake, A., Friedman, N. P., Emerson, M. J., Witzki, A. H., & Howerter, A. (2000). The unity and diversity of executive functions and their contributions to complex "frontal lobe" tasks: A latent variable analysis. *Cognitive Psychology, 41,* 49–100.

Moffitt, T. E., Arseneault, L., Belsky, D., Dickson, N., Hancox, R. J., Harrington, H., et al. (2011). A gradient of childhood self-control predicts health, wealth, and public safety. *Proceedings of the National Academy of Sciences of the United States of America, 108,* 2693–2698.

Monk, C., Fifer, W. P., Myers, M. M., Sloan, R. P., Trien, L., & Hurtado, A. (2000). Maternal stress responses and anxiety during pregnancy: Effects on fetal heart rate. *Developmental Psychobiology, 36,* 67–77.

Moses-Kolko, E. L., Bogen, D., Perel, J., Bregar, A., Uhl, K., Levin, B., et al. (2005). Neonatal signs after late in utero exposure to serotonin reuptake inhibitors: Literature review and implications for clinical applications. *JAMA, 293,* 2372–2383.

Mulder, E. J., Ververs, F. F., de Heus, R., & Visser, G. H. (2011). Selective serotonin reuptake inhibitors affect neurobehavioral development in the human fetus. *Neuropsychopharmacology, 36,* 1961–1971.

Murmu, M. S., Salomon, S., Biala, Y., Weinstock, M., Braun, K., & Bock, J. (2006). Changes of spine density and dendritic complexity in the prefrontal cortex in offspring of mothers exposed to stress during pregnancy. *European Journal of Neuroscience, 24,* 1477–1487.

Murphy, P. A. (2010). *Origins: How the nine months before birth shape the rest of our lives*. New York: Free Press.

Neuenschwander, R., Röthlisberger, M., Cimeli, P., & Roebers, C. M. (2012). How do different aspects of self-regulation predict successful adaptation to school? *Journal of Experimental Child Psychology, 113,* 353–371.

O'Connor, T. G., Ben-Shlomo, Y., Heron, J., Golding, J., Adams, D., & Glover, V. (2005). Prenatal anxiety predicts individual differences in cortisol in pre-adolescent children. *Biological Psychiatry, 58,* 211–217.

O'Connor, T. G., Heron, J., Golding, J., Beveridge, M., & Glover, V. (2002). Maternal antenatal anxiety and children's behavioural/emotional problems at 4 years: Report from the Avon longitudinal study of parents and children. *British Journal of Psychiatry, 180,* 502–508.

O'Connor, T. G., Heron, J., Golding, J., Glover, V., & Team, T. A. S. (2003). Maternal anxiety and behavioural/emotional problems in children: A test of a programming hypothesis. *Journal of Child Psychology and Psychiatry, 44,* 1025–1036.

O'Donnell, K. J., Glover, V., Jenkins, J., Browne, D., Ben-Shlomo, Y., Golding, J., et al. (2013). Prenatal maternal mood is associated with altered diurnal cortisol in adolescence. *Psychoneuroendocrinology, 38,* 1630–1638.

Oberlander, T. F., Gingrich, J. A., & Ansorge, M. S. (2009). Sustained neurobehavioral effects of exposure to SSRI antidepressants during development: Molecular to clinical evidence. *Clinical Pharmacology and Therapeutics, 86,* 672–677.

Oberlander, T. F., Grunau, R., Mayes, L., Riggs, W., Rurak, D., Papsdorf, M., et al. (2008). Hypothalamicpituitary-adrenal (HPA) axis function in 3-month old infants with prenatal selective serotonin reuptake inhibitor (SSRI) antidepressant exposure. *Early Human Development, 84,* 689–697.

Oberlander, T. F., Grunau, R. E., Fitzgerald, C., Ellwood, A. L., Misri, S., Rurak, D., et al. (2002). Prolonged prenatal psychotropic medication exposure alters neonatal acute pain response. *Pediatric Research, 51,* 443–453.

Oberlander, T. F., Grunau, R. E., Fitzgerald, C., Papsdorf, M., Rurak, D., & Riggs, W. (2005). Pain reactivity in 2-month-old infants after prenatal and postnatal serotonin reuptake inhibitor medication exposure. *Pediatrics, 115,* 411–425.

Oberlander, T. F., Misri, S., Fitzgerald, C. E., Kostaras, X., Rurak, D., & Riggs, W. (2004). Pharmacologic factors associated with transient neonatal symptoms following prenatal psychotropic medication exposure. *Journal of Clinical Psychiatry, 65,* 230–237.

Oberlander, T. F., Reebye, P., Misri, S., Papsdorf, M., Kim, J., & Grunau, R. (2007). Externalizing and attentional behaviors in children of depressed mothers treated with a selective serotonin reuptake inhibitor antidepressant during pregnancy. *Archives of Pediatrics and Adolescent Medicine, 161,* 22–29.

Oberlander, T. F., Warburton, W., Misri, S., Aghajanian, J., & Hertzman, C. (2006). Neonatal outcomes after prenatal exposure to selective serotonin reuptake inhibitor antidepressants and maternal depression using population-based linked health data. *Archives of General Psychiatry, 63,* 898–906.

Ochsner, K. N., & Gross, J. J. (2005). The cognitive control of emotion. *Trends in Cognitive Sciences, 9,* 242–249.

Pawluski, J. L., Galea, L. A. M., Brain, U., Papsdorf, M., & Oberlander, T. F. (2009). Neonatal S100B protein levels after prenatal exposure to selective serotonin reuptake inhibitors. *Pediatrics, 124,* e662–e670.

Pearson, R. M., Bornstein, M. H., Cordero, M., Scerif, G., Mahedy, L., Evans, J., et al. (2016). Maternal perinatal mental health and offspring academic achievement at age 16: The mediating role of childhood executive function. *Journal of Child Psychology and Psychiatry, 57,* 491–501.

Peters, D. A. (1990). Maternal stress increases fetal brain and neonatal cerebral cortex 5-hydroxytryptamine synthesis in rats: A possible mechanism by which stress influences brain development. *Pharmacology, Biochemestry, and Behavior, 35,* 943–947.

Pluess, M., Velders, F. P., Belsky, J., van IJzendoorn, M. H., Bakermans-Kranenburg, M. J., Jaddoe, V. W., … Tiemeier, H. (2011). Serotonin transporter polymorphism moderates effects of prenatal maternal anxiety on infant negative emotionality. *Biological Psychiatry, 69,* 520–525.

Pruessner, J. C., Dedovic, K., Khalili-Mahani, N., Engert, V., Pruessner, M., Buss, C., et al. (2008). Deactivation of the limbic system during acute psycho-social stress: Evidence from positron emission tomography and functional magnetic resonance imaging studies. *Biological Psychiatry, 63,* 234–240.

Rai, D., Lee, B. K., Dalman, C., Golding, J., Lewis, G., & Magnusson, C. (2013). Parental depression, maternal antidepressant use during pregnancy, and risk of autism spectrum disorders: Population based case-control study. *British Medical Journal, 349,* f2059.

Ramage, A. G. (2001). Central cardiovascular regulation and 5-hydroxytryptamine receptors. *Brain Research Bulletin, 56,* 425–439.

Rurak, D., Lim, K., Sanders, A., Brain, U., Riggs, W., & Oberlander, T. F. (2011). Third trimester fetal heart rate and Doppler middle cerebral artery blood flow velocity characteristics during prenatal selective serotonin reuptake inhibitor exposure. *Pediatric Research, 70,* 96–101.

Sanchez, M. M., Young, L. J., Plotsky, P. M., & Insel, T. R. (2000). Distribution of corticosteroid receptors in the rhesus brain. *The Journal of Neuroscience, 20,* 4657–4568.

Sandman, C. A., Buss, C., Head, K., & Davis, E. P. (2015). Fetal exposure to maternal depressive symptoms is associated with cortical thickness in late childhood. *Biological Psychiatry, 77,* 324–334.

Sandman, C. A., Davis, E., & Glynn, L. (2012). Prescient human fetuses thrive. *Psychological Science, 23,* 93–100.

Sapolsky, R. M., Uno, H., Rebert, C. S., & Finch, C. E. (1990). Hippocampal damage associated with prolonged glucocorticoid exposure in primates. *Journal of Neuroscience, 10,* 2897–2902.

Schneider, M. L., Roughton, E. C., Koehler, A. J., & Lubach, G. R. (1999). Growth and development following prenatal stress exposure in primates: An examination of ontogenetic vulnerability. *Child Development, 70,* 263–274.

Seckl, J. R., & Meaney, M. J. (1993). Early life events and later development of ischaemic heart disease. *Lancet, 342,* 1236.

Simons, S. S. H., Beijers, R., Cillessen, A. H. N., & de Weerth, C. (2015). Development of the cortisol circadian rhythm in the light of stress early in life. *Psychoneuroendocrinology, 62,* 292–300.

Sodhi, M. S., & Sanders-Bush, E. (2004). Serotonin and brain development. *International Revue of Neurobiology, 59,* 111–174.

Spielberger, C. D., Gorsuch, R. L., & Lushene, R. E. (1970). *STAI manual for the state-trait anxiety inventory*. Palo Alto, CA: Consulting Psychologists Press.

Stiles, J., & Jernigan, T. L. (2010). The basics of brain development. *Neuropsychology Review, 20,* 327–348.

Sundstrom, E., Kolare, S., Souverbie, F., Samuelsson, E. B., Pschera, H., Lunell, N. O., et al. (1993). Neurochemical differentiation of human bulbospinal monoaminergic neurons during the first trimester. *Brain Research. Developmental Brain Research, 75,* 1–12.

Takahashi, H., Nakashima, S., Ohama, E., Takeda, S., & Ikuta, F. (1986). Distribution of serotonin-containing cell bodies in the brainstem of the human fetus determined with immunohistochemistry using antiserotonin serum. *Brain Development, 8,* 355–365.

Talge, N. M., Neal, C., & Glover, V. (2007). Antenatal maternal stress and long-term effects on child neurodevelopment: How and why? *Journal of Child Psychology and Psychiatry and Allied Disciplines, 48,* 245–261.

Tollenaar, M. S., Beijers, R., Jansen, J., Riksen-Walraven, J. M. A., & de Weerth, C. (2011). Maternal prenatal stress and cortisol reactivity to stressors in human infants. *Stress, 14,* 53–65.

Tronick, E. Z., & Weinberg, M. K. (1997). Depressed mothers and infants: Failure to form dyadic states of consciousness. In: L. Murray & P. J. Cooper (Eds.), *Postpartum depression and child development* (pp. 54–81). New York: Guilford Press.

Van den Bergh, B. R. H., & Marcoen, A. (2004). High antenatal maternal anxiety is related to ADHD symptoms, externalizing problems, and anxiety in 8- and 9-year-olds. *Child Development, 75,* 1085–1097.

Van den Bergh, B. R. H., Mennes, M., Oosterlaan, J., Stevens, V., Stiers, P., Marcoen, A., & Lagae, L. (2005). High antenatal maternal anxiety is related to impulsivity during performance on cognitive tasks in 14- and 15-year-olds. *Neuroscience and Biobehavioral Reviews, 29*, 259–269.

Van den Bergh, B. R. H., Mennes, M., Stevens, V., Van der Meere, J., Börger, N., Stiers, P., et al. (2006). ADHD deficit as measured in adolescent boys with a continuous performance task is related to antenatal maternal anxiety. *Pediatric Research, 59,* 78–82.

Van den Bergh, B. R. H., Mulder, E. J., Mennes, M., & Glover, V. (2005b). Antenatal maternal anxiety and stress and the neurobehavioural development of the fetus and child: Links and possible mechanisms: A review. *Neuroscience and Biobehavioral Reviews, 29,* 237–258.

Van den Bergh, B. R. H., Van Calster, B., Smits, T., Van Huffel, S., & Lagae, L. (2008). Antenatal maternal anxiety is related to HPA-axis dysregulation and self-reported depressive symptoms in adolescence: A prospective study on the fetal origins of depressed mood. *Neuropsychopharmacology, 33,* 536–535.

Vänskä, M., Punamäki, R.-L., Lindblom, J. K., Tolvanen, A., Flykt, M., Unkila-Kallio, L., … Tiitinen, A. (2015). Timing of early maternal mental health and child cortisol regulation. *Infant and Child Development, (early view- online version), 25,* 461–483. doi:10.1002/icd.194

Weikum, W. M., Brain, U., Chau, C. M. Y., Grunau, R. E., Boyce, T., Diamond, A., et al. (2013). Prenatal serotonin reuptake inhibitor (SRI) antidepressant exposure and serotonin transporter promoter genotype (SLC6A4) influence executive functions at 6 years of age. *Frontiers in Cellular Neuroscience, 7,* 1–12.

Weikum, W. M., Oberlander, T. F., Hensch, T. K., & Werker, J. F. (2012). Prenatal exposure to antidepressants and depressed maternal mood alter trajectory of infant speech perception. *Proceedings of the National Academy of Sciences, 109,* 17221–17227.

Weinberg, M. K., & Tronick, E. Z. (1998). The impact of maternal psychiatric illness on infant development. *Journal of Clinical Psychiatry, 59*(Suppl 2), 53–61.

Weinstock, L., Cohen, L. S., Bailey, J. W., Blatman, R., & Rosenbaum, J. F. (2001). Obstetrical and neonatal outcome following clonazepam use during pregnancy: A case series. *Psychotherapy and Psychosomatics, 70,* 158–162.

Weinstock, M. (2001). Alterations induced by gestational stress in brain morphology and behaviour of the offspring. *Progress in Neurobiology, 65,* 427–451.

Weinstock, M. (2008). The long-term behavioural consequences of prenatal stress. *Neuroscience and Biobehavioral Reviews, 32,* 1073–1086.

Whitaker-Azmitia, P. M. (2001). Serotonin and brain development: Role in human developmental diseases. *Brain Research Bulletin, 56,* 479–485.

Whitaker-Azmitia, P. M., Druse, M., Walker, P., & Lauder, J. M. (1996). Serotonin as a developmental signal. *Behavioral Brain Research, 73,* 19–29.

Zeskind, P. S., & Stephens, L. E. (2004). Maternal selective serotonin reuptake inhibitor use during pregnancy and newborn neurobehavior. *Pediatrics, 113,* 368–375.

Chapter 7
DNA Methylation: A Mediator Between Parenting Stress and Adverse Child Development?

Rosa H. Mulder, Jolien Rijlaarsdam and Marinus H. Van IJzendoorn

Introduction

In the contemporary version of the nature versus nurture debate, it is taken for granted that the (parental) environment *as well as* the genetic makeup determines the behavior of a developing child, with the child's genome being differentially open to environmental influences. For example, in their groundbreaking gene-by-environment (G × E) study, Caspi et al. (2003) found that individuals who had experienced stressful life events were more often depressed when they carried one or two short alleles of the serotonin transporter gene (*5-HTT* or *SLC6A4*) in the serotonin-transporter-linked polymorphic region (*5-HTTLPR*). Likewise, in a first randomized controlled G × E trial, Bakermans-Kranenburg, Van IJzendoorn, Pijlman, Mesman, & Juffer, (2008) showed that changing sensitive parenting and limit setting only influenced the externalizing behavior if the child was a carrier of the dopamine D4 receptor (*DRD4*) 7-repeat allele.

However, in G × E studies, it remains unknown where and how genetics and the environment exactly interact. The field of epigenetics might suture this gap between nature and nurture (Meaney, 2010). 'Epigenetics' is a term coined by the embryologist Waddington (1939, 1956), who used it to describe the interplay of

R.H. Mulder · J. Rijlaarsdam · M.H. Van IJzendoorn (✉)
Centre for Child and Family Studies, Leiden University, Leiden, The Netherlands
e-mail: vanijzen@fsw.leidenuniv.nl

R.H. Mulder
e-mail: r.h.mulder@fsw.leidenuniv.nl

J. Rijlaarsdam
e-mail: j.rijlaarsdam@fsw.leidenuniv.nl

M.H. Van IJzendoorn
School of Pedagogical and Educational Sciences, Erasmus University Rotterdam, Rotterdam, The Netherlands

K. Deater-Deckard and R. Panneton (eds.), *Parental Stress and Early Child Development*, DOI 10.1007/978-3-319-55376-4_7

genes and external cues in the development of the omnipotent cell into a fully specialized one. A related term, epigenesis, was later used by Gilbert Gottlieb to emphasize how variation in the DNA does not simply lead to variation in functioning proteins in a one-to-one fashion, but rather contributes in a bidirectional manner with several layers to the developmental system, going from the genetic level, via the neural and behavior level all the way to the environmental level (Gottlieb & Halpern, 2002). Indeed, with modern laboratory technologies, different epigenetic mechanisms have been identified through which the environment can get 'under the skin' and act upon genetic variation to affect the transcriptional and translational processes to form genes' main product: proteins.

One of these epigenetic mechanisms is DNA methylation, involving a methyl group (CH_3) that attaches to the cytosine nucleotide in the DNA, in places where the cytosine nucleotide is situated alongside a guanine nucleotide, connected via a phosphate bridge (hence cytosine-phosphate-guanine site, or CpG site) (Klose & Bird, 2006; Law & Jacobsen, 2010). The human genome has millions of CpG sites where a methyl group might be attached, which has been found to affect the three-dimensional DNA formation so that it may hinder or facilitate transcription of the DNA (Li & Reinberg, 2011). Other mechanisms work at the level of the histones, proteins around which the chromatin is packaged. Examples would be histone acetylation, or histone methylation (Bannister & Kouzarides, 2011; Berger, 2011). Again, these histone-based mechanisms change the accessibility of the gene for transcriptional processes. Epigenetic mechanisms might also take place further into the translational process, for example, in the form of small noncoding RNA, which can affect splicing variants (Stefani & Slack, 2008).

Since DNA methylation takes place through the covalent binding of the methyl group to the cytosine nucleotide, this is the most physically stable form of epigenetics and most likely to survive the chemical treatment that takes place in the laboratory. Therefore, it is the most frequently studied form of epigenetics. It has been shown that DNA methylation indeed makes the genome more dynamic and is involved, as postulated by Waddington, in cell differentiation (Holliday & Pugh, 1996; Meissner et al., 2008), as well as in X-chromosomal inactivation in female mammals (Chow & Heard, 2009; Riggs, 1975) and in aberrant cell functioning such as cancer (Esteller & Herman, 2002). The downstream effects of DNA methylation are complex: It might functionally silence a gene by decreasing its accessibility by DNA polymerase, promote gene transcription by increasing its accessibility but could also, for example, indirectly affect transcription of genes by altering accessibility of distal regulatory regions such as enhancers or silencers (Aran, Sabato, & Hellman, 2013; Moore & Fan, 2013).

Importantly, it seems that DNA methylation can be affected by life events. In a series of experiments on rodents, Weaver and colleagues showed that early life stress, for example, maternal separation, is related to altered stress reactivity in the adult offspring, and that this effect seemed to be mediated by methylation of the promoter of the glucocorticoid receptor gene (*NR3C1* or *GR*) in the hippocampus (Weaver, Szyf, & Meaney, 2002). The binding of corticosterone (rodents) or cortisol (humans) to the glucocorticoid receptors causes negative feedback to the hypothalamic–pituitary–adrenal axis (HPA axis) and is necessary to control stress reactivity. Intriguingly, the results of Weaver, Szyf, and Meaney imply not only that DNA methylation is affected by life events, but also that it could influence gene transcription to the extent that it changes behavior into adulthood. Moreover, Weaver et al. (2004) showed that normal variation in maternal caretaking, as measured by the amount of licking and grooming, could alter methylation of the *NR3C1* promoter.

In humans, it has also been shown that major life events can modify outcomes in later life, possibly via DNA methylation. Examples can be found in the Dutch Hunger Winter Families Studies (Lumey et al., 2007), which focused on offspring conceived in the winter of 1944–45 during the Second World War, a period in which food was extremely scarce and starvation ubiquitous. In these studies, it was found that fetuses who were exposed to famine in the first trimester after conception had less methylation of the insulin-like growth factor II gene (*IGF2*) (Heijmans et al., 2008), resulting in lower birth weights, and LDL cholesterol (Tobi et al., 2014) in adulthood.

In this chapter, we examine whether DNA methylation mediates the relation between parenting stress and child development. Parenting stress is typically indicated by the recording of actual stressors, of parental psychological affliction such as depression or anxiety, and/or of a history of abuse in the child. Such stress might occur during pregnancy, as well as postnatally. Child development may be operationalized as psychological, hormonal, or neurological development. Importantly, throughout the chapter, several methodological issues will be touched upon as behavioral epigenetics is an emerging field facing a large number of problems and pitfalls.

In the following section, we review studies on the association between parenting stress and DNA methylation, prenatally and postnatally. Effects of DNA methylation cannot be separated from the genes they act upon, and we will elaborate on such epi-allelic interactions. Subsequently, we consider research on the association between DNA methylation and adverse child development, with a special emphasis on the mediation of the association between parenting stress and child development via epigenetics. In a final discussion section, we summarize our findings and address some caveats.

Epigenetic Signatures as Biomarkers of Exposure

Candidate Epi-Gene Approaches

Adversities and related stress (e.g., maternal depression and anxiety in the prenatal period) have been suggested to affect epigenetic patterns in the neonate, and differences in epigenetic signatures have been speculated to be markers of prenatal programming for postnatal life circumstances (see also Chap. 6 by Oberlander and

Neuenschwander), in accordance with the Barker hypothesis (Barker, 1990). Several studies examined the association between prenatal stress and methylation state of the *NR3C1* promotor region of the offspring. *NR3C1* has been found to co-regulate secretion and reuptake of cortisol and might thus be important for regulation of stress. In a groundbreaking study building on earlier work by Weaver et al. (2004) on rodents, McGowan et al. (2009) investigated the postmortem hippocampal brain tissues of male suicide victims with (n = 12) and without (n = 12) a history of child abuse and those of matched controls who died in car accidents (n = 12). They found that suicide victims with a history of child abuse had less GR expression and more methylation of *NR3C1* than suicide victims without a history of child abuse or controls, whereas no significant difference was found between suicide victims without a history of abuse and controls. Specifically, DNA hypermethylation was found in 3 out of 38 measured CpG sites. Moreover, it was found that within the group of suicide victims with child abuse, more DNA methylation was associated with less GR messenger RNA, as well as less GR messenger RNA overall (messenger RNA triggers the production of associated proteins downstream). These findings indicate that childhood abuse is related to DNA methylation, which decreases *NR3C1* transcription. This might lead to aberrant HPA axis functioning and dysfunctional stress regulation, rendering the affected individual more susceptible to the development of psychopathologies such as depression and anxiety, ultimately increasing the risk of suicide.

DNA methylation might also be a mechanism through which the intergenerational transmission of stress dysregulation takes place (see also Chap. 10 by Mileva-Seitz and Fleming). This hypothesis was tested by Yehuda et al. (2014), who examined *NR3C1* promoter methylation in a sample of adult offspring (without PTSD) with at least one Holocaust survivor parent (with or without PTSD) (n = 80) and demographically matched participants without parental Holocaust exposure or PTSD (n = 15). Yehuda et al. (2014) found an interaction between maternal and paternal PTSD in the prediction of offspring *NR3C1* promoter methylation. Specifically, only in the absence of maternal PTSD, offspring exposed to paternal PTSD had higher levels of *NR3C1* promoter methylation. Offspring exposed to both maternal and paternal PTSD showed lower levels of *NR3C1* promoter methylation. Interestingly, *NR3C1* promoter methylation negatively correlated with *NR3C1* expression. Furthermore, stronger cortisol suppression was related to lower DNA methylation. Replication of the rather complicated interactions in a relatively small sample is of course needed, and the results should be considered potentially fruitful hypotheses about the biological underpinnings of the intergenerational transmission of post-traumatic stress.

Thus far, we primarily discussed the association between postnatal parental stress and DNA methylation in the child. It is theorized, however, that prenatal parenting, may it be through the intake of harmful agents or through psychological stress, can have a lasting harmful impact on the child (Huizink, Mulder, & Buitelaar, 2004; Jacobson, Chiodo, Sokol, & Jacobson, 2002). Below, we discuss two studies on how prenatal psychological stress may affect *NR3C1* methylation.

In a study of 83 pregnant women, Hompes et al. (2013) assessed maternal stress each trimester and found it to be significantly associated with methylation of one specific CpG site of the *NR3C1* promoter in the cord blood of their newborns. Also, several dimensions of pregnant women's anxiety about their impending delivery predicted methylation of various CpG sites of the nerve growth factor-inducible protein A (NGFI-A) binding sites of *NR3C1* (Hompes et al., 2014, corrigendum). The study was meant to replicate the earlier results of a pioneering study by Oberlander et al. (2008) who found no multivariate association between the methylation state of 13 CpG sites in *NR3C1* with several measures for prenatal depression and anxiety in 82 mothers ($n = 46$ depressed), but did find that the methylation of 3 CpG sites was correlated with some prenatal depression and anxiety indicators. Oberlander et al.'s results were not replicated by Hompes et al. (2013) who conducted statistical analyses with corrections for multiple testing and found associations during different time windows, on different CpG sites and with different directions. In spite of these inconsistencies, it seems likely that maternal stress during pregnancy is capable of altering gene expression in offspring in ways that increase the risk of stress dysregulation at future points in their development (see also Chap. 6 by Oberlander and Neuenschwander).

In another related study, 23 mother-child dyads were assessed with retrospective reports of intimate partner violence during mothers' pregnancy and DNA methylation was extracted from blood samples when the children were 10–19 years old (Radtke et al., 2011). These authors found a significantly higher mean DNA methylation percentage in 10 CpG sites of the promotor region of *NR3C1* in those adolescents whose mothers had experienced intimate partner violence during pregnancy. However, the small number of subjects from various ethnic backgrounds and the relatively large number of statistical tests (not corrected for multiple testing) might make replication of these results difficult. Together, the results of Radtke et al. and Hompes et al. show that stress during pregnancy might affect *NR3C1* methylation of the fetus in a lasting way, but replication is needed.

Taking into account all aforementioned studies, it seems that the effect of stress on *NR3C1* promoter methylation that was initially found in rats translates into studies on humans. Following, we will briefly discuss some studies that also focus on methylation of genes other than *NR3C1*.

In a study on 57 mothers and their offspring, Braithwaite, Kundakovic, Ramchandani, Murphy, and Champagne (2015) studied the association between 2nd and 3rd trimester depressive symptoms in the mother and methylation of *NR3C1* and *BDNF* in 2-month-old offspring, while controlling for postnatal maternal depressive symptoms. They found that prenatal depressive symptoms were associated with neonatal increased *NR3C1* DNA methylation in male infants, and they also found decreased methylation of an exon upstream of the brain-derived neurotrophic factor gene (*BDNF*) in both male and female infants. In an earlier study on prenatal depression in 82 pregnant women, Devlin, Brain, Austin, and Oberlander (2010) showed associations with methylation status of *5-HTT*, but in contrast to Braithwaite et al. (2015), they did not find associations with methylation of *BDNF*.

Using a sample of 152 females, Vijayendran, Beach, Plume, Brody, and Philibert (2012) examined the associations between childhood sexual abuse and DNA methylation at 16 sites across the *5-HTT* gene in females. One out of the 16 measured CpG sites was positively associated with both genotype and sexual abuse, whereas DNA methylation of another CpG site was associated solely with sexual abuse. In a cross-sectional study, Unternaehrer et al. (2015) investigated the association between maternal care and DNA methylation of *BDNF* (one sequence including 7 CpG sites) and the oxytocin receptor gene (*OXTR*; two sequences including 6 and 17 CpG sites, respectively). They showed that university students reporting low maternal care in childhood and adolescence ($n = 45$) had higher levels of DNA methylation in the *BDNF* target sequence than students reporting high maternal care ($n = 40$). Similarly, students reporting low maternal care had higher levels of DNA methylation in the first *OXTR* target sequence but not in the second target sequence.

Together, these studies suggest that candidate genes involved in stress regulation as well those affecting other regulators of the central nervous system are affected by parenting stress. However, research driven by a priori hypotheses on genes involved can form an 'information bottleneck' (Zhu & Zhao, 2007), as it is unlikely to reveal new genes or mechanisms. Like genome-wide association studies (GWASs), epigenome-wide association studies (EWASs) are hypothesis free and cover the length of the whole genome. With the latest arrays, EWASs can gauge up to 850,000 CpG sites, in locations such as the promoter, intergenic regions, and intragenic regions. In the following paragraph, we will discuss studies that relate stressful parenting to epigenome-wide DNA methylation.

Epigenome-Wide Association Studies

In developmental and psychiatric epigenetics, the dominant approach is based on methylation patterns of candidate genes and their promotor areas. Epigenome-wide association studies (or EWASs) seem less often used, presumably because the sample sizes involved in this type of research are too small to offer sufficient power for the large numbers of CpG sites to be examined. The Illumina Infinium 450 K HumanMethylation array is often used to assess DNA methylation at 485,577 CpG sites. The array is considered a highly suitable platform for large-scale studies, but it still targets only <2% of the CpG sites present in the human genome. Nonetheless, some rather small EWASs have been conducted on pregnant women with psychiatric symptoms and possible epigenetic alterations in infant cellular function.

In a prospective study on 201 pregnant women suffering from (mainly depressive) psychiatric illness and using various medications, Schroeder et al. (2012) found no significant methylation effects across 27,578 CpG sites in the newborn cord blood. However, the authors did find an average methylation rate difference of 3% at 2 loci, tumor necrosis factor receptor subfamily 21 (*TNFRSF21*) and cholinergic receptor, nicotinic, $\alpha 1$ (*CHRNA2*), for use of antidepressant medication.

In contrast, Non, Binder, Kubzansky, and Michels (2014) compared cord blood DNA methylation in newborns of mothers not medicated during pregnancy (n = 13), of newborns of mothers using SSRIs during pregnancy (n = 22), and of unexposed newborns (n = 23), and did not find DNA methylation effects as a result of maternal depression that was treated with SSRIs. On the other hand, non-medicated prenatal depression was associated with 10 differentially methylated CpG sites, most of which had slightly lower DNA methylation rates, compared to non-depressed controls in genes clusters involved in regulation, translation, and cell division processes.

Labonté et al. (2013) took an epigenome-wide approach in brain tissue, studying DNA methylation of 400 K promoters of 25 suicide completers with a history of childhood abuse and of 16 control subjects. They found 362 promoters to be differentially methylated, about two-thirds of which were hypermethylated. In a subsample (13 suicide with abuse and 9 controls), these hypermethylated CpG sites were shown to be related to decreased expression levels. Moreover, it seemed that most of the differentially methylated promoters were in the neuronal, rather than the glial tissue of the hippocampus and that most genes of affected promoters were involved in neuronal plasticity.

Nemoda et al. (2015) also studied DNA methylation using the Illumina 450 K array and compared EWAS hits from cord blood with DNA methylation ratios in brain tissue, in children of mothers who had experienced depression. They compared the DNA methylation level of T cells in cord blood of 15 newborns with mothers with current depression, 14 with mothers with past (but not during pregnancy) depression, and 15 newborns of mothers without any history of depression. Differences of the separate depression groups versus control group were negligible, but when the two depression groups were taken together and compared with the control group, 145 differentially methylated CpG sites were found. In a comparison of hippocampal tissue of 12 males with a history of maternal depression with 50 males without a history of maternal depression, some genes were found to be differentially methylated in the brain that were also differentially methylated in the cord blood. These genes were often associated with immune function.

One of the largest studies on epigenome-wide DNA methylation patterns in newborns to date (n = 912 mother-newborn dyads) was conducted by our research group (2016) as part of the Generation R cohort study (Jaddoe et al., 2012; Kruithof et al., 2014), with a replication in the Avon Longitudinal Study of Parents and Children (Fraser et al., 2013). The aim of this study was to examine the association between a composite score of prenatal exposure to maternal stress and offspring genome-wide cord blood methylation using meta-analysis, follow-up pathway analyses, and differentially methylated regions (DMRs) analyses. The composite measure of prenatal maternal stress was based on maternal reports at several points in time during pregnancy, covering four stress domains (Rijlaarsdam et al., 2016): (i) life stress (e.g., death in family, illness, work problems), (ii) contextual stress (e.g., financial difficulties, housing problems), (iii) personal stress (e.g., psychopathology, substance abuse including alcohol and drugs), and (iv) interpersonal stress (e.g., family relationship difficulties, arguments with partner).

It was remarkable that the large meta-analysis (total $N = 1740$) across the two studies revealed no epigenome-wide associations of prenatal maternal stress exposure with neonatal differential DNA methylation. Follow-up analyses of the top hits derived from the epigenome-wide meta-analysis indicated an overrepresentation of the methyltransferase activity pathway. Methyltransferases are important in regulating gene expression and might therefore form an efficient system for feedback regulation of the response to initial environmental pressures and stress might decrease the plasticity of the genomic regulation of protein levels (Rijlaarsdam et al., 2016). However, we identified no DMRs associated with prenatal maternal stress exposure. When the two extreme top and bottom 10% scoring respondents on the prenatal stress composite were compared, no significant DNA methylation differences emerged. Three marginally significant DMRs in Generation R were not replicated in ALSPAC. Concluding, combining data from two independent population-based samples in an epigenome-wide meta-analysis, Rijlaarsdam et al. (2016) did not find large, replicable effects of prenatal maternal stress exposure on neonatal DNA methylation.

To summarize, candidate epi-gene studies indicate that parenting stress is associated with DNA methylation in the child. However, EWASs do not confirm that methylation of genes such as *NR3C1* is associated with parenting stress and employ rather lenient corrections for multiple comparisons to find associations with methylation of other genes. Here, of course, null findings trigger a large number of alternative interpretations related to the normalcy of the samples, the self-reported strains and stresses in specific periods of pregnancy, but fact is that in this study, state-of-the-art methods were used, and a built-in replication effort was conducted. Although they might disappoint high but premature expectations of significant hits in earlier, smaller studies, such replication efforts are essential in the search for robust associations, whether derived from candidate gene methylation or epigenome-wide studies. This is the reason why Rijlaarsdam et al. (2016) subtitled the paper: 'A model approach for replication.' Myriad of problems and pitfalls are inherent to EWAS including limited coverage of the genome and extremely large numbers of tests. In addition, previous studies found small effect sizes in small samples without replication in independent samples or animal model systems, which raise concerns regarding the reproducibility of the epigenetic findings in the behavioral sciences.

In summary, it is likely that a global environmental influence such as parenting stress has a global effect on many CpG sites adjacent to many genes, instead of a very localized effect on a few CpG sites. This makes it a challenge to pinpoint where parenting stress exactly affects DNA methylation. Moreover, child development is expected to be influenced by many small, pleiotropic DNA methylation effects. Furthermore, these effects on and of DNA methylation are unlikely to stand alone. Rather, it is expected that they interact with the underlying genetic code. These issues will be discussed below.

Bidirectional Effects of the Genome and Epigenome

When considering the literature on the effect of the environment on DNA methylation, one should bear in mind that in some cases, DNA methylation patterns and associations may be allele-specific (Meaburn, Schalkwyk, & Mill, 2010). Hence, DNA methylation, or the environmental effects on DNA methylation, might be affected by the genome itself. For example, Van der Knaap et al. (2015) showed in 939 adolescents that stressful life events were positively associated with methylation of *5-HTTLPR* for those with the protective *ll* variant, but not among those with the *sl/ss* variants. Van IJzendoorn, Caspers, Bakermans-Kranenburg, Beach, & Philibert, (2010) reported that methylation of the *5-HTT* gene at *5-HTTLPR* was positively associated with risk of unresolved loss or trauma in the *5-HTTLPR ll* variant but not in the *sl* and *ss* variants in 143 adoptees. The authors observed this gene by DNA methylation interaction in the absence of (epi)genetic main effects, suggesting that opposing associations canceled each other out. Together, these studies provide suggestive evidence that DNA methylation might be allele-specific, masking or revealing associations between genotype and stress exposure.

Similar to associations between stress exposure and DNA methylation, associations between DNA methylation and psychological outcomes (e.g., emotional and behavioral problems) might be allele-specific. Hence, the effect of DNA methylation on child outcomes should not be seen separately from the genome it acts upon. Ziegler et al. (2015) compared *OXTR* methylation in unmedicated 110 social anxiety patients and matched 110 controls, taking into account *OXTR* rs53576 allelic variation. They showed that *OXTR* methylation was predominant in social anxiety patients carrying the *OXTR* rs53576 A-allele. Similarly, Reiner et al. (2015) reported that, in their sample of 43 clinically depressed women and 42 healthy controls, *OXTR* rs53576 clinically depressed A-allele carriers, but not G-allele homozygotes, exhibited significantly increased *OXTR* methylation levels.

In a population-based study on 298 mother-child dyads (Mulder et al., 2017), we showed that cord blood methylation patterns of the *FKBP5* gene, which are involved in hypothalamic–pituitary–adrenal (HPA) axis functioning, increased cortisol reactivity of 14-month-old infants. This association was especially present when the infants were also T-allele carriers of rs1360780 *FKBP5, and* when infants had an insecure-resistant attachment to their mother. While the temporal organization of the study did not allow for examination of potential environmental effects on DNA methylation, this Gene × Methylation × Environment (G × M × E) study does expose some of the complexities that are involved in the study of epigenetics.

In all, we discussed how the association between parenting stress and DNA methylation may be modified by the genetic variance of the child. Furthermore, it seems that the effect of DNA methylation on child outcomes might be dependent on the genetic code as well. We will encounter more epi-allelic effects in the following section, as we discuss studies that take into account the suspected antecedents as well as the consequences of DNA methylation.

DNA Methylation as Mediation

Candidate (Epi-) Genomic Approaches

Whereas studies discussed above imply that the family environment can affect DNA methylation and that DNA methylation may influence child outcomes, studies that incorporate both the presumed precursors as well as the consequences of DNA methylation are needed to confirm that DNA methylation is a true mediator of parenting stress and child development. An early example of this approach is the Oberlander et al. (2008) study showing that maternal depressed/anxious prenatal mood was associated with methylation of NGFI-A binding site of the *NR3C1* gene, which was in turn associated with increased salivary cortisol. An important caveat, however, is that no formal mediation testing was conducted, which leaves open whether mediation was only partial or complete.

Using a longitudinal design embedded in the Avon Longitudinal Study of Parents and Children (ALSPAC), Cecil et al. (2014) demonstrated that neonates ($N = 84$) who were exposed to maternal stress (e.g., maternal psychopathology, criminal behaviors, substance use) in the prenatal period had higher methylation levels of the oxytocin receptor (*OXTR*) gene than non-exposed neonates. Higher neonatal *OXTR* methylation, in turn, showed temporal stability (from birth to 9 years of age) and was associated with callous-unemotional (CU) traits at age 13 years independent of postnatal stress exposure and associated *OXTR* methylation. Interestingly, these associations were observed exclusively in youth with low versus high internalizing problems, suggesting distinct developmental pathways to CU. However, despite this innovative path analytic model that incorporated stress exposure, *OXTR* methylation, and CU traits, no formal mediation analysis was presented.

Using data from the Generation R Study, our research group, (Rijlaarsdam et al., 2016) examined *OXTR* rs53576 allele-specific sensitivity for neonatal *OXTR* methylation in relation to both prenatal maternal stress exposure and child autistic traits at age 6 in 743 children. Specifically, we investigated the extent to which prenatal maternal stress exposure was predicted by *OXTR* methylation variation among neonates, while taking into account *OXTR* rs53576 genotype. In addition, we investigated the extent to which prenatal maternal stress exposure and neonatal *OXTR* methylation combined either additively or interactively with *OXTR* rs53576 genotype to influence child autistic traits. We demonstrated that prenatal maternal stress exposure, but not *OXTR* rs53576 genotype and *OXTR* methylation, showed a main effect on child autistic traits. Because prenatal maternal stress exposure and *OXTR* DNA methylation were unrelated across both *OXTR* rs53576 G-allele homozygous children and A-allele carriers, findings argued against a mediating role of *OXTR* methylation in the association between prenatal maternal stress exposure and child autistic traits. However, we did observe a significant *OXTR* rs53576 genotype by *OXTR* methylation interaction for child autistic traits in general and social communication problems in particular. More specifically, *OXTR* methylation levels were positively associated with social problems for *OXTR* rs53576 G-allele homozygous children but not for A-allele carriers. These results highlight the importance of incorporating epi-allelic information and support the role of both stress exposure and *OXTR* methylation in child autistic traits.

Elevated methylation of the *OXTR* CpG island is expected to decrease gene expression (Kusui et al., 2001) and subsequently levels of circulating oxytocin (Dadds et al., 2014). Evidence also suggests that the *OXTR* rs53576 A-allele is a 'risk allele' for autistic traits (Liu et al., 2010; Wermter et al., 2010; Wu et al., 2005). Thus, *OXTR* methylation may decrease the expression of the otherwise protective *OXTR* rs53576 GG-allele and elevate the risk for emotional or behavioral problems. Consequently, one would expect the emotional or behavioral problems of G-allele homozygous children to more closely resemble those of A-allele carriers. Together, these findings suggest that DNA methylation might (1) nullify the effect of the protective allele, resulting in a functionality equivalent to the risk allele or (2) mask the effect of risk alleles (Reiner et al., 2015; Van der Knaap et al., 2015; Rijlaarsdam et al., 2016; Van IJzendoorn et al., 2010; Ziegler et al., 2015).

By means of a formal mediation test, another longitudinal study embedded in ALSPAC Rijlaarsdam et al. (2016) also highlights the importance of the prenatal environment. The authors examined, for youth with early-onset persistent (EOP, $n = 83$) versus low conduct problems (CP, $n = 81$), the extent to which high-fat and high-sugar diet (prenatal, postnatal) associates with ADHD symptoms (age 7–13) via DNA methylation of the insulin-like growth factor 2 gene (*IGF2*; birth, age 7, collected from blood). Results showed a positive association between prenatal high-fat and high-sugar diet with *IGF2* DNA methylation at birth across both EOP and low CP youth. However, only for EOP youth, higher *IGF2* DNA methylation at birth predicted ADHD symptoms. Interestingly, only for EOP youth, the association between prenatal high-fat and high-sugar diet and higher ADHD symptoms was mediated by *IGF2* DNA methylation at birth independent of postnatal diet and associated *IGF2* methylation. Together, these studies support ideas focusing on prenatal maternal health as an important risk for postnatal child disease vulnerability (Barker, 1990, 2004). For example, a prenatal maternal high-fat and high-sugar diet may alter the DNA methylation status of the *IGF2* gene at birth, which in turn, may increase risk for psychiatric and health disorders as was illustrated dramatically in the pioneering Dutch Hunger Winter study (Heijmans et al., 2008).

IGF2 was also targeted in our prospective Generation R study by Bouwland-Both et al. (2015) focusing on the influence of prenatal maternal smoking on newborn birthweight via *IGF2* methylation in 506 newborns. Prenatal maternal smoking should in fact be considered a risky type of prenatal parenting that in the population-based cohort of Generation R was shown by an impressive 25% of the pregnant women who reported on their tobacco smoking habits at three time points before the birth of their child. Continued maternal prenatal smoking was inversely related to the level of DNA methylation in a differentially methylated region of *IGF2*, in a dose–response manner. A formal mediation test showed that prenatal maternal smoking led to lower birthweight via lower *IGF2* DMR methylation levels, which explained part of the variance in weight (partial mediation).

Paternal tobacco smoking did not show a similar cascade of effects (Bouwland-Both et al., 2015).

We have seen that postnatal stressors might also leave their traces in epigenetic signatures. Klengel et al. (2013) found that trauma in childhood ($n = 30$; vs. $n = 46$ controls) was related to *FKBP5* demethylation, which was exclusively the case for T carriers of the *FKBP5* rs1360780 SNP. Importantly, adult trauma did not seem to be related to *FKBP5* methylation in either the childhood trauma group, or the control group, indicating that it was especially childhood trauma and not later trauma that affected *FKBP5* methylation. Investigating the effects of *FKBP5* methylation, Klengel et al. (2013) also found that methylation of the *FKBP5* gene attenuated the response to dexamethasone administration, indicating that methylation of the *FKBP5* gene can affect stress reactivity. This study shows us both sides of the equation: childhood trauma may affect DNA methylation, and DNA methylation might have long-term effects on psychobiological functioning. However, no formal test of mediation was conducted.

Demonstrating the feasibility of DNA methylation mediation testing, Beach, Brody, Todorov, Gunter, and Philibert (2011) examined in 155 women whether methylation of the *5-HTT* promoter mediated the association between childhood sexual abuse and symptoms of antisocial personality disorder in adulthood, by contrasting models with direct and indirect pathways between the three variables. First, they found that childhood sexual abuse was related to antisocial personality disorder, that childhood sexual abuse was related to *5-HTT* promoter hypermethylation, and that *5-HTT* hypermethylation was associated with antisocial personality disorder. Importantly, in a second step, they showed that a model with a direct path from sexual abuse to antisocial personality disorder differed significantly from a model with only the indirect paths, via *5-HTT* methylation, included. Therefore, it was concluded that the association between childhood sexual abuse and antisocial personality disorder was mediated by *5-HTT* promoter methylation.

In summary, these candidate epi-gene studies substantiate the idea that DNA methylation can be a mediator between parenting stress and child outcomes and that its role is often dependent upon the genetic code itself. In the next paragraph, we will explore whether such candidate epi-gene associations also emerge in EWASs.

Epigenome-Wide Association Studies (EWASs)

In EWAS on 169 participants with and without PTSD, Mehta et al. (2013) found that PTSD patients with a history of childhood trauma ($n = 32$) and PTSD patients without childhood trauma but otherwise matched on adult trauma ($n = 29$) had dissimilar genome expression profiles, suggesting that converging clinical syndromes can arise from different genetic transcription profiles. Further analysis showed that the PTSD group with child abuse especially had differential DNA methylation in gene expression networks involved in CNS development, among others, while the PTSD group without child abuse especially had differential methylation in gene expression networks involved in apoptosis and growth rate. Importantly, the genes associated with these two expression profiles were tested for DNA methylation within each group versus controls (PTSD but no trauma, or trauma but no PTSD, respectively). It was found that much more (up to 12 times) of the variance of the genetic transcripts was explained by variance in DNA methylation in the PTSD group that had experienced childhood trauma than in the PTSD group that had only experienced trauma in adulthood. It seems that childhood abuse may have a long-lasting effect on psychosocial functioning, possibly through the effect on DNA methylation (see also McGowan et al., 2009) and that the traumatic experiences associated with the development of PTSD are in particular related to methylomic changes when they happen early in life. However, formal mediation tests were not reported.

In another small EWAS on 83 males who were 60 years or older, Khulan et al. (2014) studied DNA methylation differences between participants who were separated from their families for about two years during the Second World War at the age of 5 years, and a group of non-separated men. Ten years later, a psychological follow-up was performed. Earlier research in the Helsinki Birth Cohort Study already had shown that separated individuals have a higher prevalence of psychological problems, altered cortisol reactivity, and poorer cognitive control (Pesonen et al., 2010, 2013; Räikkönen et al., 2011). However, no difference in DNA methylation was found between separated and non-separated men.

Earlier, we discussed how allelic variation should be taken into account when investigating associations of DNA methylation with child development. In EWASs, this would of course lead to major statistical power issues. However, Chen et al. (2015) did take into account the variation of one particular SNP in their EWAS in the Singaporean GUSTO birth cohort ($n = 237$). In this study, Chen et al. examined the associations between prenatal maternal anxiety, epigenome-wide methylation, and neonatal brain volumes, while taking *BDNF* genotype into account. Maternal prenatal anxiety was found to be related to methylation of a SNP-dependent way; for infants with methione (Met/Met) genotype, methylation of more CpG sites was related to maternal prenatal anxiety than in infants with Met/valine (Val) and Val/Val genotypes. In a second step, they examined the association between epigenome-wide methylation and neonatal brain volumes. It was found that DNA methylation was associated with the volumetrics of several brain areas, again in a *BDNF* SNP-dependent way. Unfortunately, it remains unclear to what extent CpG sites implicated in prenatal maternal anxiety corresponded to the CpG sites related to neonatal brain volumes, thereby precluding strong inferences on the role of DNA methylation as a mediator between prenatal maternal anxiety and neonatal brain volumes.

Altogether, the results from candidate epi-gene studies and EWASs offer support for the notion that epigenetics, in the form of DNA methylation, can mediate the association between parenting stress and child outcomes. Interestingly, genes that appear differentially methylated in candidate epi-gene studies do not necessarily appear among the hits in the EWASs discussed. One reason for this might be that EWASs are still underpowered to find the effects that are observed in candidate studies. However, this discrepancy might also confirm the idea that the hypothesis-driven approach of candidate epi-gene studies creates an 'information bottleneck.' The human DNA contains over 20,000 genes and focusing on the DNA methylation of only a few seems far-fetched. These and other methodological issues will be elaborated upon in the following section, before coming to a final conclusion.

Caveats and Conclusions

Reliability and Validity of DNA Methylation Measurement

While the number of studies on DNA methylation in developmental and family psychology is increasing (Coll, 2016), pivotal questions regarding the reliability and validity of DNA methylation indicators in human research remain unanswered. In fact, basic research on these essential characteristics of any adequate measure has been neglected. Several issues should be mentioned here.

First, it is not clear which markers of DNA methylation are stable over what periods of time (trait-like indicators) and which markers can change rapidly depending on momentary endogenous or exogenous changes (state-like markers). For parenting and developmental studies, this is crucial information, as we are mostly interested in influences of parenting on long-term and more persistent, trait-like changes in the child's development. Regarding epigenome-wide array analyses, large parts of the epigenome as assessed by the Illumina approach are stable by definition because it pertains to CpG sites that show no methylation at all or, in contrast, show maximum methylation (with a confidence interval indicating imprecision of measurement) which may inflate epigenomic stability figures. Nevertheless, Lévesque et al. (2014) found that more than half of the probes measured with the 450 K Illumina were unstable over a 3–6 months' time period in young adolescents. In contrast, Wang et al. (2012) analyzed the methylome of newborns and found that only 5% of CpG sites made a true shift from methylated to unmethylated, or vice versa, within the first 2 years of life.

CpG sites of interest to developmentalists can potentially vary due to environmental pressures but at the same time should not show short-term volatility. In a small sample of adults, we found that at some genes, such as *DRD4* or *5-HTT*, almost all indicators of reliability across time were satisfactory. In contrast, at *BDNF*, many probes showed poor reliability especially in blood spots (Greenwood et al., 2017, in prep.). Talens et al. (2010) found some evidence for stable DNA methylation patterns in peripheral blood over a period of one to two decades in CpG sites of eight genes, of young to middle-aged individuals. Taken together, these results seem to indicate that DNA methylation can be stable over a prolonged period of time, but the disparity in age range, array methods, and definition of temporal stability makes it impossible to draw firm conclusions before more systematic reliability studies become available.

Second, tissue is the issue. The central question for parenting and developmental research is the link between DNA methylation markers derived from peripheral tissue and methylation patterns in behaviorally relevant regions of the brain. Because in humans brain DNA methylation patterns are nearly inaccessible ante mortem, very few studies have looked into the association with peripheral DNA methylation, with somewhat disappointing results. For example, Hannon, Lunnon, Schalkwyk, and Mill (2015) examined interindividual methylomic variation across blood, cortex, and cerebellum and found that the majority of DNA methylation derived from whole blood was not a strong predictor of variation in the brain, although the relation with cortical regions appeared to be stronger than with the cerebellum. DNA methylation of only about 1% of CpG sites was strongly correlated between blood and brain, and about 6% are moderately correlated.

DNA methylation patterns derived from blood may, however, not be the most valid indicator of methylation in the brain, not only because of the blood–brain barrier but also because of the heterogeneity of cellular composition of blood samples that might be corrected for in various ways (Houseman et al., 2012). Buccal tissue has been used rather frequently as a source of information about methylation levels because it is less invasive compared to blood sampling. Buccal epithelial tissue has been argued to be less heterogeneous than blood cells and to be 'closer' to brain tissue in a developmental sense (Lowe et al., 2013). Without going into technical details, we found better test–retest reliability figures for DNA methylation levels established in buccal cells than for blood or blood spots (Greenwood et al. 2016, in prep). Of course, some part of DNA methylation stability may depend on the heritability of DNA methylation levels as suggested by rather strong associations between some genotypes and DNA methylation level (Gaunt et al., 2016) but it would be premature to conclude that DNA methylation is in fact determined by variations in structural DNA and thus potentially completely genotypic instead of (endo-)phenotypic.

Reproducibility

In the behavioral and biomedical sciences, the problem of reproducibility of research has been discussed quite vigorously, starting with the (in-)famous Ioannidis (2005) paper on 'Why most published research findings are false.' The replication controversies around candidate G × E studies seem to be still ongoing (Bosker et al., 2011; Caspi, Hariri, Holmes, Uher, & Moffit, 2010; Duncan & Keller, 2011; Gage, Davey Smith, Ware, Flint, & Munafò, 2016) with considerable emphasis on the need for large sample sizes and built-in replication or meta-analysis efforts, parallel to current practices in the GWAS area. For DNA methylation studies based on the selection of one or few candidate genes for which DNA methylation data are collected, the issue of statistical power, and thus the problem of reproducibility, may be aggravated because the number of tests might increase considerably compared to the few tests with bi-allelic candidate genes. The advantage, though, which also comes up in the candidate gene versus GWAS debate, is the theory-guided hypothesis testing approach for which the functionality of hyper- or hypo-methylation might already have been established (Mehta et al., 2013). Factor analysis to reduce the number of CpG sites to a few dimensions might also be helpful (Mulder et al., 2017; Rijlaarsdam et al., 2016). Last but not least, meta-analyses to synthesize a large number of small candidate gene methylation studies are indispensable.

Epigenome-wide association studies (EWASs) suffer from power issues similar to the hypothesis-free approach of GWAS, and certainly even more so in comparison with candidate epigenetic approaches, simply because of the large number of CpG sites interrogated by the standard Illumina 450 K, a problem that might become exacerbated by the new Illumina 850 K chip. Alternative methods of significance testing (e.g., permutation testing) are important as well as robust statistical corrections for multiple testing, and analyses that account for dependence of CpG sites in differentially methylated regions (Rakyan, Down, Balding, & Beck, 2011) and through bump hunter (Choudalakis, 2011; Jaffe et al., 2012) or block finder (Hansen et al., 2011). Nevertheless, EWAS results will be difficult to replicate because of the small effect sizes to be expected and the large number of tests on a relatively small number of subjects (Rijlaarsdam et al., 2016). Therefore, the replication of EWAS findings in independent studies are needed before more definite conclusions can be reached and large consortia such as the Pregnancy and Childhood Epigenetics (PACE) consortium are badly needed. As an example, in the PACE consortium with 16 cohort studies, Joubert et al. (2016) identified more than 6000 differentially methylated CpG sites in newborns in relation to prenatal maternal smoking, with nearly half of the sites not previously associated with smoking and DNA methylation in either newborns or adults.

Causality

The large majority of human DNA methylation studies are correlational—whether conducted with a retrospective, concurrent, or prospective design with regard to the timing of assessment of biological tissue, and the predictors and outcomes of interest. This design is beset with the problems of confounding, spurious associations because of unmeasured third factors, and reversed causality. In this respect, epigenetics is not different from any other epidemiological approach (Mill & Heijmans, 2013). One of the statistical means to address the question of causality is through mediation modeling, preferably based on longitudinal study designs (MacKinnon, Fairchild, & Fritz, 2007; Selig & Preacher, 2009). Full mediation provides insights into the cascade from environmental determinants through mediating DNA methylation changes to some developmental outcome. In the foregoing sections, we emphasized the need for mediation analyses to shed light on the role of DNA methylation in the association between environmental input and behavioral output, but only few studies successfully probed this mediation mechanism. DNA methylation should be considered a mechanism instead of endpoint of child development determined by prenatal adversities or the ultimate determinant of later developmental outcomes. Crucial is the combination of stressful (prenatal) parenting influencing child development mediated by DNA methylation.

Of course, for inferring causality, no design can beat real experiments with randomized assignment of subjects to experimental manipulation and control group (for an excellent example on nonhuman primates, see Provençal et al., 2012). The number of quasi-experimental studies on DNA methylation is increasing as methylation signatures have been used as indicators of symptom improvement in psychotherapy of combat veterans with PTSD (Yehuda et al., 2013), as markers of therapeutic success in a matched-controls design with clinically depressed in-patients (Reiner et al., 2015) or in a pre/posttest only design (Eley et al., 2012), in studies of cognitive behavior therapy with anxious individuals (Eley et al., 2012; Roberts et al., 2014), and in studies of foster care based on a randomized control design turned into a correlational approach (Non et al., 2016).

These are important exploratory advances in the field of therapygenetics (Eley et al., 2012) because they suggest that DNA methylation may not only change for the worse, but with the right intervention, also for the better. At the least, these preliminary results do suggest the usefulness of DNA methylation as a biomarker, with which one might be able to gauge responsiveness to therapy. However, the quasi-experiments need to be followed by genuine experiments similar to randomized G × E interventions. We initiated experimental human candidate G × E research more than 10 years ago (Bakermans-Kranenburg & Van IJzendoorn, 2006) and recently showed that the statistical power of experimental candidate G × E is some 13 times higher than the regular correlational candidate G × E studies (Bakermans-Kranenburg & Van IJzendoorn, 2015). Such experiments also adequately prevent gene–environment correlations from confounding the G × E results. The same might be true for DNA methylation studies in which DNA methylation changes are considered proximal outcomes or mediators of subsequent behavioral changes as a consequence of the intervention.

DNA methylation may be a crucial component of genetic differential susceptibility that explains why interventions usually show disappointingly small effects on child development. Differential susceptibility theory suggests that some children are more susceptible to the environment, for better *and* for worse, than their peers without a susceptible genotype. We found that dopamine- and serotonin-related genes are involved in differential susceptibility to parenting and speculated that DNA methylation might play a role in G × E interactions leading to Gene × Methylation × Environment interplay (G × M × E; Bakermans-Kranenburg & Van IJzendoorn, 2015). DNA methylation may modulate adaptation to a changing environment and make the organism less dependent on its structural DNA. A prime example is the crucial role of DNA methylation in genetically identical apomictic dandelions that adapt to a great variety of ecological niches only due to epigenetic changes superimposed on an asexually inherited fixed genotype

(Verhoeven, Jansen, Van Dijk, & Biere, 2010). Genetic markers of differential susceptibility in humans might in part reflect allelic differences coding for degree of plasticity of DNA methylation that make some individuals less adaptive to adverse (prenatal) circumstances and thus dispose them to sub-optimal development, whereas these same individuals may benefit more from benign environments compared to their peers with more flexible epi-allelic characteristics.

Conclusion and Future Directions

We presented some evidence for the exciting hypothesis that distressed parenting can affect DNA methylation of the offspring, which in turn through regulating the expression of genes may influence behavioral development. DNA methylation is one of the epigenetic mechanisms that holds great promise for the unification of the fields of nature- and nurture-centered research. We also argued, however, that research on behavioral epigenetics in humans often fails to ascertain the reproducibility of its results, using unreliable and invalid measures and samples that are too small, often also failing to address the question of mediation and causality. We did not touch on the million dollar question of the transgenerational transmission (see also Chap. 10 by Mileva-Seitz and Fleming) of DNA methylation—epigenetic heritability through the germline—potentially explaining the transmission of (abusive or positive) parenting across generations. Whereas in some plant species (Holeski, Jander, & Agrawal, 2012; Verhoeven et al., 2010) and in rodents (Bohacek et al., 2015), this transgenerational transmission of epigenetic signatures has been experimentally illustrated; in humans, it still is one of the most challenging and outstanding issues to be addressed in a rigorous manner. For a Lamarckian cry of victory, it is way too early.

Looking ahead, whereas many questions regarding DNA methylation specifically and epigenetics in general have been left unanswered, its possible applications are titillating. Since the research discussed in the current chapter seems to indicate that stressful parenting can affect the epigenetic profile of the developing child in a detrimental way, one wonders whether positive parenting or intervention might influence the child's epigenetics beneficially. In a study in adult rats performed by Weaver et al. (2005), methyl supplementation was able to reverse *NR3C1* methylation and stress responses induced by experienced maternal stress early in life. Also, in a study performed by Roberts et al. (2014), it was shown that children with anxiety disorders who responded well to cognitive behavior therapy had an increase in DNA methylation of a CpG site upstream of *5-HTT*, whereas methylation of this CpG site decreased in non-responding children. Even though we cannot be certain that the change in DNA methylation is a functional one, its possible use as a diagnostic tool is intriguing. We are evidently a long way from using epigenetics validly in a therapeutic setting, but a continuous investment in epigenetic research may bring us closer to understanding the intricacies of the interplay of genes, the environment, and the developing child.

Acknowledgements Marinus van IJzendoorn is a member of the Consortium on Individual Development which is funded through the Gravitation program of the Dutch Ministry of Education, Culture, and Science and the Netherlands Organisation for Scientific Research (NWO grant number 024.001.003). Additional funding was provided by the Netherlands Organisation for Scientific Research (NWO SPINOZA prize). Jolien Rijlaarsdam was supported by a research award from The Netherlands Organisation for Scientific Research (NWO VICI, grant no. 453-09-003) to Marian Bakermans-Kranenburg. Last, the authors would like to thank Wichor Bramer, biomedical information specialist, for his assistance with the literature search strategy.

References

Aran, D., Sabato, S., & Hellman, A. (2013). DNA methylation of distal regulatory sites characterizes dysregulation of cancer genes. *Genome Biology, 14*(3), 1.

Bakermans-Kranenburg, M. J., & Van IJzendoorn, M. H. (2015). The hidden efficacy of interventions: Gene × environment experiments from a differential susceptibility perspective. *Annual Review of Psychology, 66*, 381–409.

Bakermans-Kranenburg, M. J., & Van IJzendoorn, M. H. (2006). Gene-environment interaction of the dopamine D4 receptor (DRD4) and observed maternal insensitivity predicting externalizing behavior in preschoolers. *Developmental Psychobiology, 48*(5), 406–409.

Bakermans-Kranenburg, M. J., Van IJzendoorn, M. H., Pijlman, F. T. A., Mesman, J., & Juffer, F. (2008). Experimental evidence for differential susceptibility: Dopamine D4 receptor polymorphism (DRD4 VNTR) moderates intervention effects on toddlers' externalizing behavior in a randomized controlled trial. *Developmental Psychology, 44*(1), 293.

Bannister, A. J., & Kouzarides, T. (2011). Regulation of chromatin by histone modifications. *Cell Research, 21*(3), 381–395.

Barker, D. J. (1990). The fetal and infant origins of adult disease. *BMJ. British Medical Journal, 301*(6761), 1111.

Barker, D. J. P. (2004). The developmental origins of adult disease. *Journal of the American College of Nutrition, 23*(6), 588S–595S.

Beach, S. R. H., Brody, G. H., Todorov, A. A., Gunter, T. D., & Philibert, R. A. (2011). Methylation at 5HTT mediates the impact of child sex abuse on women's antisocial behavior: An examination of the iowa adoptee sample. *Psychosomatic Medicine, 73*(1), 83–87.

Berger, A. (2011). Individual differences in self-regulation. *Self-regulation: Brain, congition and development.* Washington, DC: American Psychologica Association, (pp 61–90).

Bohacek, J., Farinelli, M., Mirante, O., Steiner, G., Gapp, K., Coiret, G., … & Mansuy, I. M. (2015). Pathological brain plasticity and cognition in the offspring of males subjected to postnatal traumatic stress. *Molecular Psychiatry, 20*(5), 621–631.

Bosker, F. J., Hartman, C. A., Nolte, I. M., Prins, B. P., Terpstra, P., Posthuma, D., … & Hoogendijk, W. J. (2011). Poor replication of candidate genes for major depressive disorder using genome-wide association data. *Molecular Psychiatry, 16*(5), 516–532.

Bouwland-Both, M. I., Van Mil, N. H., Tolhoek, C. P., Stolk, L., Eilers, P. H. C., Verbiest, M. M. P. J., … & Van IJzendoorn, M. H. (2015). Prenatal parental tobacco smoking, gene specific DNA methylation, and newborns size: The Generation R study. *Clinical Epigenetics, 7*(1), 1.

Braithwaite, E. C., Kundakovic, M., Ramchandani, P. G., Murphy, S. E., & Champagne, F. A. (2015). Maternal prenatal depressive symptoms predict infant NR3C1 1F and BDNF IV DNA methylation. *Epigenetics, 10*(5), 408–417.

Caspi, A., Hariri, A. R., Holmes, A., Uher, R., & Moffitt, T. E. (2010). Genetic sensitivity to the environment: The case of the serotonin transporter gene and its implications for studying complex diseases and traits. *Focus, 8*(3), 398–416.

Caspi, A., Sugden, K., Moffitt, T. E., Taylor, A., Craig, I. W., Harrington, H., … & Braithwaite, A. (2003). Influence of life stress on depression: Moderation by a polymorphism in the 5-HTT gene. *Science, 301*(5631), 386–389.

Cecil, C. A. M., Lysenko, L. J., Jaffee, S. R., Pingault, J. B., Smith, R. G., Relton, C. L., … & Barker, E. D. (2014). Environmental risk, Oxytocin Receptor Gene (OXTR) methylation and youth callous-unemotional traits: A 13-year longitudinal study. *Molecular Psychiatry.*

Chen, L., Pan, H., Tuan, T. A., Teh, A. L., MacIsaac, J. L., Mah, S. M., … & Holbrook, J. D. (2015). Brain-derived neurotrophic factor (BDNF) Val66Met polymorphism influences the association of the methylome with maternal anxiety and neonatal brain volumes. *Development and Psychopathology, 27*(1), 137–150.

Choudalakis, G. (2011). On hypothesis testing, trials factor, hypertests and the BumpHunter. arXiv preprint arXiv:1101.0390.

Chow, J., & Heard, E. (2009). X inactivation and the complexities of silencing a sex chromosome. *Current Opinion in Cell Biology, 21*(3), 359–366.

Coll, C. G. (Ed). (2016). Epigenetics, child behavior and development: Unraveling the gene-environment interaction [Special Issue]. *Child Development, 87*(1).

Dadds, M. R., Moul, C., Cauchi, A., Dobson-Stone, C., Hawes, D. J., Brennan, J., et al. (2014). Methylation of the oxytocin receptor gene and oxytocin blood levels in the development of psychopathy. *Development and Psychopathology, 26*(1), 33–40.

Devlin, A. M., Brain, U., Austin, J., & Oberlander, T. F. (2010). Prenatal exposure to maternal depressed mood and the MTHFR C677T variant affect SLC6A4 methylation in infants at birth. *PLoS ONE, 5*(8), e12201.

Duncan, L. E., & Keller, M. C. (2011). A critical review of the first 10 years of candidate gene-by-environment interaction research in psychiatry. *American Journal of Psychiatry, 168* (10), 1041–1049.

Eley, T. C., Hudson, J. L., Creswell, C., Tropeano, M., Lester, K. J., Cooper, P., … & Rapee, R. M. (2012). Therapygenetics: The 5HTTLPR and response to psychological therapy. *Molecular Psychiatry, 17*(3), 236.

Esteller, M., & Herman, J. G. (2002). Cancer as an epigenetic disease: DNA methylation and chromatin alterations in human tumours. *The Journal of Pathology, 196*(1), 1–7.

Fraser, A., Macdonald-Wallis, C., Tilling, K., Boyd, A., Golding, J., Smith, G. D., … & Ring, S. (2013). Cohort profile: The Avon Longitudinal Study of Parents and Children: ALSPAC mothers cohort. *International Journal of Epidemiology,42*(1), 97–110.

Gage, S. H., Smith, G. D., Ware, J. J., Flint, J., & Munafò, M. R. (2016). G = E: What GWAS can tell us about the environment. *PLoS Genetics, 12*(2), e1005765.

Gaunt, T. R., Shihab, H. A., Hemani, G., Min, J. L., Woodward, G., Lyttleton, … & Relton, C. L. (2016). Systematic identification of genetic influences on methylation across the human life course. *Genome Biology, 17*, 61.

Gottlieb, G., & Halpern, C. T. (2002). A relational view of causality in normal and abnormal development. *Development and Psychopathology, 14*, 421–435.

Hannon, E., Lunnon, K., Schalkwyk, L., & Mill, J. (2015). Interindividual methylomic variation across blood, cortex, and cerebellum: Implications for epigenetic studies of neurological and neuropsychiatric phenotypes. *Epigenetics, 10*(11), 1024–1032.

Hansen, K. D., Timp, W., Bravo, H. C., Sabunciyan, S., Langmead, B., McDonald, O. G., … & Diep, D. (2011). Increased methylation variation in epigenetic domains across cancer types. *Nature Genetics, 43*(8), 768–775.

Heijmans, B. T., Tobi, E. W., Stein, A. D., Putter, H., Blauw, G. J., Susser, E. S., … & Lumey, L. H. (2008). Persistent epigenetic differences associated with prenatal exposure to famine in humans. *Proceedings of the National Academy of Sciences, 105*(44), 17046–17049.

Holeski, L. M., Jander, G., & Agrawal, A. A. (2012). Transgenerational defense induction and epigenetic inheritance in plants. *Trends in Ecology & Evolution, 27*(11), 618–626.

Holliday, R., & Pugh, J. E. (1996). DNA modification mechanisms and gene activity during development. *Cold Spring Harbor Monograph Archive, 32*, 639–645.

Hompes, T., Izzi, B., Gellens, E., Morreels, M., Fieuws, S., Pexsters, A., … & Claes, S. (2014). Corrigendum to "Investigating the influence of maternal cortisol and emotional state during pregnancy on the DNA methylation status of the glucocorticoid receptor gene (NR3C1) promoter region in cord blood" [Journal of Psychiatric Research 47 880–91]. *Journal of Psychiatric Research, 56*(1), 165–167.

Hompes, T., Izzi, B., Gellens, E., Morreels, M., Fieuws, S., Pexsters, A., … & Claes, S. (2013). Investigating the influence of maternal cortisol and emotional state during pregnancy on the DNA methylation status of the glucocorticoid receptor gene (NR3C1) promoter region in cord blood. *Journa of Psychiatric Research, 47*(7), 880–891.

Houseman, E. A., Accomando, W. P., Koestler, D. C., Christensen, B. C., Marsit, C. J., Nelson, H. H., … & Kelsey, K. T. (2012). DNA methylation arrays as surrogate measures of cell mixture distribution. *BMC Bioinformatics, 13*(1), 1–16.

Huizink, A. C., Mulder, E. J., & Buitelaar, J. K. (2004). Prenatal stress and risk for psychopathology: Specific effects or induction of general susceptibility? *Psychological Bulletin, 130*(1), 115–142.

Ioannidis, J. P. A. (2005). Why most published research findings are false. *PLoS Med, 2*(8), e124.

Jacobson, S. W., Chiodo, L. M., Sokol, R. J., & Jacobson, J. L. (2002). Validity of maternal report of prenatal alcohol, cocaine, and smoking in relation to neurobehavioral outcome. *Pediatrics, 109*(5), 815–825.

Jaddoe, V. W., Van Duijn, C. M., Franco, O. H., Van der Heijden, A. J., Van IJzendoorn, M. H., de Jongste, J. C., … & Hofman, A. (2012). The Generation R Study: Design and cohort update 2012. *European Journal of Epidemiology, 27*(9), 739–756.

Jaffe, A. E., Murakami, P., Lee, H., Leek, J. T., Fallin, M. D., Feinberg, A. P., et al. (2012). Bump hunting to identify differentially methylated regions in epigenetic epidemiology studies. *International Journal of Epidemiology, 41*(1), 200–209.

Joubert, B. R., Felix, J. F., Yousefi, P., Bakulski, K. M., Just, A. C., Breton, C., … & Xu, C.-J. (2016). DNA methylation in newborns and maternal smoking in pregnancy: Genome-wide consortium meta-analysis. *The American Journal of Human Genetics, 98*(4), 680–696.

Khulan, B., Manning, J. R., Dunbar, D. R., Seckl, J. R., Raikkonen, K., Eriksson, J. G., & Drake, A. J. (2014). Epigenomic profiling of men exposed to early-life stress reveals DNA methylation differences in association with current mental state. *Translational Psychiatry, 4*(9).

Klengel, T., Mehta, D., Anacker, C., Rex-Haffner, M., Pruessner, J. C., Pariante, C. M., … & Binder, E. B. (2013). Allele-specific FKBP5 DNA demethylation mediates gene-childhood trauma interactions. *Nature Neuroscience, 16*(1), 33–41.

Klose, R. J., & Bird, A. P. (2006). Genomic DNA methylation: The mark and its mediators. *Trends in Biochemical Sciences, 31*(2), 89–97.

Kruithof, C. J., Kooijman, M. N., Van Duijn, C. M., Franco, O. H., de Jongste, J. C., Klaver, C. C. W., … & Rings, E. H. H. M. (2014). The Generation R study: Biobank update 2015. *European Journal of Epidemiology, 29*(12), 911–927.

Kusui, C., Kimura, T., Ogita, K., Nakamura, H., Matsumura, Y., Koyama, M., … & Murata, Y. (2001). DNA methylation of the human oxytocin receptor gene promoter regulates tissue-specific gene suppression. *Biochemical and Biophysical Research Communications, 289*(3), 681–686.

Labonté, B., Suderman, M., Maussion, G., Lopez, J. P., Navarro-Sanchez, L., Yerko, V., … & Turecki, G. (2013). Genome-wide methylation changes in the brains of suicide completers. *American Journal of Psychiatry, 170*(5), 511–520.

Law, J. A., & Jacobsen, S. E. (2010). Establishing, maintaining and modifying DNA methylation patterns in plants and animals. *Nature Reviews Genetics, 11*(3), 204–220.

Lévesque, M. L., Casey, K. F., Szyf, M., Ismaylova, E., Ly, V., Verner, M.-P., … & Dionne, G. (2014). Genome-wide DNA methylation variability in adolescent monozygotic twins followed since birth. *Epigenetics, 9*(10), 1410–1422.

Li, G., & Reinberg, D. (2011). Chromatin higher-order structures and gene regulation. *Current Opinion in Genetics & Development, 21*(2), 175–186.

Liu, X., Kawamura, Y., Shimada, T., Otowa, T., Koishi, S., Sugiyama, T., … & Tochigi, M. (2010). Association of the oxytocin receptor (OXTR) gene polymorphisms with autism spectrum disorder (ASD) in the Japanese population. *Journal of Human Genetics, 55*(3), 137–141.

Lowe, R., Gemma, C., Beyan, H., Hawa, M. I., Bazeos, A., Leslie, R. D., … & Ramagopalan, S. V. (2013). Buccals are likely to be a more informative surrogate tissue than blood for epigenome-wide association studies. *Epigenetics, 8*(4), 445–454.

Lumey, L. H., Stein, A. D., Kahn, H. S., Van der Pal-de, K. M., Blauw, G. J., Zybert, P. A., et al. (2007). Cohort profile: The Dutch Hunger Winter families study. *International Journal of Epidemiology, 36*(6), 1196–1204.

MacKinnon, D. P., Fairchild, A. J., & Fritz, M. S. (2007). Mediation analysis. *Annual Review of Psychology, 58,* 593.

McGowan, P. O., Sasaki, A., D'Alessio, A. C., Dymov, S., Labonté, B., Szyf, M., … & Meaney, M. J. (2009). Epigenetic regulation of the glucocorticoid receptor in human brain associates with childhood abuse. *Nature Neurosciencee, 12*(3), 342–348.

Meaburn, E. L., Schalkwyk, L. C., & Mill, J. (2010). Allele-specific methylation in the human genome: Implications for genetic studies of complex disease. *Epigenetics, 5*(7), 578–582.

Meaney, M. J. (2010). Epigenetics and the biological definition of gene × environment interactions. *Child Development, 81*(1), 41–79.

Mehta, D., Klengel, T., Conneely, K. N., Smith, A. K., Altmann, A., Pace, T. W., … & Binder, E. B. (2013). Childhood maltreatment is associated with distinct genomic and epigenetic profiles in posttraumatic stress disorder. *Proceedings of the National Academy of Sciences, 110*(20), 8302–8307.

Meissner, A., Mikkelsen, T. S., Gu, H., Wernig, M., Hanna, J., Sivachenko, A., … & Jaffe, D. B. (2008). Genome-scale DNA methylation maps of pluripotent and differentiated cells. *Nature, 454*(7205), 766–770.

Mill, J., & Heijmans, B. T. (2013). From promises to practical strategies in epigenetic epidemiology. *Nature Reviews Genetics, 14*(8), 585–594.

Moore, L. D., Le, T., & Fan, G. (2013). DNA methylation and its basic function. *Neuropsychopharmacology Reviews, 38,* 23–38.

Mulder, R. H., Rijlaarsdam, J., Luijk, M. P. C. M., Verhulst, F. C., Felix, J. F., Tiemeier, H., Bakermans-Kranenburg M. J., & Van IJzendoorn, M. H. (2017). Methylation matters: FK506 binding protein 51 (*FKBP5*) methylation moderates the associations of *FKBP5* genotype and resistant attachment with stress regulation. *Development and Psychopathology*, *29*, 491–503.

Nemoda, Z., Massart, R., Suderman, M., Hallett, M., Li, T., Coote, M., … & Szyf, M. (2015). Maternal depression is associated with DNA methylation changes in cord blood T lymphocytes and adult hippocampi. *Translational Psychiatry, 5,* e545.

Non, A. L., Binder, A. M., Kubzansky, L. D., & Michels, K. B. (2014). Genome-wide DNA methylation in neonates exposed to maternal depression, anxiety, or SSRI medication during pregnancy. *Epigenetics, 9*(7), 964–972.

Non, A. L., Hollister, B. M., Humphreys, K. L., Childebayeva, A., Esteves, K., Zeanah, C. H., … & Drury, S. S. (2016). DNA methylation at stress-related genes is associated with exposure to early life institutionalization. *American Journal of Physical Anthropology.*

Oberlander, T. F., Weinberg, J., Papsdorf, M., Grunau, R., Misri, S., & Devlin, A. M. (2008). Prenatal exposure to maternal depression, neonatal methylation of human glucocorticoid receptor gene (NR3C1) and infant cortisol stress responses. *Epigenetics, 3*(2), 97–106.

Pesonen, A.-K., Eriksson, J. G., Heinonen, K., Kajantie, E., Tuovinen, S., Alastalo, H., … & Barker, D. J. P. (2013). Cognitive ability and decline after early life stress exposure. *Neurobiology of Aging, 34*(6), 1674–1679.

Pesonen, A.-K., Räikkönen, K., Feldt, K., Heinonen, K., Osmond, C., Phillips, D. I. W., … & Kajantie, E. (2010). Childhood separation experience predicts HPA axis hormonal responses in late adulthood: A natural experiment of World War II. *Psychoneuroendocrinology, 35*(5), 758–767.

Provençal, N., Suderman, M. J., Guillemin, C., Massart, R., Ruggiero, A., Wang, D., … & Côté, S. M. (2012). The signature of maternal rearing in the methylome in rhesus macaque prefrontal cortex and T cells. *The Journal of Neuroscience, 32*(44), 15626–15642.

Radtke, K. M., Ruf, M., Gunter, H. M., Dohrmann, K., Schauer, M., Meyer, A., et al. (2011). Transgenerational impact of intimate partner violence on methylation in the promoter of the glucocorticoid receptor. *Translational Psychiatry, 1,* e21.

Räikkönen, K., Lahti, M., Heinonen, K., Pesonen, A.-K., Wahlbeck, K., Kajantie, E., … & Eriksson, J. G. (2011). Risk of severe mental disorders in adults separated temporarily from their parents in childhood: The Helsinki birth cohort study. *Journal of Psychiatric Research, 45* (3), 332–338.

Rakyan, V. K., Down, T. A., Balding, D. J., & Beck, S. (2011). Epigenome-wide association studies for common human diseases. *Nature Reviews Genetics, 12*(8), 529–541.

Reiner, I., Van, I. M. H., Bakermans-Kranenburg, M. J., Bleich, S., Beutel, M., & Frieling, H. (2015). Methylation of the oxytocin receptor gene in clinically depressed patients compared to controls: The role of OXTR rs53576 genotype. *Journal of Psychiatric Research, 65,* 9–15.

Riggs, A. D. (1975). X inactivation, differentiation, and DNA methylation. *Cytogenetic and Genome Research, 14*(1), 9–25.

Rijlaarsdam, J., Cecil, A. M., Walton, E., Mesirow, M. S. C., Relton, C. T., Gaunt, T. R., … & Barker, E. D. (2016). Prenatal unhealthy diet, insulin-like growth factor 2 gene (IGF2) methylation and attention deficit hyperactivity disorder (ADHD) symptoms for early-onset conduct problem youth. *The Journal of Child Psychology and Psychiatry.*

Rijlaarsdam, J., Pappa, I., Walton, E., Bakermans-Kranenburg, M. J., Mileva-Seitz, V. R., Rippe, R. C. A., … & Felix, J. F. (2016). An epigenome-wide association meta-analysis of prenatal maternal stress in neonates: A model approach for replication. *Epigenetics, 11*(2), 140–149.

Rijlaarsdam, J., Van IJzendoorn, M. H., Verhulst, F. C., Jaddoe, W. V., Felix, J. F., Tiemeier, H., & Bakermans-Kranenburg, M. J. (2016). Prenatal stress exposure, oxytocin receptor gene (OXTR) methylation and child autistic traits: The moderating role of OXTR rs53576 genotype. *Autism Research.*

Roberts, S., Lester, K. J., Hudson, J. L., Rapee, R. M., Creswell, C., Cooper, P. J., … & Eley, T. C. (2014). Serotonin tranporter methylation and response to cognitive behaviour therapy in children with anxiety disorders. *Translational Psychiatry, 4*(9), e444.

Schroeder, J. W., Smith, A. K., Brennan, P. A., Conneely, K. N., Kilaru, V., Knight, B. T., … & Stowe, Z. N. (2012). DNA methylation in neonates born to women receiving psychiatric care. *Epigenetics, 7*(4), 409–414.

Selig, J. P., & Preacher, K. J. (2009). Mediation models for longitudinal data in developmental research. *Research in Human Development, 6*(2), 144–164.

Stefani, G., & Slack, F. J. (2008). Small non-coding RNAs in animal development. *Nature Reviews Molecular Cell Biology, 9*(3), 219–230.

Talens, R. P., Boomsma, D. I., Tobi, E. W., Kremer, D., Jukema, J. W., Willemsen, G., … & Heijmans, B. T. (2010). Variation, patterns, and temporal stability of DNA methylation: Considerations for epigenetic epidemiology. *The FASEB Journal, 24*(9), 3135–3144.

Tobi, E. W., Goeman, J. J., Monajemi, R., Gu, H., Putter, H., Zhang, Y., … & Müller, F. (2014). DNA methylation signatures link prenatal famine exposure to growth and metabolism. *Nature Communications, 5.*

Unternaehrer, E., Meyer, A. H., Burkhardt, S. C., Dempster, E., Staehli, S., Theill, N., … & Meinlschmidt, G. (2015). Childhood maternal care is associated with DNA methylation of the genes for brain-derived neurotrophic factor (BDNF) and oxytocin receptor (OXTR) in peripheral blood cells in adult men and women. *Stress,* 1–11.

Van der Knaap, L. J., Riese, H., Hudziak, J. J., Verbiest, M. M., Verhulst, F. C., Oldehinkel, A. J., et al. (2015). Adverse life events and allele-specific methylation of the serotonin transporter gene (SLC6A4) in adolescents: The TRAILS study. *Psychosomatic Medicine, 77*(3), 246–255.

Van IJzendoorn, M. H., Caspers, K., Bakermans-Kranenburg, M. J., Beach, S. R., & Philibert, R. (2010). Methylation matters: Interaction between methylation density and serotonin transporter genotype predicts unresolved loss or trauma. *Biological Psychiatry, 68*(5), 405–407.

Verhoeven, K. J. F., Jansen, J. J., Van Dijk, P. J., & Biere, A. (2010). Stress-induced DNA methylation changes and their heritability in asexual dandelions. *New Phytologist, 185*(4), 1108–1118.

Vijayendran, M., Beach, S. R., Plume, J. M., Brody, G. H., & Philibert, R. A. (2012). Effects of genotype and child abuse on DNA methylation and gene expression at the serotonin transporter. *Frontiers in Psychiatry, 3,* 55.

Waddington, C. H. (1939). An introduction to modern genetics. *An Introduction to Modern Genetics.*

Waddington, C. H. (1956). *Principles of embryology*. London: George Allen & Unwin Ltd.

Wang, D., Liu, X., Zhou, Y., Xie, H., Hong, X., Tsai, H. J., … & Wang, X. (2012). Individual variation and longitudinal pattern of genome-wide DNA methylation from birth to the first two years of life. *Epigenetics, 7*(6), 594–605.

Weaver, I. C. G., Cervoni, N., Champagne, F. A., D'Alessio, A. C., Sharma, S., Seckl, J. R., … & Meaney, M. J. (2004). Epigenetic programming by maternal behavior. *Nature Neuroscience, 7* (8), 847–854.

Weaver, I. C. G., Champagne, F. A., Brown, S. E., Dymov, S., Sharma, S., Meaney, M. J., et al. (2005). Reversal of maternal programming of stress responses in adult offspring through methyl supplementation: Altering epigenetic marking through later life. *Journal of Neuroscience, 25*(47), 11045–11054.

Weaver, I. C. G., Szyf, M., & Meaney, M. J. (2002). From maternal care to gene expression: DNA methylation and the maternal programming of stress responses. *Endocrine Research, 28*(4), 699.

Wermter, A. K., Kamp-Becker, I., Hesse, P., Schulte-Körne, G., Strauch, K., & Remschmidt, H. (2010). Evidence for the involvement of genetic variation in the oxytocin receptor gene (OXTR) in the etiology of autistic disorders on high-functioning level. *American Journal of Medical Genetics Part B: Neuropsychiatric Genetics, 153*(2), 629–639.

Wu, S., Jia, M., Ruan, Y., Liu, J., Guo, Y., Shuang, M., … & Zhang, D. (2005). Positive association of the oxytocin receptor gene (OXTR) with autism in the Chinese Han population. *Biological Psychiatry, 58*(1), 74–77.

Yehuda, R., Daskalakis, N. P., Desarnaud, F., Makotkine, I., Lehrner, A. L., Koch, E., … & Bierer, L. M. (2013). Epigenetic biomarkers as predictors and correlates of symptom improvement following psychotherapy in combat veterans with PTSD. *Frontiers in Psychiatry, 4,* 118.

Yehuda, R., Daskalakis, N. P., Lehrner, A., Desarnaud, F., Bader, H. N., Makotkine, I., … & Meaney, M. J. (2014). Influences of maternal and paternal PTSD on epigenetic regulation of the glucocorticoid receptor gene in Holocaust survivor offspring. *American Journal of Psychiatry, 171*(8), 872–880.

Zhu, M., & Zhao, S. (2007). Candidate gene identification approach: Progress and challenges. *Internaltional Journal of Biological Sciences, 3*(7), 420–427.

Ziegler, C., Dannlowski, U., Bräuer, D., Stevens, S., Laeger, I., Wittmann, H., … & Domschke, K. (2015). Oxytocin receptor gene methylation: Converging multilevel evidence for a role in social anxiety. *Neuropsychopharmacology, 40*(6), 1528–1538.

Chapter 8
Poverty, Parent Stress, and Emerging Executive Functions in Young Children

Eric D. Finegood and Clancy Blair

Executive functions are higher-order cognitive abilities that guide complex goal-directed behaviors. They support decision-making, problem solving, reasoning, planning, and abstract thinking (Diamond, 2013; Zelazo, 2015). As such, these abilities are crucial to many aspects of daily functioning—especially, in those moments of our lives that require us to suppress or inhibit impulses, to flexibly shift our attention or our mindset from one position to another, or to maintain and work with information in our memory. Primarily understood to comprise the cognitive domain of self-regulation, executive functions are important for success in school (Blair, 2002; Blair & Razza, 2007); they not only help students to use numbers and apply concepts, but they also help them to be less impulsive and to focus their attention toward attaining goals. Executive function abilities are also associated with health and success throughout life (McClelland, Acock, Piccinin, Rhea, & Stallings, 2013). For instance, children who exhibit higher self-control, in which executive function is implied, tend to be more financially secure as adults, tend to have fewer run-ins with law enforcement, are less likely to use and abuse substances and more likely to enjoy better overall health as adults (Moffitt, Poulton, & Caspi, 2013).

One point that is becoming increasingly clear is that our experiences in early life have a significant influence on the development of our executive functions. This relation has to do, in part, with the effects of early life experiences on the neural and physiological substrates that underlie and support executive functions. For instance, children who experience high amounts of stress, such as children in high-poverty homes, tend to show deficits in executive functions (e.g., Hackman & Farah, 2009)

E.D. Finegood (✉) · C. Blair
Department of Applied Psychology, New York University, 627 Broadway, Floor 8, New York, NY 10012, USA
e-mail: edf237@nyu.edu

K. Deater-Deckard and R. Panneton (eds.), *Parental Stress and Early Child Development*, DOI 10.1007/978-3-319-55376-4_8

as well as alterations to brain areas that support executive function abilities (e.g., prefrontal cortex; Hanson et al., 2013; Noble et al., 2015) and the stress response systems (e.g., the hypothalamic pituitary adrenal axis; Blair et al., 2011a) known to be involved in regulating executive functions. To be clear, evidence in support of associations among poverty, stress, and executive function does not in any way indicate that the brains of children and families in poverty are damaged or irremediably altered. In contrast, the data indicate that brain and behavior are responding exactly as would be expected in a high stress, high-poverty environment (Blair & Raver, 2016). Stress tunes the brain and the body to be more reactive and less reflective, less likely to engage the executive functions (Arnsten, 2009). Greater reactivity and less reflection are generally advantageous in high stress contexts though not without specific disadvantages. In part, this is seen in data indicating that to some extent, effects of early experience on child executive functions and early brain development are mediated through early *caregiving* and the relationship with the primary caregiver. For instance, studies are beginning to identify specific parenting behaviors that are positively correlated with executive function development in children. These behaviors include the use of verbal "scaffolding" techniques to assist children during problem solving and patterns of interaction in which parents are warm and responsive (e.g., Bernier, Carlson, & Whipple, 2010; Blair et al., 2011a). Notably, however, children and families are embedded within and stratified across socioeconomic contexts and the hardships that disadvantaged families face may be associated with parents' perceptions of stress and disrupted family functioning (see Nomaguchi & Milkie, Chap. 3). The social, economic, and institutional constraints that confront families in poverty increase stress and pressure in parents, often making it difficult for them to engage in the types of early caregiving known to support children's executive function development (McLoyd, 1998). Consequently, children's development in poverty is more likely to be shaped in ways that are appropriate for that context; that is, to be less reflective and more reactive and responsive to immediate and unpredictable aspects of the environment (Blair & Raver, 2012). In theory, poverty-related stressors shape the proximal caregiving environments of children, and this may be a primary mechanism through which the broader experience of poverty influences the development of children's executive functions.

This chapter has a number of specific aims. The first aim is to briefly review some of the neurobiological foundations of executive functions and the developmental trajectory of these skills across the childhood years. The second aim is to outline what is known about the relation between poverty and executive function development in children. In doing so, we attempt to leverage what is known from neuroscience and developmental psychology about the neurophysiological and behavioral mechanisms of this relation to better understand the means through which poverty gets "under the skin" to influence children's executive function development. The third aim is to highlight the extent to which aspects of executive function development, and the development of the neurophysiological systems supporting executive functions, are socially mediated in early life. Studies of humans and non-human animals enhance our understanding of the ways in which the caregiving environment in general and early life experiences with parents in particular shape the developmental trajectories of executive functions and early self-regulation at several levels. The fourth aim is to place family processes and the proximal caregiving environments of children within larger socioecological contexts that include the communities and neighborhoods that families reside in—not only to consider the effects of these larger contexts on children's self-regulation development, but also the effects on parent well-being and family functioning. Lastly, we address how the context of poverty and experiences of early life adversity affect caregivers at neural and physiological levels and consider the extent to which these effects represent mechanisms through which the context of poverty and environmental stress influence parents' interactions with their children and ultimately, their children's self-regulation development. Understanding the ways in which poverty-related stress influences parents at psychobiological and behavioral levels is crucial from the perspective of designing and assessing targeted interventions to support parents and families and to reduce stress at multiple levels.

Executive Functions: Development and Neurophysiological Foundations

Executive functions comprise three distinct but related domains of functioning—attention shifting, working memory, and inhibition (Blair & Ursache, 2011; Friedman et al., 2006; Miyake et al., 2000; Wager, Jonides, & Reading, 2004). Attention switching or the ability to shift one's mental set involves the ability to flexibly switch attention between multiple competing tasks, or, within a task or problem, the ability to easily switch one's mental set between multiple operations or rules. A common task to assess this ability in children is the Dimensional Change Card Sort (DCCS; Zelazo, 2006) in which children are asked to sort several cards according to one dimension (e.g., shape) until a "post-switch" phase in which children are asked to sort according to a different dimension (e.g., color). Difficulties in mental set or attention shifting manifest as erroneous perseverative responses in which children fail to make the switch in the sorting rule. Working memory is the ability to hold in mind and to actively manipulate task-relevant information (Baddeley & Hitch, 1974). In one working memory task (Willoughby, Blair, Wirth, & Greenberg, 2010), children are presented with a line drawing of a house, inside of which is a drawing of an animal (e.g., a fish) and a colored dot (e.g., a blue dot). Next, the animal and colored dot disappear leaving only the drawing of the empty house, at which point children are asked to recall which animal was in the house (or, in another condition, are asked to recall which color was in this house). Successful completion of this task requires children to hold both pieces of information (i.e., the type of animal and the color of the dot) in memory, but to bring only one of these pieces of information to mind. Inhibition involves one's ability to inhibit a dominant response in favor of a sub-dominant response (Miyake et al., 2000). A common task for assessing this in children is the Day-Night task (Gerstadt, Hong, & Diamond, 1994) in which children are instructed to say "day" when shown a picture of a moon and to say "night" when shown a picture of a sun. Successful completion of this task involves the ability to overcome the dominant impulse to answer congruently with the picture scene.

An extensive neuropsychological literature has established that executive functions are supported by the prefrontal cortex (PFC) of the brain (see Fuster, 2015). The developmental course of the PFC is somewhat distinct from other areas of the human brain in that it experiences an enormous amount of synaptic growth and development in the first years of life but does not reach maturity until much later in young adulthood (Huttenlocher, 2002). Consistent with this, children show rapid improvements in executive function abilities throughout the toddler, preschool, and early childhood years (Diamond, 2006) and continue showing improvement (albeit at a slower rate) throughout adolescence and young adulthood (De Luca & Leventer, 2008; Zelazo, Craik, & Booth, 2004). The prolonged developmental course of the PFC also makes this brain area especially amenable to environmental influence, that is, to experiential input.

The PFC has long been considered the cognitive control center of the brain—the part of the brain that exerts "top-down" control over our behavior and mind, helping us to organize our thoughts and actions in ways that are volitional, intentional, and goal-directed. Importantly, however, PFC activity is modulated by neurochemicals produced in the brainstem and the limbic system—structures and neural systems both phylogenetically and ontogenetically older than the PFC. These neural systems and their chemical mediators (e.g., glucocorticoids and catecholamines) serve critical bodily functions including visceral and metabolic regulation, sympathetic nervous activity, and attentional processes, and are key players in the body's stress response to perceived environmental threat. As a product of this integrated system, executive functions are organized in a bi-directional manner by both "top–down" (intentional/reflective) and "bottom-up" (automatic/reactive) processes that are ultimately shaped by acute and chronic experiences (Blair & Ursache, 2011). Glucocorticoids (i.e., cortisol in humans) and catecholamines (i.e., norepinephrine and dopamine) exert influence on the PFC in an inverted-U shaped function. For example, it has been shown that executive functions are optimized and that synaptic potentiation in the PFC is at its highest when glucocorticoids and catecholamines are circulating at moderate levels—both under- and over-activation of adrenergic, dopaminergic, and endocrine pathways in the contexts of sleepiness and acute stress, respectively, has been associated with decrements in executive functioning and decreased cell communication in the PFC (Arnsten, 2009; de Kloet, Oitzl, & Joëls, 1999; Lupien, Maheu, Tu, Fiocco, & Schramek, 2007). Chronic exposure to adversity in early life (i.e., early experiences that engender high amounts of stress) has been associated with long-term alterations to these neural and physiological systems, and this has consequences for executive function development in children.

Poverty and Executive Function Development

Children living in poverty often endure an enormous amount of stress as a result of the psychosocial and physical environments in which they grow up. Children from poor families are more likely than children from non-poor families to be exposed to violence both in and out of their homes and are more likely to be exposed to pollutants and toxins, and the neighborhoods that their families reside in are often substandard (Evans, 2004). Eviction is a frequently occurring stress exposure associated with poverty leading to increased material hardship, job loss, homelessness, psychological distress, and increased and prolonged poverty and residential instability. Rates of eviction in high-poverty neighborhoods in major metropolitan areas are extremely high, disproportionately affecting women and children (Desmond, 2012). Especially, relevant to the current volume, children from poor families, as a consequence of the aforementioned stressors, also tend to have interactions with parents that are less warm and supportive, experience high amounts of household chaos and instability in caregivers, and their home learning environments tend to be poorer in terms of the psychosocial and material resources they have available to them for learning and success in school (Bradley & Corwyn, 2002; Bradley, Corwyn, McAdoo, & Coll, 2001; Brooks-Gunn, Duncan, & Aber, 1997; Duncan & Brooks-Gunn, 2000; Evans, 2004; Foster & Brooks-Gunn, 2009). A number of studies have indicated that the neural systems supporting executive functions are among the most negatively affected by the stress of poverty (Noble et al., 2015; Noble, McCandliss, & Farah, 2007). Consistent with these effects, differences in executive functioning have been observed across the socioeconomic spectrum. Associations between socioeconomic status (SES) and executive functions have been explored in a number of studies with preschool-aged children (e.g., Blair et al., 2011b; Carlson, Mandell, & Wiliams, 2004; Hughes & Ensor, 2005, 2009; Rhoades, Greenberg, Lanza, & Blair, 2011), after the transition to school (e.g., Engel, Santos, & Gathercole, 2008; Hughes, Ensor, Wilson, & Graham, 2009; Mezzacappa, 2004; Noble et al., 2007; Noble, Norman, & Farah, 2005), and during later childhood (e.g., Ardila, Rosselli, Matute, & Guajardo, 2005; Evans, 2003; Evans & English, 2002; Evans, Gonnella, Marcynyszyn, Gentile, & Salpekar, 2005; Farah et al., 2006; Hackman, Gallop, Evans, & Farah, 2015; Sarsour et al., 2011). Together, these studies suggest that children from lower SES families show reduced executive function abilities relative to children from higher-SES families, on average (but see Engel et al., 2008 for an exception).

In terms of executive function development or change across childhood, several recent longitudinal studies have assessed the extent to which SES is associated with children's rate of executive function growth. Studies suggest that while children from lower SES families perform worse on measures of executive function than their higher-SES counterparts, findings relating SES to children's rate of executive function growth are mixed. Whereas some prior studies have found preliminary evidence that static measures of SES did not predict change in executive functions over time (Hackman et al., 2014, 2015; Hughes et al., 2009), changes in the socioeconomic circumstances of families across time have been associated with children's rate of growth in executive functions across childhood. Specifically, reductions in family income across the elementary school years have been associated with reduced growth in executive functions across that time (Hackman et al., 2015). In the context of deep poverty, it may be the instability associated with high-income volatility that is most damaging to executive function development during childhood. In a large population-based sample of children and families in predominantly low-income and rural communities, other factors including the amount of time per week that children spend out of highly chaotic homes have been positively associated with executive function abilities (Berry et al., 2016) and Kuhn, Willoughby, Vernon-Feagans, Blair, and The Family Life Project Key Investigator (2016) found that children's rate of vocabulary growth was associated with child executive function at age 3 years and with the trajectory of executive function from age 3 to age 5.

There are multiple potential explanations for the robust association between SES and children's executive function development. Evidence is mounting to suggest that poverty and early life adversity have long-term effects on the physiological stress response systems that regulate prefrontal activity and executive functions. One such physiological system associated with environmental stress is the hypothalamic pituitary adrenal (HPA) axis. In response to a perceived environmental threat, for instance, the HPA axis releases the glucocorticoid hormone cortisol into the bloodstream where it mobilizes energy stores to prepare the body for action. In the brain, high levels of glucocorticoids signal the need to be *reactive* rather than *reflective*—as it may be more advantageous in a moment of acute stress to direct one's energy toward quick attentional processes and visceral functions rather than toward slower and more reflective or planful processes. The prolonged release of glucocorticoids under conditions of chronic stress, however, can have toxic effects on the brain and body—a state known as allostatic load (McEwen, 2000), in which individuals show under- or over-arousal and general dysregulation of this stress regulation system. Growing up in poverty has been linked with alterations in the functioning of the HPA axis that are consistent with the notion of allostatic load. Studies have shown, for instance, that low-SES children evidence higher baseline levels of cortisol (Evans & English, 2002; Lupien, King, Meaney, & McEwen, 2000, 2001) as well as more dysregulated daily rhythms of HPA axis activity than higher-SES children (Wolf, Nicholls, & Chen, 2008). Other studies have found evidence for patterns of under-activation of the HPA axis associated with the context of poverty (Badanes, Watamura, & Hankin, 2011; Chen & Paterson, 2006; Kliewer, Reid-Quiñones, Shields, & Foutz, 2008; Kraft & Luecken, 2009). These discrepant findings reflect the fact that poverty and poverty-related stress are not one-dimensional. It may be that under-activation of the HPA axis is associated with exposure to severe forms of early life adversity including child abuse, neglect, and maltreatment (Gunnar & Donzella, 2002). In fact, children raised in low-SES families are at a higher risk for experiencing these severe forms of adversity and whether the HPA axis evidences under- or over-activation as a function of early life adversity likely has to do with the particular form, chronicity, and severity of the stress exposure (Badanes, Watamura, & Hankin, 2011; Gunnar & Donzella, 2002). Moreover, the timing of stress exposure in a child's life (whether stress occurs prenatally, post-natally, or later in childhood) may also play a role in the extent of influence that glucocorticoids including cortisol have on prefrontal cortex and self-regulation development (Neuenschwander & Oberlander, Chap. 6).

Children in poverty tend to be exposed to more daily stressors than their middle-income counterparts, and because of this, measuring the multiple risks that children are exposed to may be a better predictor of their physiological and neurocognitive functioning than their poverty status alone (Evans & English, 2002; Sameroff & Fiese, 2000). Indeed, the number of psychosocial and physical environmental risks that a child is exposed to (i.e., exposure to crowded households, noise, violence, family turmoil, and separation from family) has been shown to be positively associated with measures of children's allostatic load—increased levels of circulating glucocorticoids and catecholamines in their bodies (Evans, 2003). Furthermore, Evans and colleagues (2003; Evans and English 2002) have shown that the number of poverty-related psychosocial and physical risk factors that children face in their environments is associated with children's ability to delay gratification at age nine. Thus, it may not be exposure to income poverty, per se, that is damaging to children's emerging self-regulation, but rather, children's overexposure to extreme or to "toxic" stressors in the context of poverty that is damaging (Evans, 2004; Felitti et al., 1998; Repetti, Taylor, & Seeman, 2002; Shonkoff, Boyce, & McEwen, 2009).

Models of chronicity of income poverty exposure (Duncan & Brooks-Gunn, 1997, 2000; McLoyd, 1990) are also helpful in clarifying the relation between poverty and executive function and self-regulation development in children. For instance, chronicity of poverty exposure before the age of four (defined as the number of years since birth that a child has lived in a home that was at or below the United States poverty line) has been negatively associated with executive function at four years of age (Raver, Blair, Willoughby, & The Family Life Project Key Investigators, 2013). In their analysis, Raver et al. (2013) showed that children's executive functions at age four were decreased by a tenth of a standard deviation with each additional year of life lived at or below the U.S. poverty line. Similarly, Evans and colleagues have shown that the proportion of time lived below the U.S. poverty line during childhood is negatively associated with working memory (Evans & Schamberg, 2009) and positively associated with measures of allostatic load (Evans & Kim, 2012) at age seventeen. Thus, evidence is converging to show that living in poverty for longer periods confers more risk to emerging executive functions in children and that this relation is likely mediated, in part, by the effects of poverty-related stress exposure on the physiological systems that modulate executive functions.

Poverty exposure has also been associated with structural and functional characteristics of the brain that support and regulate executive functions. In terms of brain structure, low SES has been shown to be associated with cortical thinning of regions of the frontal lobes including the anterior cingulate cortex (ACC; Lawson,

Duda, Avants, Wu, & Farah, 2013), an area of the medial prefrontal cortex involved in error detection and monitoring (Luu & Tucker, 2004). Cortical thinning reflects the relative thickness of gray matter in regions of the cerebral cortex and has been associated with cognitive ability and aging processes. In addition to objective measures of SES (e.g., family income and parental education), Gianaros et al. (2007) showed that a person's subjective perception of their own SES relative to others was associated with the volume of the ACC. That is, individuals who perceived themselves as being of a lower social status relative to others in the USA evidenced reduced gray matter volume in the ACC. Low SES in childhood has also been associated with structural brain architecture of the amygdala and hippocampus in adolescence (Luby et al., 2013; Noble, Houston, Kan, & Sowell, 2012), which has implications for children's neurocognitive development given that the amygdala and hippocampus are key players in the limbic system of the brain—a primary "bottom-up" influence on executive functions.

In terms of brain function, Kim et al. (2013) used functional magnetic resonance imaging (fMRI) to show that poverty exposure in childhood was associated prospectively with reduced prefrontal and increased amygdala activity during an effortful regulation task at age 24 years. Furthermore, exposure to cumulative stress during childhood and adolescence mediated this relation. Increased amygdala activity in young adulthood would suggest a developmental process in which self-regulatory structures and circuits of the brain are being shaped over time to a more *reactive* as opposed to *reflective* phenotype. Others have used methodologies including diffusion tensor imaging and shown that educational attainment is associated with increased white matter integrity in adolescence, which, in turn, mediated the relation between educational attainment and cognitive control abilities (Noble, Korgaonkar, Grieve, & Brickman, 2013). Taken together, evidence is mounting to suggest that poverty-related stress influences the structural and functional development of neural systems involved in error detection and active goal maintenance, memory, threat detection, and general information processing. Consistent with a bi-directional psychobiological model of executive function development, the effects of chronic stress on lower-order or "bottom-up" neural systems undermine the positive development of higher-order reflective cognitions including executive functions.

At this point, it is well established that poverty and low-resource environments are associated with decrements in children's executive functions and cognitive control abilities. That these effects are detectable at both neurophysiological and behavioral levels during early childhood and also prospectively at later ages supports the idea that early life experiences have long-term consequences for self-regulation across the lifespan. What are the critical ingredients of the early life experience that are responsible for this? Parents and other caregivers are the primary socializing agents of young children—and the caregiving environment in general constitutes the child's most proximal environment. As such, one leading hypothesis is that the proximal caregiving environment mediates the effects of more distal contexts on children's self-regulation development. In the context of poverty, for instance, parents and their behaviors are hypothesized to be critical mediators of the relation between adverse environmental conditions and child outcomes. Such a model has considerable theoretical and empirical support (Blair & Raver, 2012; Bradley & Corwyn, 2002; Conger & Donnellan, 2007; Duncan & Brooks-Gunn, 1997; McLoyd, 1998; Repetti, Taylor, & Seeman, 2002; Sastry, 2015; Wadsworth & Ahlkvist, 2015; see also Crnic & Ross, Chap. 11). The idea that poverty-related stress could affect child development *through* intermediary effects on the caregiving environments of children, including caregiver language (Kuhn et al., 2016), is important because it suggests the power of families and other forms of care to buffer or exacerbate the negative effects of poverty on children's executive function development.

Quality of Early Caregiving and Executive Functions

The most striking empirical examples of the importance of families and early rearing environments in self-regulation development come from circumstances in which children are raised in the absence of stable parental caregivers. Studies of institutionalized Romanian orphans have been especially informative in this respect (Carlson & Earls, 1997; Gunnar & Donzella, 2002; Nelson, Bos, Gunnar, & Sonuga-Barke, 2011; Zeanah et al., 2003). Children reared in these settings experience higher amounts of neglect and maternal deprivation (Zeanah et al., 2003), which has effects on the development of children's stress physiology (Carlson & Earls, 1997; for a comprehensive review, see Gunnar & Donzella, 2002). In a large randomized control trial of Romanian orphans (Zeanah et al., 2003), it was shown that institutionalized children displayed blunted HPA axis reactivity and regulation to psychosocial stress compared to children randomly assigned to foster care and to children who were raised at home (McLaughlin et al., 2015). Critically, however, the authors showed that the positive effects of foster care on HPA axis reactivity and regulation were only present for those children who were randomly assigned to foster care before they turned 2 years old. That is, placement into foster care was only effective in mitigating the blunting effects of institutionalization on HPA axis reactivity and regulation if it occurred very early in a child's life. The experimental nature of this study design (i.e., institutionalized orphans were *randomly assigned* to either foster care placement or to remain in institutionalized care as usual) helps researchers draw inferences regarding the true effect of the caregiving environment on self-regulatory systems in contexts of adversity. This type of study design is a notable strength given that nearly all other human work in this area of study is correlational and therefore suffers from some form of selection bias (i.e., in the case of non-random assignment of orphans into foster care, for instance, those orphans placed into foster care may be different in some ways than those not placed into foster care).

Experimental work conducted with non-human animals has also been particularly beneficial in this respect. That early rearing experiences influence the biobehavioral development of offspring has long been shown in non-human animal research. The importance of the primary attachment figure, the mother, for the development of well-regulated psychophysiological development is particularly evident in non-human primate studies of maternal deprivation (for review see Stevens, Leckman, Coplan, & Suomi, 2009; Suomi, 1997). As well, experiments with non-human primates that induced environmental stress by creating situations in which access to food was unpredictable caused significant amounts of stress in parents, which not only disrupted parent-infant interactions, but also had negative consequences for long-term psychophysiological and self-regulatory development of offspring (Coplan et al., 1996; Stevens et al., 2009). Research with rodents has also shown that individual variation in prototypical maternal behaviors (i.e., licking and grooming of pups as well as arched-back nursing) is a primary cause of stress physiological development in rodent offspring and that the effects of the caregiving environment on development persist into adulthood (Meaney, 2001). In a series of cross-fostering experiments, Meaney and colleagues showed that offspring who were reared by mothers expressing high amounts of maternal care displayed more well-regulated behavioral and more efficient physiological stress responses as adults than offspring who were reared by mothers who expressed low amounts of care (Caldji et al., 1998; Francis, Diorio, Liu, & Meaney, 1999; Liu et al., 1997). Recent work has shown that these effects of the early caregiving environment on biobehavioral development are mediated by an organism's epigenome, that part of the genome responsible for gene expression or the dynamic turning "on" and "off" of genes that allows an organism to be highly adaptable to their specific environmental conditions (Provençal et al., 2012; Weaver et al., 2004).

Human studies of more normative early rearing environments have also been informative for exploring the extent to which social environments shape the physiological systems associated with executive functions in children. In the Family Life Project (FLP), a prospective longitudinal sample of children and families in predominantly low-income and rural communities in the USA, instability in the number of caregivers in the home—specifically, more adult exists from the home—was associated with higher resting cortisol levels in children as early as 15 months of age, and this association persisted (and grew in magnitude) over the child's first four years (Blair et al., 2011a). This effect was present even when controlling for ethnicity, SES, parental perceptions of material hardship, and an observed behavioral measure of maternal sensitivity—itself a variable that was uniquely associated with resting levels of cortisol. In another analysis from the FLP, infants and toddlers of mothers who displayed high levels of engagement with their children during parent–child interactions showed more efficient HPA axis regulation in response to an emotion induction procedure than did infants and toddlers of mothers who displayed less engagement with their children (Blair et al., 2008). In terms of relations between SES, parenting, stress physiology, and early executive function development in children, analyses of this sample have also provided evidence that both maternal sensitivity and children's resting levels of cortisol mediate the relation between family SES and children's executive functions at age three (Blair et al., 2011b). Together, the human and animal work provide evidence that early exposure to chronic stress in the caregiving environment shapes the regulation of stress physiology associated with executive function development.

Consistent with theory regarding the development of self-regulation more generally (Kopp, 1982), children's very early control abilities begin by being primarily externally regulated through the actions of parents and other caregivers. As development progresses, experiential input becomes internalized and emotional, attentional, and also executive processes mature and become increasingly *self*-regulated. It has been shown that parental scaffolding, or the process by which parents actively support and organize the problem solving of their children (Wood, Bruner, & Ross, 1976), is associated with children's executive function concurrently at two years of age (Bibok, Carpendale, & Müller, 2009) and longitudinally at four years of age (Hughes & Ensor, 2009). One mechanism through which parental scaffolding may have effects on higher-order cognitions including executive functioning is through children's verbal competencies. Indeed, studies have shown that parental scaffolding at two years of age had positive effects on children's executive function at age four via positive effects on children's verbal ability (Hammond, Müller, Carpendale, Bibok, & Liebermann-Finestone, 2012). Similarly, Landry, Miller-Loncar, Smith and Swank (2002) have shown that verbal scaffolding in parents of 3-year olds was positively associated with children's executive function at six years of age. Again, as implied in the analysis of Kuhn et al. (2016) described previously, this effect was mediated by gains in children's language and nonverbal skills, which were supported by parents' use of scaffolding. Thus, parental verbal scaffolding during problem solving may increase children's capacity for language, which, in turn, may serve to organize their later self-directed problem-solving abilities and executive functions.

In addition to scaffolding, maternal sensitivity (i.e., a concept describing the extent to which a mother is able to interpret meaning and respond appropriately and contingently to her child's cues; Ainsworth, Blehar, Waters, & Wall, 1978) has been associated with children's executive function measured at 18, 26, and 36 months of age (Bernier, Carlson, Deschênes, & Matte-Gagné, 2012; Bernier, Carlson, & Whipple, 2010). Longitudinally, maternal sensitivity assessed at one year of age has been associated with children's executive function two years later (Rochette & Bernier, 2014). Using Family Life Project data, Blair et al. (2011b) found that observed measures of both maternal negativity (intrusiveness and negative regard for child) and maternal sensitivity in the child's first two years made unique contributions to children's executive function at three years of age. Furthermore, each domain of observed parenting behavior statistically mediated the association between parent education and children's executive function, suggesting that the proximal caregiving environment of children acted as an intermediary in the broader relation between families' SES and children's executive function at age three. With respect to educational outcomes in children, it has been shown that maternal sensitivity observed across the first three years of life was associated with preschoolers' delay of gratification abilities, which in turn, partially mediated the relation between maternal sensitivity and school readiness (Razza & Raymond, 2013). Together, these studies provide evidence that the caregiving environment of children is especially important for supporting early self-regulation and success in school.

Research has also begun to address questions regarding the relation between the caregiving environment and growth or change in executive functions across childhood. In a novel approach to modeling change in parenting behaviors and growth in executive functioning from three to five years of age, Blair, Raver, and Berry (2014) employed a cross-lagged latent change score model to explore the potential for bi-directional effects between caregiving and change (i.e., growth) in child executive function across childhood. This analysis showed that higher maternal sensitivity observed at three years of age predicted increased growth in child executive functions from three to five years of age. Furthermore, the authors showed that higher child executive function at three years of age predicted less decline in observed maternal sensitivity from three to five years of child age. This is consistent with a transactional model of early regulation (Sameroff & Fiese, 2000) where both parent and child characteristics are observed to contribute meaningfully to each other's development in a process of co-regulation. Here, it is notable that previously cited studies (Hackman et al., 2014, 2015; Hughes et al., 2009) found no relations between family SES and children's executive function growth across early childhood, which suggests a unique contribution of the early caregiving environment, as opposed to more distal family socioeconomic factors, in predicting longitudinal change and growth in executive functions across childhood.

Parenting and Child Development in Context

Parenting behaviors and caregiving environments are embedded within families and socioeconomic contexts, and the early caregiving environment may be one mechanism through which the broader context of poverty confers risk to children's emerging executive functions. Parents living in poverty experience higher amounts of psychological distress, depression, more marital discord and increased risk of intimate partner violence, and more negative life events compared to non-poor parents (McLoyd, 1990). These factors can increase parenting stress and reduce parents' capacity for warm and sensitive caregiving with their children—rendering their interactions with children harsher than those observed in families experiencing far less daily stress (Cassells & Evans, Chap. 2; Duncan & Brooks-Gunn, 2000). These realities have the potential to disrupt family functioning and to negatively affect children's development (Conger & Conger, 2002; Conger & Donnellan, 2007; Conger & Elder, 1994). Poverty also limits the extent to which parents are able to invest in the social capital of their children (i.e., to provide a rich home learning environment by buying books or cognitively stimulating toys, paying for tutoring, and visiting museums; Becker & Tomes, 1994; Conger & Donnellan, 2007; Haveman & Wolfe, 1994). In the context of deep poverty, parents' investments are often necessarily directed more toward survival goals (Conger & Donnellan, 2007). Such conditions can undermine the development of executive functions. For instance, having fewer learning resources in the home has been shown to be associated with slower growth in inhibitory control and cognitive flexibility during the preschool years (Clark et al., 2013) and both the home learning environment and parental responsiveness have been shown to mediate relations between family SES and inhibitory control and working memory at nine years of age (Sarsour et al., 2011). One recent study showed that aspects of the home learning environment mediated the effects of family SES on children's executive function and planning ability (i.e., a skill highly associated with executive function) and that maternal sensitivity mediated the relation between family SES and children's planning ability (Hackman et al., 2015). Findings from these studies suggest that the home caregiving environment—characterized by both the provision of learning materials/experiences as well as the parenting behaviors that a child is exposed to—may be seen as both a consequence of parent stress processes in the context of poverty as well as an antecedent of neurocognitive outcomes in children including executive functions.

It is important to acknowledge that family processes and the proximal caregiving environment are embedded within larger socioecological contexts that influence stress processes in parents. For instance, the communities and neighborhoods that poor families reside in tend to be inferior to those of wealthier families in terms of infrastructure and services and disadvantaged neighborhoods often have higher instances of violence than do more advantaged neighborhoods (Brooks-Gunn, Duncan, & Aber, 1997; Duncan & Brooks-Gunn, 2000; Evans, 2004; Foster & Brooks-Gunn, 2009), and there is evidence that residential segregation by family income is increasing (Bischoff & Reardon, 2014). How does neighborhood stress permeate the family unit? Parents' perceptions of high neighborhood stress, that is, of poor services available in their community, of high unemployment and drug use, of low social cohesion, and of economic disadvantage, have been associated with increased psychological distress in parents as well as with negative interactions with adolescents (Gutman, McLoyd, & Tokoyawa, 2005). Mothers' perceptions of neighborhood danger are also associated with less maternal warmth toward adolescent children (Gonzales et al., 2011), and a study using public crime report data showed that residential proximity to recent homicides in Chicago communities was associated with higher distress in parents—a potential mechanism through which community violence may be transmitted indirectly to children (Sharkey, Tirado-Strayer, Papachristos, & Raver, 2012).

There are also recent findings suggesting that the neighborhood context may be associated with the development of stress response physiology at the individual level. For instance, high neighborhood stress measured both objectively (e.g., using U.S. Census data) and subjectively (e.g., perceptions of neighborhood disorder and safety) have been associated with flatter diurnal HPA activity in adults—indicating dysregulation of stress systems involved in self-regulation within neighborhood contexts of high stress (Karb, Elliott, Dowd, & Morenoff, 2012). Concentrated neighborhood disadvantage has also been associated with heightened resting cortisol levels (Rudolph et al., 2014) and with increased HPA reactivity to psychosocial stress in adolescents (Hackman, Betancourt, Brodsky, Hurt, & Farah,

2012). Others have found lower neighborhood SES to be associated with lower cortisol levels in children (Dulin-Keita, Casazza, Fernandez, Goran, & Gower, 2012) and adolescents (Chen & Paterson, 2006). One study found no association between neighborhood SES and HPA activity (Kapuku, Treiber, & Davis, 2002). These studies provide preliminary evidence that the broader neighborhood context may be associated with developing stress physiology over and above the proximal family-level environment. The small number of studies and the inconsistencies in the findings (i.e., neighborhood-level stress and disadvantage have been associated with both over- and under-activation of HPA axis), however, suggests that the exact relation between the neighborhood context and this stress response system is not yet fully understood and suggests an area for future research. Discrepant findings are likely due to inconsistencies in the measurement of neighborhood-level stress and disadvantage across studies, differences in the extent of stress that children face in their home environments and if and how the home environment is measured across studies, differences in the developmental ages of participants in previous studies, and differences in the exact measure of HPA activity across studies. Clarifying these terms will aid in understanding the true relation, if any, between the neighborhood context and the development of this stress response system. In terms of relations between neighborhood characteristics and children's executive function development, one recent study found no relation between concentrated neighborhood disadvantage and children's working memory at age ten, nor between concentrated neighborhood disadvantage and children's growth in working memory through age fourteen, controlling for family socioeconomic status (Hackman et al., 2014).

Families living in poor neighborhoods are also exposed to more violence than those living in non-poor neighborhoods (Brooks-Gunn et al., 1997). Results from a recent study suggest that aspects of preschoolers' self-regulation may be compromised when exposed to local violence in their community. Specifically, Sharkey, Tirado-Strayer, Papachristos, and Raver (2012) matched data on preschoolers' self-regulation with Chicago Police homicide records and found that children who were recently exposed to community violence (operationalized as residing within 2500 feet of a homicide that occurred within seven days of testing) displayed worse impulse control and attention and scored worse on pre-academic skills measures including early vocabulary and math than children who were not recently exposed to violence. There were no significant effects of exposure to community violence on executive function or effortful control. These effects may have consequences for children's success in school. As evidence of this, in a study of a different sample, Sharkey (2010) found that living in the proximity of a homicide taking place within seven days prior to testing was associated with lower reading and vocabulary scores in African–American students. Although the very limited number of studies that have assessed relations between the neighborhood context and children's executive functions have found no evidence of such a relation, findings from these studies do suggest that aspects of the neighborhood context may be associated with more "bottom-up" aspects of self-regulation in children including their stress response physiology and attentional processes.

In addition to the effects of environmental stress on family processes and self-regulatory outcomes in children, poverty-related stress may also be associated with the neurophysiological and cognitive regulation of parents themselves (Barrett & Fleming, 2011; see also Mileva-Seitz & Fleming, Chap. 10). Consistent with findings indicating the early and long-lasting social regulation of the developing HPA axis, research has shown that adult mothers who reported having experienced early life adversity show heightened and dysregulated patterns of diurnal HPA axis activity compared to mothers who reported no early life adversity (Gonzalez, Jenkins, Steiner, & Fleming, 2009). The relation between stress exposure and parents' HPA axis regulation is important given that regulation of the maternal HPA axis has been associated with variation in maternal caregiving behaviors in humans. For instance, increased cortisol levels in mothers have been associated with more fatigue and negative mood (Krpan, Coombs, Zinga, Steiner, & Fleming, 2005) and with less observed maternal sensitivity and more intrusive behaviors in the first six months of the postpartum period (Mills-Koonce et al., 2009; Thompson & Trevathan, 2008). Higher maternal cortisol levels have also been associated with lower levels of maternal sensitivity observed across the first two postpartum years (Finegood et al., 2016). Using functional magnetic resonance imaging (fMRI) to assess regional brain activity associated with aspects of the parent experience, new research has shown that mothers' neural response to baby-cry stimuli in key regulatory areas of the brain are correlated with measures of observed maternal sensitivity (Kim et al., 2011; Musser, Kaiser-Laurent, & Ablow, 2012; Swain, 2011), suggesting that parenting behaviors are organized by psychobiological processes operating at multiple levels. Retrospective reports of the quality of parental care that one received during childhood have also been shown to predict adult mothers' grey matter density in several key self-regulatory regions of the brain and, as well, are predictive of mothers' functional neural responses to baby cries (Kim et al., 2009), suggesting a potential neural mechanism through which early experiences with caregivers shape the development of the parental brain and indirectly affect parenting behaviors and child outcomes—a potential means through which stress may be transmitted across generations (see Mileva-Seitz & Fleming, Chap. 10).

Consistent with the observed effects of environmental stress on adult stress physiology as well as on the structure and function of brain areas involved in self-regulation, a number of recent studies have noted relations between maternal executive function and maternal behaviors with children (Chico, Gonzalez, Ali, Steiner, & Fleming, 2014; Cuevas et al., 2014; Deater-Deckard, Sewell, Petrill, & Thompson, 2010; Deater-Deckard, Wang, Chen, & Bell, 2012). Indeed, one study has shown that both maternal HPA axis activity and maternal executive function fully mediate the relation between mothers' exposure to early life adversity and maternal sensitivity in adulthood (Gonzalez, Jenkins, Steiner, & Fleming, 2012). The evidence suggests that parent stress associated with the strains of poverty and early life adversity is associated with alterations to the neurophysiological systems that underlie the parental brain, which supports parents' own cognitive self-regulation as well as the organization of their interactions with children.

Conclusions and Future Directions

In this chapter, we have overviewed some of the neurobiological foundations of executive functions and the developmental trajectory of these skills across the childhood years. We outlined what is known regarding the relation between poverty and executive function development in children and some of the specific neurobiological mechanisms of this relation—specifically emphasizing research suggesting that the caregiving environment is a primary mediator of the relation between the socioeconomic conditions of families and children's neurocognitive development. In doing so, we considered several aspects of the caregiving environment that may be affected by the context of poverty (e.g., parents' behaviors with children, the home learning environment, and parents' own cognitive and biobehavioral regulation) that are presumed to shape children's neurocognitive growth.

The relation between stress exposure in early life and children's executive function development is moderate and robust across a large number of studies. The specific mechanisms of this relation remain somewhat unclear, however, even after the large amount of studies conducted on this topic. This is because almost all of the findings from the human research discussed herein are derived from non-experimental correlational studies, which suffer from selection bias, limiting the extent of inference that may be drawn with respect to casual mechanisms. Descriptive correlational studies preclude the ability to conclusively say, for instance, that poverty *causes* changes in the caregiving environments of children, which, in turn, shape the trajectories of children's neurocognitive development. With this in mind, more non-human experimental work is needed to understand the causal links between low-resource environments, specific caregiving environments, and neurophysiological and behavioral outcomes in offspring. Non-human animal models are extremely useful from a causal inference perspective because they allow for the experimental manipulation of environmental stress, for instance, which helps to clarify the role that low-resources play in shaping parenting behaviors (Raineki, Moriceau, & Sullivan, 2010). Furthermore, experimental manipulation of the caregiving environment itself in animal models, through either induction of environmental stress (Raineki et al., 2010) or through cross-fostering procedures (Meaney, 2001) and the observation of subsequent changes to neural, physiological, and behavioral outcomes in offspring are necessary steps in estimating the true and potentially multifaceted role that the caregiving environment plays in early self-regulation development of offspring.

Of course, non-human animal studies are limited in their translation to human ecology and development. Particularly, when these studies are used to model cognitive abilities such as executive functions. As such, it is important to note that there have been a small number of randomized controlled trials conducted with humans in low-income settings that have directly targeted the caregiving environment (e.g., by focusing on enhancing parents' competencies and supporting parent–child relationships) and shown positive effects in terms of boosting maternal responsiveness and cognitive, socioemotional, and language development in infants (Landry, Smith, & Swank, 2006; Landry, Smith, Swank, & Guttentag, 2008). Other parenting programs have been successful in reducing attention deficit hyperactivity disorder symptoms in preschoolers at risk for conduct problems (Bor, Sanders, & Markie-Dadds, 2002; Jones, Daley, Hutchings, Bywater, & Eames, 2007) and in improving the functioning of neural systems involved in early attention processes in children (Neville et al., 2013). Parenting interventions have also had positive effects on HPA axis regulation in preschoolers at high risk of conduct problems (Brotman et al., 2007) and enhanced foster care interventions have had positive effects on HPA axis regulation in children in foster care (Dozier, Peloso, Lewis, Laurenceau, & Levine, 2008; Fisher, Gunnar, Dozier, Bruce, & Pears, 2006; Fisher, Stoolmiller, Gunnar, & Burraston, 2007). These studies are promising and provide necessary experimental evidence for the role of the caregiving environment in shaping infants and preschoolers' early self-regulation. Experimental studies that test intervention effects on direct assessments of children's early executive functions as well as on related aspects of stress physiology, neural functioning, and behavior are needed to more firmly establish the causal mechanisms and the multifaceted nature of children's early self-regulation development in the context of adversity.

The field would also benefit from more studies that measure and model multiple component stress processes in low-income parents. In particular, it would be beneficial to test which forms of stress are most responsible for the relation between poverty and parenting behaviors. Is it, for instance, parenting stress (i.e., stress having to do with the parenting role in particular) that is most responsible for the relation between the context of poverty and reductions in maternal sensitivity (see Crnic & Ross, Chap. 11)? Is the relation more strongly accounted for by other stress processes in these contexts (e.g., perceptions of material hardship, marital conflict, violence exposure, or psychopathology)? What about aspects of parents' cognitive and neurophysiological regulation that have been shown to be associated not only with stress exposure in early life but also with parenting behaviors? How do the unique or interactive effects of multiple coordinated stress processes come to organize parental executive functions and HPA axis activity, as well as the functional and structural components of the parental brain? The answers to these questions would benefit policy and early intervention immensely.

Given that children and families are embedded within sociocultural contexts, future research that aims to understand the influence of context on family functioning and child development would benefit from widening the concept of disadvantage to consider people's individual subjective and/or relative experiences of hardship rather than focusing on absolute levels of disadvantage (e.g., income and education) alone. For instance, one recent study (Ursache, Noble, & Blair, 2015) showed that both objective family SES and parents' subjective perceptions of relative social status were uniquely associated with children's executive functions measured at age nine. Children who were from poorer families or whose parents rated themselves as being of lower social status performed worse on executive function tasks. Additionally, the authors noted a significant negative association between parents' perceptions of stress and their children's cortisol levels, although neither objective family SES nor parents' subjective social status was associated with children's cortisol levels. Little is currently known about the mechanisms through which these effects on children's executive function might occur, but it is likely that perceptions of low status increase stress in parents which may influence their interactions with their children. No studies to date have directly tested these questions, although the field would benefit greatly from such approaches. Additionally, given the interconnectedness of social class and race, perceptions of discrimination may be another factor relevant to understanding stress processes in parents and family functioning in the context of adversity. For instance, one recent study found relations between mothers' perceptions of daily racial discrimination and their children's birthweight (Earnshaw et al., 2013).

A similarly beneficial approach may be to examine macrocontextual factors—aligned with a social epidemiological perspective on relations between social class and health—as they relate to family functioning, proximal family stress processes and to child self-regulation development in particular. Incorporating measures of regional income inequality or of social stratification of families using U.S. Census data, in addition to family-level measures of SES, may be particularly beneficial to understanding the etiology of family stress processes in the context of adversity given recent evidence suggesting that the link between SES and health is stronger in geographic contexts characterized by higher income inequality (Wilkinson & Pickett, 2006), that individual health is worse when relative income deprivation is high (Kondo, Kawachi, Subramanian, Takeda, & Yamagata, 2008), and that psychosocial comparative processes are associated with alterations to individual-level stress systems that partially explain mortality and morbidity in human and non-human primates (Sapolsky, 2005). It may be that proximal family stress processes and children's emerging self-regulation abilities evidence similar etiologic and developmental patterns to those found for physical health outcomes, and/or that family stress processes and children's emerging self-regulation abilities are mechanisms of the association between SES and physical health.

Further examination of the specific mechanisms that explain the association between the socioeconomic conditions of families and children's emerging self-regulation and executive functions is warranted. An abundance of descriptive, correlational research and theory suggests that aspects of the caregiving environment of children may be partially responsible for this association, but we note the need for more experimental studies that not only test the malleability of parenting behaviors and caregiving environments in the context of poverty, but also that test the extent to which children's early self-regulation including their executive functions and supporting attentional and neurophysiological processes are amenable to family-based intervention and concomitant changes to the caregiving environment.

References

Ainsworth, M. D., Blehar, M. C., Waters, E., & Wall, S. (1978). *Patterns of attachment: A psychological study of the strange situation*. Oxford, England: Lawrence Erlbaum.

Ardila, A., Rosselli, M., Matute, E., & Guajardo, S. (2005). The influence of the parents' educational level on the development of executive functions. *Developmental Neuropsychology, 28*(1), 539–560.

Arnsten, A. F. T. (2009). Stress signalling pathways that impair prefrontal cortex structure and function. *Nature Reviews Neuroscience, 10*(6), 410–422. doi:10.1038/nrn2648.

Badanes, L. S., Watamura, S. E., & Hankin, B. L. (2011). Hypocortisolism as a potential marker of allostatic load in children: Associations with family risk and internalizing disorders. *Development and Psychopathology, 23,* 881–896. doi:10.1017/S095457941100037X.

Baddeley, A. D., & Hitch, G. (1974). Working memory. In G. H. Bower (Ed.), *The psychology of learning and motivation: Advances in research and theory* (Vol. 8, pp. 47–89). New York, NY: Academic Press.

Barrett, J., & Fleming, A. S. (2011). Annual research review: All mothers are not created equal: Neural and psychobiological perspectives on mothering and the importance of individual differences. *Journal of Child Psychology and Psychiatry, 52*(4), 368–397. doi:10.1111/j.1469-7610.2010.02306.x.

Becker, G. S., & Tomes, N. (1994). Human capital and the rise and fall of families. In G. S. Becker (Ed.), *Human capital: A theoretical and empirical analysis with special reference to education* (3rd ed., pp. 257–298). Chicago, Il: The University of Chicago Press.

Bernier, A., Carlson, S. M., Deschênes, M., & Matte-Gagné, C. (2012). Social factors in the development of early executive functioning: A closer look at the caregiving environment. *Developmental Science, 15*(1), 12–24. doi:10.1111/j.1467-7687.2011.01093.x.

Bernier, A., Carlson, S. M., & Whipple, N. (2010). From external regulation to self-regulation: Early parenting precursors of young children's executive functioning. *Child Development, 81*(1), 326–339. doi:10.1111/j.1467-8624.2009.01397.x.

Berry, D., Blair, C., Willoughby, M., Garrett-peters, P., Vernon-Feagans, L., Mills-koonce, W. R., & The Family Life Project Key Investigators. (2016). Household chaos and children's cognitive and socio-emotional development in early childhood: Does childcare play a buffering role? *Early Childhood Research Quarterly, 34,* 115–127. doi:10.1016/j.ecresq.2015.09.003.

Bibok, M. B., Carpendale, J. I. M., & Müller, U. (2009). Parental scaffolding and the development of executive function. In C. Lewis & J. I. M. Carpendale (Eds.), Social interaction and the development of executive function. *New directions in child and adolescent development* (Vol. 123, pp. 17–34).

Bischoff, K., & Reardon, S. F. (2014). Residential segregation by income, 1970–2009. In J. R. Logan (Ed.), *Diversity and disparities: America enters a new Century* (pp. 208–233). New York, NY: Russell Sage Foundation.

Blair, C. (2002). School readiness: Integrating cognition and emotion in a neurobiological conceptualization of children's functioning at school entry. *American Psychologist, 57*(2), 111–127. doi:10.1037//0003-066X.57.2.111.

Blair, C., Granger, D. A., Willoughby, M., Mills-Koonce, R., Cox, M., Greenberg, M. T., … Family Life Project Key Investigators. (2011). Salivary cortisol mediates effects of poverty and parenting on executive functions in early childhood. *Child Development, 82*(6), 1970–1984. doi:10.1111/j.1467-8624.2011.01643.x.

Blair, C., Granger, D. A., Kivlighan, K. T., Mills-Koonce, R., Willoughby, M., Greenberg, M. T., … & The Family Life Project Investigators. (2008). Maternal and child contributions to cortisol response to emotional arousal in young children from low-income, rural communities. *Developmental Psychology, 44*(4), 1095–1109. doi:10.1037/0012-1649.44.4.1095.

Blair, C., & Raver, C. C. (2012). Child development in the context of adversity: Experiential canalization of brain and behavior. *American Psychologist, 67*(4), 309–318. doi:10.1037/a0027493.

Blair, C., & Raver, C. C. (2016). Poverty, stress, and brain development: New directions for prevention and intervention. *Academic Pediatrics, 16*(3), S30–S36. doi:10.1016/j.acap.2016.01.010.

Blair, C., Raver, C. C., Berry, D. J., & the Family Life Project Investigators. (2014). Two approaches to estimating the effect of parenting on the development of executive function in early childhood. *Developmental Psychology, 50*(2), 554–565. doi:10.1037/a0033647.

Blair, C., Raver, C. C., Granger, D., Mills-Koonce, R., Hibel, L., & The Family Life Project Key Investigators. (2011). Allostasis and allostatic load in the context of poverty in early childhood. *Development and Psychopathology, 23*(3), 845–857. doi:10.1017/S0954579411000344.

Blair, C., & Razza, R. P. (2007). Relating effortful control, executive function, and false belief understanding to emerging math and literacy ability in kindergarten. *Child Development, 78*(2), 647–663. doi:10.1111/j.1467-8624.2007.01019.x.

Blair, C., & Ursache, A. (2011). A bidirectional model of executive functions and self-regulation. In K. D. Vohs & R. F. Baumeister (Eds.), *Handbook of self-regulation: Research, theory, and applications* (pp. 300–320). New York: The Guilford Press.

Bor, W., Sanders, M. R., & Markie-Dadds, C. (2002). The effects of the Triple-P-Positive parenting program on preschooler children with co-occurring disruptive behavior and attential/hyperactive difficulties. *Journal of Abnormal Child Psychology, 30*(6), 571–587.

Bradley, R. H., & Corwyn, R. F. (2002). Socioeconomic status and child development. *Annual Review of Psychology, 53,* 371–399. doi:10.1146/annurev.psych.53.100901.135233.

Bradley, R. H., Corwyn, R. F., McAdoo, H. P., & Coll, C. G. (2001). The home environments of children in the United States part I: Variations by age, ethnicity, and poverty status. *Child Development, 72*(6), 1844–1867. doi:10.1111/1467-8624.t01-1-00382.

Brooks-Gunn, J., Duncan, G. J., & Aber, J. L. (Eds.). (1997). *Neighborhood poverty: Context and consequences for children.* New York, NY: Russell Sage Foundation.

Brotman, L. M., Gouley, K. K., Huang, K.-Y., Kamboukos, D., Fratto, C., & Pine, D. S. (2007). Effects of a psychosocial family-based preventive intervention on cortisol response to a social challenge in preschoolers at high risk for antisocial behavior. *Archives of General Psychiatry, 64*(10), 1172–1179. doi:10.1001/archpsyc.64.10.1172.

Caldji, C., Tannenbaum, B., Sharma, S., Francis, D. D., Plotsky, P. M., & Meaney, M. J. (1998). Maternal care during infancy regulates the development of neural systems mediating the expression of fearfulness in the rat. *Proceedings of the National Academy of Sciences of the United States of America, 95*(9), 5335–5340. doi:10.1073/pnas.95.9.5335.

Carlson, M., & Earls, F. (1997). Psychological and neuroendocrinological sequelae of early social deprivation in institutionalized children in Romania. *Annals of the New York Academy of Sciences, 807,* 419–428.

Carlson, S. M., Mandell, D. J., & Wiliams, L. (2004). Executive function and theory of mind: Stability and prediction from ages 2 to 3. *Developmental Psychology, 40*(6), 1105–1122.

Chen, E., & Paterson, L. Q. (2006). Neighborhood, family, and subjective socioeconomic status: How do they relate to adolescent health? *Health Psychology, 25*(6), 704–714. doi:10.1037/0278-6133.25.6.704.

Chico, E., Gonzalez, A., Ali, N., Steiner, M., & Fleming, A. S. (2014). Executive function and mothering: Challenges faced by teenage mothers. *Developmental Psychobiology, 56*(5), 1027–1035. doi:10.1002/dev.21185.

Clark, C. A. C., Sheffield, T. D., Chevalier, N., Nelson, J. M., Wiebe, S. A., & Espy, K. A. (2013). Charting early trajectories of executive control with the shape school. *Developmental Psychology, 49*(8), 1481–1493. doi:10.1037/a0030578.

Conger, R. D., & Conger, K. J. (2002). Resilience in Midwestern families: Selected findings from the first decade of a prospective, longitudinal study. *Journal of Marriage and Family, 64*(2), 361–373. doi:10.1111/j.1741-3737.2002.00361.x.

Conger, R. D., & Donnellan, M. B. (2007). An interactionist perspective on the socioeconomic context of human development. *Annual Review of Psychology, 58,* 175–199.

Conger, R. D., & Elder, G. H. (1994). *Families in troubled times: Adapting to change in rural America.* Hawthorn, NY: Aldine de Gruyter.

Coplan, J. D., Andrews, M. W., Rosenblum, L. A., Owens, M. J., Friedman, S., Gorman, J. M., et al. (1996). Persistent elevations of cerebrospinal fluid concentrations of corticotropin-releasing factor in adult nonhuman primates exposed to early-life stressors: Implications for the pathophysiology of mood and anxiety disorders. *Proceedings of the National Academy of Sciences of the United States of America, 93,* 1619–1623.

Cuevas, K., Deater-Deckard, K., Kim-Spoon, J., Watson, A. J., Morasch, K. C., & Bell, M. A. (2014). What's mom got to do with it? Contributions of maternal executive function and caregiving to the development of executive function across early childhood. *Developmental Science, 17*(2), 224–238. doi:10.1111/desc.12073.

de Kloet, E. R., Oitzl, M. S., & Joëls, M. (1999). Stress and cognition: Are corticosteroids good or bad guys? *Trends in Neurosciences, 22*(10), 422–426. doi:10.1016/S0166-2236(99)01438-1.

De Luca, C. R., & Leventer, R. J. (2008). Developmental trajectories of executive functions across the lifespan. In V. Anderson, R. Jacobs, & P. J. Anderson (Eds.), *Executive functions and the frontal lobes: A lifespan perspective* (pp. 23–56). New York, NY: Taylor and Francis.

Deater-Deckard, K., Sewell, M. D., Petrill, S. A., & Thompson, L. A. (2010). Maternal working memory and reactive negativity in parenting. *Psychological Science, 21*(1), 75–79. doi:10.1177/0956797609354073.

Deater-Deckard, K., Wang, Z., Chen, N., & Bell, M. A. (2012). Maternal executive function, harsh parenting, and child conduct problems. *Journal of Child Psychology and Psychiatry, 53*(10), 1084–1091. doi:10.1111/j.1469-7610.2012.02582.x.

Desmond, M. (2012). Eviction and the reproduction of urban poverty. *American Journal of Sociology, 118*(1), 88–133.

Diamond, A. (2006). The early development of executive functions. In E. Bialystok & F. I. M. Craik (Eds.), *Lifespan cognition: Mechanisms of change* (pp. 70–95). New York, NY: Oxford University Press.

Diamond, A. (2013). Executive functions. *The Annual Review of Psychology, 64,* 135–168. doi:10.1146/annurev-psych-113011-143750.

Dozier, M., Peloso, E., Lewis, E., Laurenceau, J.-P., & Levine, S. (2008). Effects of an attachment-based intervention on the cortisol production of infants and toddlers in foster care. *Development and Psychopathology, 20*(3), 845–859. doi:10.1017/S0954579408000400.

Dulin-Keita, A., Casazza, K., Fernandez, J. R., Goran, M. I., & Gower, B. (2012). Do neighbourhoods matter? Neighbourhood disorder and long-term trends in serum cortisol levels. *Journal of Epidemiology and Community Health, 66*(1), 24–29. doi:10.1136/jech.2009.092676.

Duncan, G. J., & Brooks-Gunn, J. (Eds.). (1997). *Consequences of growing up poor*. New York, NY: Russell Sage Foundation.

Duncan, G. J., & Brooks-Gunn, J. (2000). Family poverty, welfare reform, and child development. *Child Development, 71*(1), 188–196.

Earnshaw, V. A., Rosenthal, L., Lewis, J. B., Stasko, E. C., Tobin, J. N., Lewis, T. T., … Ickovics, J. R. (2013). Maternal experiences with everyday discrimination and infant birth weight: A test of mediators and moderators among young, urban women of color. *Annals of Behavioral Medicine, 45*(1), 13–23. doi:10.1007/s12160-012-9404-3

Engel, P. M. J., Santos, F. H., & Gathercole, S. E. (2008). Are working memory measures free of socioeconomic influence? *Journal of Speech, Language, and Hearing Research, 51,* 1580–1587.

Evans, G. W. (2003). A multimethodological analysis of cumulative risk and allostatic load among rural children. *Developmental Psychology, 39*(5), 924–933. doi:10.1037/0012-1649.39.5.924.

Evans, G. W. (2004). The environment of childhood poverty. *American Psychologist, 59*(2), 77–92. doi:10.1037/0003-066X.59.2.77.

Evans, G. W., & English, K. (2002). The environment of poverty: Multiple stressor exposure, psychophysiological stress, and socioemotional adjustment. *Child Development, 73*(4), 1238–1248.

Evans, G. W., Gonnella, C., Marcynyszyn, L. A., Gentile, L., & Salpekar, N. (2005). The role of chaos in poverty and children's socioemotional adjustment. *Psychological Science, 16*(7), 560–565. doi:10.1111/j.0956-7976.2005.01575.x.

Evans, G. W., & Kim, P. (2012). childhood poverty and young adults' allostatic load: The mediating role of childhood cumulative risk exposure. *Psychological Science, 23*(9), 979–983. doi:10.1177/0956797612441218.

Evans, G. W., & Schamberg, M. A. (2009). Childhood poverty, chronic stress, and adult working memory. *Proceedings of the National Academy of Sciences, 106*(16), 6545–6549. doi:10.1073/pnas.0811910106.

Farah, M. J., Shera, D. M., Savage, J. H., Betancourt, L., Giannetta, J. M., Brodsky, N. L., … Hurt, H. (2006). Childhood poverty: Specific associations with neurocognitive development. *Brain Research, 1110*, 166–174. doi:10.1016/j.brainres.2006.06.072

Felitti, V. J., Anda, R. F., Nordenberg, D., Williamson, D. F., Spitz, A. M., Edwards, V., … Marks, J. S. (1998). Relationship of childhood abuse and household dysfunction to many of the leading causes of death in adults: The adverse childhood experiences (ACE) study. *American Journal of Preventive Medicine, 14*(4), 245–258. doi:10.1016/S0749-3797(98)00017-8

Finegood, E. D., Blair, C., Granger, D. A., Hibel, L. C., Mills-Koonce, R., & The Family Life Project Key Investigators. (2016). Psychobiological influences on maternal sensitivity in the context of adversity. *Developmental Psychology, 52*(7), 1073–1087. doi:10.1037/dev0000123.

Fisher, P. A., Gunnar, M. R., Dozier, M., Bruce, J., & Pears, K. C. (2006). Effects of therapeutic interventions for foster children on behavioral problems, caregiver attachment, and stress regulatory neural systems. *Annals of the New York Academy of Sciences, 1094*, 215–225. doi:10.1196/annals.1376.023.

Fisher, P. A., Stoolmiller, M., Gunnar, M. R., & Burraston, B. O. (2007). Effects of a therapeutic intervention for foster preschoolers on diurnal cortisol activity. *Psychoneuroendocrinology, 32*, 892–905. doi:10.1016/j.psyneuen.2007.06.008.

Foster, H., & Brooks-Gunn, J. (2009). Toward a stress process model of children's exposure to physical family and community violence. *Clinical Child and Family Psychology Review, 12*, 71–94. doi:10.1007/s10567-009-0049-0.

Francis, D., Diorio, J., Liu, D., & Meaney, M. J. (1999). Nongenomic transmission across generations of maternal behavior and stress responses in the rat. *Science, 286*(5442), 1155–1158. doi:10.1126/science.286.5442.1155.

Friedman, N. P., Miyake, A., Corley, R. P., Young, S. E., DeFries, J. C., & Hewitt, J. K. (2006). Not all executive functions are related to intelligence. *Psychological Science, 17*(2), 172–179. doi:10.1111/j.1467-9280.2006.01681.x.

Fuster, J. M. (2015). *The prefrontal cortex* (5th ed.). London, UK: Academic Press.

Gerstadt, C. L., Hong, Y. J., & Diamond, A. (1994). The relationship between cognition and action: performance of children 3.5–7 years old on a Stroop- like day-night test. *Cognition, 53*, 129–153.

Gianaros, P. J., Horenstein, J. A., Cohen, S., Matthews, K. A., Brown, S. M., Flory, J. D., … Hariri, A. R. (2007). Perigenual anterior cingulate morphology covaries with perceived social standing. *Social Cognitive and Affective Neuroscience*, *2*(3), 161–173. doi:10.1093/scan/nsm013

Gonzales, N. A., Coxe, S., Roosa, M. W., White, R. M. B., Knight, G. P., Zeiders, K. H., et al. (2011). Economic hardship, neighborhood context, and parenting: Prospective effects on Mexican-American adolescent's mental health. *American Journal of Community Psychology, 47*(1), 98–113. doi:10.1007/s10464-010-9366-1.

Gonzalez, A., Jenkins, J. M., Steiner, M., & Fleming, A. S. (2009). The relation between early life adversity, cortisol awakening response and diurnal salivary cortisol levels in postpartum women. *Psychoneuroendocrinology, 34*(1), 76–86.

Gonzalez, A., Jenkins, J. M., Steiner, M., & Fleming, A. S. (2012). Maternal early life experiences and parenting: The mediating role of cortisol and executive function. *Journal of the American Academy of Child and Adolescent Psychiatry, 51*(7), 673–682. doi:10.1016/j.jaac.2012.04.003.

Gunnar, M. R., & Donzella, B. (2002). Social regulation of the cortisol levels in early human development. *Psychoneuroendocrinology, 27*, 199–220. doi:10.1016/S0306-4530(01)00045-2.

Gutman, L. M., McLoyd, V. C., & Tokoyawa, T. (2005). Financial strain, neighborhood stress, parenting behaviors, and adolescent adjustment in urban African American families. *Journal of Research on Adolescence, 15*(4), 425–449.

Hackman, D. A., Betancourt, L. M., Brodsky, N. L., Hurt, H., & Farah, M. J. (2012). Neighborhood disadvantage and adolescent stress reactivity. *Frontiers in Human Neuroscience, 6*(277), 1–11. doi:10.3389/fnhum.2012.00277.

Hackman, D. A., Betancourt, L. M., Gallop, R., Romer, D., Brodsky, N. L., Hurt, H., et al. (2014). Mapping the trajectory of socioeconomic disparity in working memory: Parental and neighborhood factors. *Child Development, 85*(4), 1433–1445. doi:10.1111/cdev.12242.

Hackman, D. A., & Farah, M. J. (2009). Socioeconomic status and the developing brain. *Trends in Cognitive Sciences, 13*(2), 65–73. doi:10.1016/j.tics.2008.11.003.

Hackman, D. A., Gallop, R., Evans, G. W., & Farah, M. J. (2015). Socioeconomic status and executive function: Developmental trajectories and mediation. *Developmental Science, 18*(5), 686–702.

Hammond, S. I., Müller, U., Carpendale, J. I. M., Bibok, M. B., & Liebermann-Finestone, D. P. (2012). The effects of parental scaffolding on preschoolers' executive function. *Developmental Psychology, 48*(1), 271–281.

Hanson, J. L., Hair, N., Shen, D. G., Shi, F., Gilmore, J. H., Wolfe, B. L., et al. (2013). Family poverty affects the rate of human infant brain growth. *PLoS ONE, 8*(12), e80954. doi:10.1371/journal.pone.0080954.

Haveman, R. H., & Wolfe, B. (1994). *Succeeding generations: On the effects of investments in children*. New York, NY: Russell Sage Foundation.

Hughes, C., & Ensor, R. A. (2005). executive function and theory of mind in 2 year olds: A family affair? *Developmental Neuropsychology, 28*(2), 645–668.

Hughes, C., & Ensor, R. A. (2009). How do families help or hinder the emergence of early executive function? In C. Lewis & J. L. M. Carpendale (Eds.), Social interaction and the development of executive function. *New Directions in Child and Adolescent Development, 123*, 35–50.

Hughes, C., Ensor, R., Wilson, A., & Graham, A. (2009). Tracking executive function across the transition to school: A latent variable approach. *Developmental Neuropsychology, 35*(1), 20–36. doi:10.1080/87565640903325691.

Huttenlocher, P. R. (2002). *Neural plasticity: The effects of environment on the development of the cerebral cortex*. Cambridge, MA: Harvard University Press.

Jones, K., Daley, D., Hutchings, J., Bywater, T., & Eames, C. (2007). Efficacy of the incredible years basic parent training programme as an early intervention for children with conduct disorder and ADHD. *Child: Care Health and Development, 33*, 749–756.

Kapuku, G. K., Treiber, F. A., & Davis, H. C. (2002). Relationships among socioeconomic status, stress induced changes in cortisol, and blood pressure in African American males. *Annals of Behavioral Medicine, 24*(4), 320–325.

Karb, R. A., Elliott, M. R., Dowd, J. B., & Morenoff, J. D. (2012). Neighborhood-level stressors, social support, and diurnal patterns of cortisol: The Chicago community adult health study. *Social Science and Medicine, 75*(6), 1038–1047. doi:10.1016/j.socscimed.2012.03.031.

Kim, P., Evans, G. W., Angstadt, M., Ho, S. S., Sripada, C. S., & Swain, J. E. … Phan, K. L. (2013). Effects of childhood poverty and chronic stress on emotion regulatory brain function in adulthood. *Proceedings of the National Academy of Sciences, 110*(46), 18442–18447. doi:10.1073/pnas.1308240110

Kim, P., Feldman, R., Mayes, L. C., Eicher, V., Thompson, N., Leckman, J. F., et al. (2011). Breastfeeding, brain activation to own infant cry, and maternal sensitivity. *Journal of Child Psychology and Psychiatry, 52*(8), 907–915. doi:10.1111/j.1469-7610.2011.02406.x.

Kim, P., Leckman, J. F., Mayes, L. C., Newman, M., Feldman, R., & Swain, J. E. (2009). Perceived quality of maternal care in childhood and structure and function of mothers' brain. *Developmental Science, 13*(4), 662–673. doi:10.1111/j.1467-7687.2009.00923.x.

Kliewer, W., Reid-Quiñones, K., Shields, B. J., & Foutz, L. (2008). Multiple risks, emotion regulation skill, and cortisol in low-income African American youth: A prospective study. *Journal of Black Psychology, 35*(1), 24–43. doi:10.1177/0095798408323355.

Kondo, N., Kawachi, I., Subramanian, S. V., Takeda, Y., & Yamagata, Z. (2008). Do social comparisons explain the association between income inequality and health? Relative deprivation and perceived health among male and female Japanese individuals. *Social Science and Medicine, 67*(6), 982–987. doi:10.1016/j.socscimed.2008.06.002.

Kopp, C. B. (1982). Antecedents of self-regulation: A developmental perspective. *Developmental Psychology, 18*(2), 199–214.

Kraft, A. J., & Luecken, L. J. (2009). Childhood parental divorce and cortisol in young adulthood: Evidence for mediation by family income. *Psychoneuroendocrinology, 34,* 1363–1369. doi:10.1016/j.psyneuen.2009.04.008.

Krpan, K. M., Coombs, R., Zinga, D., Steiner, M., & Fleming, A. S. (2005). Experiential and hormonal correlates of maternal behavior in teen and adult mothers. *Hormones and Behavior, 47*(1), 112–122. doi:10.1016/j.yhbeh.2004.08.006.

Kuhn, L. J., Willoughby, M. T., Vernon-Feagans, L., Blair, C. B., & The Family Life Project Key Investigators. (2016). The contribution of children's time-specific and longitudinal expressive language skills on developmental trajectories of executive function. *Journal of Experimental Child Psychology, 148,* 20–34. doi:10.1016/j.jecp.2016.03.008.

Landry, S. H., Miller-Loncar, C. L., Smith, K. E., & Swank, P. R. (2002). The role of early parenting in children's development of executive processes. *Developmental Neuropsychology, 21*(1), 15–41.

Landry, S. H., Smith, K. E., & Swank, P. R. (2006). Responsive parenting: establishing early foundations for social, communication, and independent problem-solving skills. *Developmental Psychology, 42*(4), 627–642. doi:10.1037/0012-1649.42.4.627.

Landry, S. H., Smith, K. E., Swank, P. R., & Guttentag, C. (2008). A responsive parenting intervention: The optimal timing across early childhood for impacting maternal behaviors and child outcomes. *Developmental Psychology, 44*(5), 1335–1353.

Lawson, G. M., Duda, J. T., Avants, B. B., Wu, J., & Farah, M. J. (2013). Associations between children's socioeconomic status and prefrontal cortical thickness. *Developmental Science, 16* (5), 641–652. doi:10.1111/desc.12096.

Liu, D., Diorio, J., Tannenbaum, B., Caldji, C., Francis, D., Freedman, A., … Meaney, M. J. (1997). Maternal care, hippocampal glucocorticoid receptors, and hypthalamic-pituitary-adrenal responses to stress. *Science, 277*(5332), 1659–1662. doi:10.1126/science.277.5332.1659

Luby, J., Belden, A., Botteron, K., Marrus, N., Harms, M. P., Babb, C., … Barch, D. (2013). The effects of poverty on childhood brain development. The mediating effect of caregiving and stressful life events. *JAMA Pediatrics, 167*(12), 1135–1142. doi:10.1001/jamapediatrics.2013.3139

Lupien, S. J., King, S., Meaney, M. J., & McEwen, B. S. (2001). Can poverty get under your skin? Basal cortisol levels and cognitive function in children from low and high socioeconomic status. *Development and Psychopathology, 13,* 653–676.

Lupien, S. J., King, S., Meaney, M. J., & McEwen, B. S. (2000). Child's stress hormone levels correlate with mother's socioeconomic status and depressive state. *Biological Psychiatry, 48,* 976–980. doi:10.1016/S0006-3223(00)00965-3.

Lupien, S. J., Maheu, F., Tu, M., Fiocco, A., & Schramek, T. E. (2007). The effects of stress and stress hormones on human cognition: Implications for the field of brain and cognition. *Brain and Cognition, 65,* 209–237. doi:10.1016/j.bandc.2007.02.007.

Luu, P., & Tucker, D. M. (2004). Self-regulation by the medial frontal cortex: Limbic representation of motive set-points. In M. Beauregard (Ed.), *Consciousness, emotional self-regulation and the brain* (pp. 123–161). Amsterdam: John Bejamins.

McClelland, M. M., Acock, A. C., Piccinin, A., Rhea, S. A., & Stallings, M. C. (2013). Relations between preschool attention span-persistence and age 25 educational outcomes. *Early Childhood Research Quarterly, 28*(2), 314–324. doi:10.1016/j.ecresq.2012.07.008.

McEwen, B. S. (2000). Allostasis and allostatic load: Implications for neuropsychopharmacology. *Neuropsychopharmacology, 22*(2), 108–124. doi:10.1016/S0893-133X(99)00129-3.

McLaughlin, K. A., Sheridan, M. A., Tibu, F., Fox, N. A., Zeanah, C. H., & Nelson, C. A. (2015). Causal effects of the early caregiving environment on development of stress response systems in children. *Proceedings of the National Academy of Sciences, 112*(18), 5637–5642. doi:10.1073/pnas.1423363112.

McLoyd, V. C. (1990). The impact of economic hardship on black families and children: Psychological distress, parenting, and socioemotional development. *Child Development, 61,* 311–346.

McLoyd, V. C. (1998). Socioeconomic disadvantage and child development. *The American Psychologist, 53*(2), 185–204. doi:10.1037/0003-066X.53.2.185.

Meaney, M. J. (2001). Maternal care, gene expression, and the transmission of individual differences in stress reactivity across generations. *Annual Reviews Neuroscience, 24,* 1161–1192.

Mezzacappa, E. (2004). Alerting, orienting, and executive attention: Developmental properties and sociodemographic correlates in an epidemiological sample of young, urban children. *Child Development, 75*(5), 1373–1386.

Mills-Koonce, W. R., Propper, C., Gariepy, J. L., Barnett, M., Moore, G. A., Calkins, S., et al. (2009). Psychophysiological correlates of parenting behavior in mothers of young children. *Developmental Psychobiology, 51*(8), 650–661. doi:10.1002/dev.20400.

Miyake, A., Friedman, N. P., Emerson, M. J., Witzki, A. H., Howerter, A., & Wager, T. D. (2000). The unity and diversity of executive functions and their contributions to complex "frontal lobe" tasks: A latent variable analysis. *Cognitive Psychology, 41*(1), 49–100. doi:10.1006/cogp.1999.0734.

Moffitt, T. E., Poulton, R., & Caspi, A. (2013). Lifelong impact of early self-control. *American Scientist, 101*(5), 352–359. doi:10.1511/2013.104.352.

Musser, E. D., Kaiser-Laurent, H., & Ablow, J. C. (2012). The neural correlates of maternal sensitivity: An fMRI study. *Developmental Cognitive Neuroscience, 2*(4), 428–436. doi:10.1016/j.dcn.2012.04.003.

Nelson, C. A., Bos, K., Gunnar, M. R., & Sonuga-Barke, E. J. S. (2011). V. The neurobiological toll of early human deprivation. *Monographs of the Society for Research in Child Development, 76*(4), 127–146. doi:10.1111/j.1540-5834.2011.00630.x.

Neville, H. J., Stevens, C., Pakulak, E., Bell, T. A., Fanning, J., Klein, S., et al. (2013). Family-based training program improves brain function, cognition, and behavior in lower socioeconomic status preschoolers. *Proceedings of the National Academy of Sciences of the United States of America, 110*(29), 12138–12143. doi:10.1073/pnas.1304437110.

Noble, K. G., Houston, S. M., Brito, N. H., Bartsch, H., Kan, E., Kuperman, J. M., … Sowell, E. R. (2015). Family income, parental education and brain structure in children and adolescents. *Nature Neuroscience, 18*(5), 773–778. doi:10.1038/nn.3983

Noble, K. G., Houston, S. M., Kan, E., & Sowell, E. R. (2012). Neural correlates of socioeconomic status in the developing human brain. *Developmental Science, 15*(4), 516–527. doi:10.1111/j.1467-7687.2012.01147.x.

Noble, K. G., Korgaonkar, M. S., Grieve, S. M., & Brickman, A. M. (2013). Higher education is an age-independent predictor of white matter integrity and cognitive control in late adolescence. *Developmental Science, 16*(5), 653–664. doi:10.1111/desc.12077.

Noble, K. G., McCandliss, B. D., & Farah, M. J. (2007). Socioeconomic gradients predict individual differences in neurocognitive abilities. *Developmental Science, 10*(4), 464–480. doi:10.1111/j.1467-7687.2007.00600.x.

Noble, K. G., Norman, M. F., & Farah, M. J. (2005). Neurocognitive correlates of socioeconomic status in kindergarten children. *Developmental Science, 8*(1), 74–87.

Provençal, N., Suderman, M. J., Guillemin, C., Massart, R., Ruggiero, A., Wang, D., … Szyf, M. (2012). The signature of maternal rearing in the methylome in rhesus macaque prefrontal cortex and T cells. *The Journal of Neuroscience, 32*(44), 15626–42. doi:10.1523/JNEUROSCI.1470-12.2012

Raineki, C., Moriceau, S., & Sullivan, R. M. (2010). Developing a neurobehavioral animal model of infant attachment to an abusive caregiver. *Biological Psychiatry, 67*(12), 1137–1145. doi:10.1016/j.biopsych.2009.12.019.

Raver, C. C., Blair, C., Willoughby, M., & The Family Life Project Key Investigators. (2013). Poverty as a predictor of 4-year-olds' executive function: New perspectives on models of differential susceptibility. *Developmental Psychology, 49*(2), 292–304.

Razza, R. A., & Raymond, K. (2013). Associations among maternal behavior, delay of gratification, and school readiness across the early childhood years. *Social Development, 22*(1), 180–196. doi:10.1111/j.1467-9507.2012.00665.x.

Repetti, R. L., Taylor, S. E., & Seeman, T. E. (2002). Risky families: Family social environments and the mental and physical health of offspring. *Psychological Bulletin, 128*(2), 330–366. doi:10.1037//0033-2909.128.2.330.

Rhoades, B. L., Greenberg, M. T., Lanza, S. T., & Blair, C. (2011). Demographic and familial predictors of early executive function development: Contribution of a person-centered perspective. *Journal of Experimental Child Psychology, 108*, 638–662.

Rochette, É., & Bernier, A. (2014). Parenting, family socioeconomic status, and child executive functioning: A longitudinal study. *Merrill-Palmer Quarterly, 60*(4), 431–460.

Rudolph, K. E., Gary S., W., Stuart, E. A., Glass, T. A., Marques, A. H., Duncko, R., & Merikangas, K. R. (2014). The association between cortisol and neighborhood disadvantage in a U.S. population-based sample of adolescents. *Health & Place, 25*, 68–77. doi:10.1016/j.healthplace.2013.11.001

Sameroff, A. J., & Fiese, B. H. (2000). Transactional regulation: The developmental ecology of early intervention. In J. P. Shonkoff & S. J. Meisels (Eds.), *Handbook of early childhood intervention* (pp. 135–159). Cambridge, UK: Cambridge University Press. doi:10.1017/CBO9780511529320.009

Sapolsky, R. M. (2005). The influence of social hierarchy on primate health. *Science, 308*(5722), 648–652. doi:10.1126/science.1106477.

Sarsour, K., Sheridan, M., Jutte, D., Nuru-Jeter, A., Hinshaw, S., & Boyce, W. T. (2011). Family socioeconomic status and child executive functions: The roles of language, home environment, and single parenthood. *Journal of the International Neuropsychological Society, 17*(1), 120–132. doi:10.1017/S1355617710001335.

Sastry, N. (2015). Stressful life experiences and contexts: The effects on parents and parenting. In P. R. Amato et al., (Eds.), *Families in an era of increasing inequality. National Symposium on Family Issues* (Vol. 5, pp. 105–111). Switzerland: Springer.

Sharkey, P. (2010). The acute effect of local homicides on children's cognitive performance. *Proceedings of the National Academy of Sciences, 107*(26), 11733–11738.

Sharkey, P. T., Tirado-Strayer, N., Papachristos, A. V., & Raver, C. C. (2012). The effect of local violence on children's attention and impulse control. *American Journal of Public Health, 102* (12), 2287–2293. doi:10.2105/AJPH.2012.300789.

Shonkoff, J. P., Boyce, W. T., & McEwen, B. S. (2009). Neuroscience, molecular biology, and the childhood roots of health disparities. *Journal of the American Medical Association, 301*(21), 2252–2259. doi:10.1001/jama.2009.754.

Stevens, H. E., Leckman, J. F., Coplan, J. D., & Suomi, S. J. (2009). Risk and resilience: Early manipulation of macaque social experience and persistent behavioral and neurophysiological outcomes. *Journal of the American Academy of Child and Adolescent Psychiatry, 48*(2), 114–127. doi:10.1097/CHI.0b013e318193064c.

Suomi, S. J. (1997). Early determinants of behaviour: Evidence from primate studies. *British Medical Bulletin, 53*(1), 170–184.

Swain, J. E. (2011). The human parental brain: In vivo neuroimaging. *Progress in Neuro-Psychopharmacology and Biological Psychiatry, 35*(5), 1242–1254. doi:10.1016/j.pnpbp.2010.10.017.

Thompson, L. A., & Trevathan, W. R. (2008). Cortisol reactivity, maternal sensitivity, and learning in 3-month-old infants. *Infant Behavior and Development, 31*(1), 92–106. doi:10.1016/j.infbeh.2007.07.007.

Ursache, A., Noble, K. G., & Blair, C. (2015). Socioeconomic status, subjective social status, and perceived stress: Associations with stress physiology and executive functioning. *Behavioral Medicine, 41*(3), 145–154. doi:10.1080/08964289.2015.1024604.

Wadsworth, M. E., & Ahlkvist, J. A. (2015). Inequality begins outside the home: Putting parental educational investments into context. In P. R. Amato et al. (Eds.), *Families in an era of increasing inequality. National Symposium on Family Issues* (Vol. 5, pp. 95–103). Switzerland: Springer.

Wager, T. D., Jonides, J., & Reading, S. (2004). Neuroimaging studies of shifting attention: A meta-analysis. *NeuroImage, 22,* 1679–1693. doi:10.1016/j.neuroimage.2004.03.052.

Weaver, I. C. G., Cervoni, N., Champagne, F. A., D'Alessio, A. C., Sharma, S., Seckl, J. R., … Meaney, M. J. (2004). Epigenetic programming by maternal behavior. *Nature Neuroscience, 7* (8), 847–854. doi:10.1038/nn1276

Wilkinson, R. G., & Pickett, K. E. (2006). Income inequality and population health: A review and explanation of the evidence. *Social Science and Medicine, 62*(7), 1768–1784. doi:10.1016/j.socscimed.2005.08.036.

Willoughby, M. T., Blair, C. B., Wirth, R. J., Greenberg, M. & The Family Life Project Investigators. (2010). The measurement of executive function at age 3 years: Psychometric properties and criterion validity of a new battery of tasks. *Psychological Assessment, 22*(2), 306–317. doi:10.1037/a0018708.

Wolf, J. M., Nicholls, E., & Chen, E. (2008). Chronic stress, salivary cortisol, and α-amylase in children with asthma and healthy children. *Biological Psychology, 78,* 20–28. doi:10.1016/j.biopsycho.2007.12.004.

Wood, D., Bruner, J. S., & Ross, G. (1976). The role of tutoring in problem solving. *Journal of Child Psychology and Psychiatry, 17*(2), 89–100. doi:10.1111/j.1469-7610.1976.tb00381.x.

Zeanah, C. H., Nelson, C. A., Fox, N. A., Smyke, A. T., Marshall, P., Parker, S. W., et al. (2003). Designing research to study the effects of institutionalization on brain and behavioral development: The Bucharest early intervention project. *Development and Psychopathology, 15,* 885–907.

Zelazo, P. D. (2006). The dimensional change card sort (DCCS): A method of assessing executive function in children. *Nature Protocols, 1*(1), 297–301. doi:10.1038/nprot.2006.46.

Zelazo, P. D. (2015). Executive function: Reflection, iterative reprocessing, complexity, and the developing brain. *Developmental Review, 38,* 55–68. doi:10.1016/j.dr.2015.07.001.

Zelazo, P. D., Craik, F. I. M., & Booth, L. (2004). Executive function across the life span. *Acta Psychologica, 115,* 167–183. doi:10.1016/j.actpsy.2003.12.005.

Chapter 9
Child Maltreatment: Consequences, Mechanisms, and Implications for Parenting

Brian T. Leitzke and Seth D. Pollak

The Center for Disease Control (CDC) defines child maltreatment as "any act or series of acts of commission or omission by a parent or other caregiver that results in harm, potential for harm, or threat of harm to a child" (Leeb, Paulozzi, Melanson, Simon, & Arias, 2008). Acts of commission include physical, sexual, and psychological or emotional abuse while acts of omission include failures to provide for and supervise children such as neglect and exposure to violent environments. Researchers who study the impact and outcomes of child maltreatment typically discuss child maltreatment using these terms. Of note, issues such as "emotional maltreatment" are difficult to measure, but likely co-occur with all other forms of maltreatment, and children frequently experience more than one type of abuse (Vachon, Krueger, Rogosch, & Cicchetti, 2015).

There is a lack of clarity over whether the subtypes of maltreatment differ in severity or outcome. Early research on the effects of child maltreatment included heterogeneous samples of maltreated children, including those who had experienced neglect, sexual abuse, witnessing domestic violence, and a host of other adverse conditions. Researchers reasoned that each of these circumstances likely resulted in different kinds of effects on a variety of neurodevelopmental systems. For example, the experience of severe threat exposure among physically abused children could have different developmental sequelae as contrasted with the outcomes that might result from the isolation and lack of care afforded to neglected children. Indeed, research found that children who experienced primarily physical abuse had patterns of emotion recognition that were quite distinct from those of children who suffered primarily from caregiving neglect (Pollak, Cicchetti, Hornung, & Reed, 2000). Children in the former group were more likely to develop

B.T. Leitzke (✉) · S.D. Pollak
University of Wisconsin—Madison, Madison, USA
e-mail: btleitzke@wisc.edu

S.D. Pollak
e-mail: spollak@wisc.edu

K. Deater-Deckard and R. Panneton (eds.), *Parental Stress and Early Child Development*, DOI 10.1007/978-3-319-55376-4_9

hyper-vigilance to threat cues, whereas children in the latter group were more likely to have difficulty differentiating various emotional signals. Yet, there are also ways in which different kinds of early adversity appear to have similar developmental effects. For example, research has found that children in other risk groups have problems that appear more similar. As an example, neurocognitive delays tied to behavioral problems have been observed among physically abused children, children who experienced early neglect, children reared in institutionalized settings (Hanson et al., 2013a; Pollak et al., 2010; Sheridan, Fox, & Zeanah, 2012), and children raised in very-low-income families (Hanson et al., 2013b; see also Cassell & Evans, Chap. 2, regarding poverty and parenting stress). Regardless of these similarities and differences, it is clear that child maltreatment is associated with numerous negative outcomes.

Lifetime Consequences of Child Maltreatment

Several large-scale studies have been conducted to determine the prevalence and impact of child maltreatment. A retrospective study in the USA and a longitudinal study in New Zealand are some of the largest attempts at clarifying the scope of child maltreatment. The Adverse Childhood Experiences (ACE) study was a collaboration between the CDC and a large integrated healthcare consortium designed to examine the associations between adverse childhood experiences (e.g., traumatic events such as maltreatment) and later life outcomes (Felitti, Vincent, Anda, & Robert, 1998). The largest of its kind, the ACE study demonstrated the role of early environmental circumstances on health and behavior outcomes. Surveying over 17,000 people, Felitti et al. (1998) found over two-thirds of them reported at least one incident of childhood trauma and the more traumatic experiences one had, the greater their risk was for developing a host of problems. These problems included a greater risk for heart, lung, and liver disease; several types of psychopathology; unsafe sexual behaviors; suicide attempts; and a markedly lower health-related quality of life (Felitti et al., 1998). The Dunedin Study in New Zealand found similar results following nearly 1000 individuals longitudinally and assessing them every 3–6 years from birth to most recently age 38 (Poulton, Moffitt, & Silva, 2015). This study revealed that those with a history of adverse childhood experiences (e.g., physical and sexual abuse, poverty, loss of parent) were at greater risk for PTSD (Koenen, Moffitt, Poulton, Martin, & Caspi, 2007), risky sexual behaviors (Ramrakha, Bell, Paul, & Dickson, 2007), depression and high levels of inflammation, and age-related disease (Danese et al., 2009).

In addition to these studies, other research has found child maltreatment to be associated with higher rates of criminality, violence, incarceration (Fang & Corso, 2007; Thornberry, Henry, Ireland, & Smith, 2010), and abuse toward one's own children (Widom & Maxfield, 2001, see also Mileva-Seitz & Fleming, Chap. 10). Further, new cases of child maltreatment are believed to rack up a *total lifetime economic burden* of over $500 billion due to elevated rates of unemployment and a strain on the health care and prison systems (Fang, Brown, Florence, & Mercy, 2012). While the evidence is clear that child maltreatment leads to a host of negative consequences, it is not yet clear how these early experiences have such a profound influence on our social, emotional, and psychological functioning.

Investigating the Mechanisms Behind the Impact of Child Maltreatment on Development

As illustrated in the ACE and Dunedin studies, past research on the effects of child abuse largely comprised correlational methods and behavioral observations. This formative research played an important role, both in demonstrating the degree to which maltreatment had a lasting impact on child development, but also in beginning to map the wide range of domains affected by child abuse. More recent emphases in developmental psychopathology now focus on elucidating the specific developmental processes affected by child abuse and neglect that may lead to maladaptive behavior. This newer approach mirrors significant changes in the way many developmentalists now conceptualize psychopathology. For example, cutting-edge researchers in the field of child maltreatment now tend to deemphasize distinctions between what would have previously been construed as mental versus physical disorders. There is also a renewed emphasis among researchers on the interactions between persons and their environments. These types of developmentally informed approaches have begun to permit tests of novel hypotheses about the biological conduits across levels of analysis, such as *bidirectional* influences between the biology of the individual and that individual's social environment (see also Finegood & Blair, Chap. 8).

Researchers in the field are now attempting to understand the associations between brain–behavior relationships and how perturbations in these links lead to maladaptive behaviors. Researchers continue to study issues such as dysregulation of mood, but increasingly they construe their topics more broadly than diagnostic categories such as "anxiety" or "depression." This emphasis on broader processes, such as emotion regulatory behaviors or emotion–cognition interactions, reflects a major trend in the field to focus on maladaptive processes of change. One reason for this change in emphasis is that it is now apparent that development is best characterized by probabilistic pathways rather than by linear causality (this perspective is also clearly evident in the other chapters in this volume). There has been no evidence that early adversity leads ineluctably to any one form of pathology. Rather, social and biological challenges initiate processes that may more likely lead to pathology if that maladaptive pathway continues to be supported. In this regard, developmental psychopathologists are attempting to frame questions differently. In the past, researchers in the field may have posed questions such as "what psychiatric diagnoses are maltreated children likely to develop?" But current research questions may be framed more about what is it about a child's early experience that places the child on one developmental pathway versus another. We might ask: "What constrains the individual's ability to alter these pathways," or "during which developmental time periods or under which circumstances are opportunities for change the greatest?"

Another recent trend has been for researchers to consider "biomarkers" associated with various forms of pathology. The use of biomarkers in psychopathology research has been an attempt to reconcile the extant diagnostic taxonomies of mental health problems with knowledge about underlying biological systems. These biomarker approaches harness technological advances that allow scientists to assay aspects of brain function, genetic and epigenetic markers, and neuropeptide actions on physiology and social behavior (as a few examples). In many ways, these biomarker approaches are beginning to bridge levels of analysis by linking, for example, behavioral regulation with a specific biological substrate such as a hormonal marker. The laudable goal of such approaches is to highlight either key pathogenic features or index responsiveness to treatment at levels of analysis that are more proximal to neurological activity.

At present, however, no individual biomarker has yet emerged as a discrete, causal entity that has been shown to account for a sufficient proportion of variance in normative behavior or psychopathology. Nor has any single biomarker been shown to be sensitive or specific to a behavioral disorder. In isolation, biomarkers (whether of functional brain activities, hormonal assays, interpersonal behaviors, and genetic markers—even detailed interpersonal observations or cognitive test scores) are merely *correlates* of behavior problems. In contrast, certain developmental approaches seek to understand the *processes* by which these components have emerged and become integrated across biological, psychological, and social contexts over the individual's life course.

It has been well documented that child maltreatment predicts both unfavorable mental health outcomes and poor responsiveness to mental health treatment (Nanni, Uher, & Danese, 2014). Studies of the neuroscience of attention, executive functioning, and emotion regulation serve to highlight connections between biological systems of domains of behavioral development relevant to the problems experienced by maltreated children. There is developmental evidence that an important facet of risk for maltreated children involves altered neural processing of social stimuli, which broadly impairs their regulatory processes. This research both informs our understanding of the emergence of health problems in children and adults and also sheds light on understanding principles of normative development. In this manner, we increase understanding of how is it that children's social experiences subsequently shape their thoughts, feelings, biology, and behavior. Importantly for this chapter, we believe that a child's social experiences are intricately involved with their parents, both in terms of direct relationships with parents and also via the parent's role as arbiter of other social experiences. This approach has been applied to understanding both internalizing and externalizing types of problem behaviors.

One study sought to understand potential mechanisms that might underlie the association between parent's interactions with their children and children's behaviors and physiology (Shackman & Pollak, 2014). This study found that physically abused children showed greater negative affect and aggression after experiencing an acute, laboratory stressor. Further, these negative emotions were associated with greater aggressive behavior toward children's peers. This association, however, was only present among children who exhibited greater attention to angry faces. These findings demonstrate the impact of child maltreatment on emotional attention that influences children's regulation of emotion and aggression. Another study that examined the relationship between child maltreatment and children's behavior found that children who had been abused tended to exhibit aggressive behaviors (Bernard, Zwerling, & Dozier, 2015). However, this was only true for children who showed little to no change in diurnal cortisol from when they awoke to when they went to sleep. These findings suggest a relationship between maltreatment and dysregulated distress reactivity that may have implications for the development of emotion regulation. Along these lines, dysregulation in stress reactivity was found to mediate the relationship between child maltreatment and the later emergence of externalizing behaviors in a longitudinal study spanning from middle to high school (Heleniak, Jenness, Vander Stoep, McCauley, & McLaughlin, 2015). Such difficulties in emotion regulation place children at greater risk for developing externalizing behavior disorders, have implications for children's social competence, and may negatively influence children's relationships and interactions with their parents.

Yet child maltreatment is not solely associated with any one kind of behavioral problem. Besides externalizing disorders, some children who experienced early maltreatment are at heightened risk for mood disorders. Though not all individuals who experience maltreatment develop depression or anxiety, there are a few factors that appear to be predictive of such outcomes. Recent longitudinal research analyzing mechanisms supporting the relationship between child maltreatment and mood disorders found that children with a greater number of allegations of maltreatment or who are perceived as unpopular in school have a greater chance of developing symptoms of depression and anxiety (Lauterbach & Armour, 2015). Additionally, children whose parents engage in psychologically abusive behaviors such as teasing, name-calling, and intentionally embarrassing also show increases in depressive symptomatology (Paul & Eckenrode, 2015).

One clue about the ways in which the early experience of maltreatment may lead to depression may also be found in observations of these children's attention bias for emotional cues (Pollak et al., 2000). A recent study reported that maltreated children showed attentional biases to depression-relevant cues in certain conditions: first, after they had experienced a sad emotional state, and second, if they tended to have high levels of stable cognitive patterns of rumination (Romens & Pollak, 2011). These cognitive patterns may identify which maltreated children are most likely to exhibit biased attention for sad cues and be at heightened risk for depression. The phenomenon of rumination—passively and repetitively dwelling on and questioning negative feelings in response to distress—is a known risk factor for the development of psychopathology, especially depression (Nolen-Hoeksema, Wisco, & Lyubomirsky, 2008). Recent research in a community sample of 9–14-year-olds showed it was common for youth to focus on an interpersonal stressor for a brief period of time after experiencing it—thus, some rumination appears to be normal and even useful after an interpersonal challenge. Yet about 10% of the youth continued to ruminate for a long period of time after the stressor ended (Hilt & Pollak, 2013). Although most participants were able to disengage from their ruminative thinking, those individuals who continued to ruminate showed attentional biases away from positive stimuli (Hilt & Pollak, 2013). Thus, these children actively avoided environmental cues that might have helped them regain a positive mood state and recover from the stressful event. Similarly, rumination in adolescents is associated with difficulty inhibiting negative information when switching from processing of negative to positive information (Hilt, Leitzke, & Pollak, 2014). The ruminative process is difficult to stop once it has begun. But relatively straightforward interventions, such as brief periods of distraction or mindfulness, appear to be helpful in getting children out of ruminative states (Hilt & Pollak, 2012) and thus may be useful components of interventions for maltreated children.

Also of concern for maltreated children are not just internalizing and externalizing psychopathology, but also subclinical problems that decrease children's quality of life. These include issues such as emotion regulatory difficulties, problems with social competence, factors that interfere with optimal scholastic/school performance, as well as components that affect physical health. A focus on these broader issues reflects the increasingly broad view of the whole child, rather than psychiatric diagnoses in particular. Indeed, children with healthy social information processing abilities (e.g., interpreting social situations appropriately, identifying/regulating emotions, and flexibly selecting/engaging in appropriate social behaviors) tend to be more skilled in initiating and maintaining positive relationships, rely on behaviors that are more pro-social, are more socially accepted by peers, and have more satisfactory friendships (Burgess, Wojslawowicz, Rubin, Rose-Krasnor, & Booth-LaForce, 2006; Fraser et al., 2005; Lemerise & Arsenio, 2000; Quiggle, Garber, & Panak, 1992).

An unintended effect of focusing on underlying biological and cognitive processes versus discrete disorders has been a blurring of traditional disciplinary boundaries. Methods and concepts from fields such as psychiatry, psychology, and pediatrics have come into greater contact with those from internal medicine, immunology, endocrinology, epidemiology/population health, and genetics. For example, research on children's responses to trauma and stress still includes issues such as anxious and aggressive symptoms, but also now includes foci such as sleep, physical growth and bone density, allergy/asthma, infectious disease, and cancer vulnerability (Danese, 2014; Kiecolt-Glaser et al., 2011; Miller, Chen, & Parker, 2011; Shirtcliff, Coe, & Pollak, 2009; Shonkoff, Garner, & the Committee on Psychosocial, Developmental, and Behavioral Pediatrics, 2012; Taylor, Way, & Seeman, 2011). Several large cross-sectional studies have reported relations between child maltreatment and adult health outcomes such as heart disease, cancer, and chronic diseases of the lungs and liver (Gilbert et al., 2009). Today, mental health problems are being understood and linked with indicators of physical health, eroding the distinction between mental and physical ailments. Thus, how researchers approach issues pertaining to child maltreatment and developmental sequelae will benefit from a greater focus on underlying processes and mechanisms (e.g., perception, learning, and problem solving).

Child Maltreatment and Learning Processes

Learning theory provides an account of the emergence of behavior that helps explain how individuals optimize their control of, or adjustment to, an environment. To use learning successfully in complex social situations, individuals are confronted with a difficult task: They must derive efficient representations of the environment from sensory inputs and use these to generalize past experience to new situations. Remarkably, humans and other animals seem to solve these types of problems efficiently through a combination of reinforcement learning and hierarchical sensory processing systems (Schultz, Dayan, & Montague, 1997). Therefore, it is possible that the social information processing difficulties that have been observed in maltreated children could reflect developmental variations in basic associative learning.

Associative learning is when one event or stimulus becomes linked to another event or stimulus through an individual's experience. Such processes can be adaptive when they facilitate the child's accurate prediction of future events on the basis of relevant cues (Gottfried, O'Doherty, & Dolan, 2003; Wasserman & Miller, 1997). When learning proceeds adaptively, it facilitates useful behavioral responses and coping strategies for children. As learning becomes more elaborated, children are able to learn both simple associations and also relationships between stimuli, enabling the formation of general rules or categories that can help guide them through a variety of social experiences (Call, 2001). One component of associative learning, reward processing, provides a useful window into understanding the multiple levels of impact that child abuse and neglect can have on social development.

Rodent studies provide a great deal of information about the neurobiology of socio-emotional behavior. For example, experimental disruption of reward circuitry in the brain prevents mice pups from emitting vocalizations when removed from their mothers; such a disturbance interferes with brain reward systems and also prevents mice from showing a preference for their own mothers (Moles, Kieffer, & D'Amato, 2004). This association also works in the opposite direction: When attachment to the parent is disrupted, other aspects of the animals' reward systems are also affected. Thus, animals with disrupted attachments to their parents also have abnormal responses to novelty, altered appetitive conditioning, and unusually high sensitivity to dopamine antagonists, and reactivity to other drug administrations (for review, see Bakermans-Kranenburg & Van IJzendoorn, 2011; Matthews & Robbins, 2003).

A rich body of evidence across a variety of methods and levels of analyses indicates that aspects of associative learning can be compromised or promoted by environmental experiences. This evidence includes studies that manipulated the rearing environments of monkeys (Capitanio, 1984; Mason & Capitanio, 1988; Mason & Kenney, 1974). Seminal experiments by Papoušek and Papoušek found that exposing infants to response contingent stimulation (as signaled by multicolored lights) affected their learning and their emotional behavior (Papoušek & Papoušek, 2008). Conversely, non-contingent stimulation impaired infant learning (Bigelow & DeCoste, 2003; DeCasper & Carstens, 1981). All of these results suggest that environmental experiences can powerfully shape these learning systems, which would have major implications for behavior.

There are many ways in which an abusive family environment might influence a child's associative learning processes. Past studies of physically abusive parents have shown them to be some combination of impulsive, emotionally volatile, inconsistent in their parenting, and less verbal in discussing/explaining emotional states with their children (Bousha & Twentyman, 1984; Lyons-Ruth & Block, 1996; Oldershaw, Walters, & Hall, 1986; Rohrbeck & Twentyman, 1986; Shackman et al., 2010; Shipman et al., 2007; Timmons & Margolin, 2014). In these ways, children who have suffered from physical abuse are exposed to inconsistent or poorly conveyed emotional signals in their environments.

The abusive adults who ought to be responsible for their children's care tend to convey non-normative emotional displays. Yet these social interactions with primary caregivers are the primary basis upon which these children begin to learn about their social environment. All of these experiences may create a challenging learning environment, making it especially difficult for a child to understand the associations between their behavior and later outcomes. Also, such conditions likely direct children to learn and base their behavior upon aberrant outcomes such as physical violence, which are not typical of most parent–child relationships. This highlights the importance of understanding the role of learning in children's social and emotional development. Understanding the mechanisms underlying learning will help disentangle whether children from aberrant social environments exhibit maladaptive learning processes or more global deficits in learning. Research examining attention and the neural underpinnings of learning in abused children may be particularly helpful in elucidating the relationship between children's environment and learning.

Child Maltreatment and the Development of Attentional Systems Underlying Learning

Children who have been physically abused become adept at recognizing cues of anger and hostility (Ardizzi et al., 2015; Briggs-Gowan et al., 2015; Cicchetti & Curtis, 2005; Curtis & Cicchetti, 2011; da Silva Ferreira, Crippa, & de Lima Osório, 2014; Gibb, McGeary, & Beevers, 2015; Pollak, Vardi, Putzer Bechner, & Curtin, 2005; Shackman & Pollak, 2014; Shackman, Shackman, & Pollak, 2007).

These patterns reflect ways in which children learn to direct their attention to salient and meaningful information in the environment. This type of attention to threat cues in the environment subsequently affects the way children come to construe their social worlds. As an illustration, one study found that 5-year-old abused children tended to believe that almost any kind of interpersonal situation could result in an adult becoming angry; in contrast, most non-abused children saw anger as likely only in particular interpersonal circumstances (Perlman, Kalish, & Pollak, 2008).

These findings have raised new questions about how probabilistic information about other people's behaviors becomes instantiated in children's thinking. Given that children have a limited processing capacity and that there are limitless aspects of the world that can be attended to at any given moment, it may be the case that abused children prioritize negative social cues at the expense of positive cues. For example, when viewing emotional facial expressions, abused children identified as having attachment anxiety exhibit an attentional bias away from facial expressions depicting happiness (Davis et al., 2014). Consistent with this view, on a probabilistic reward task most children respond quickly as their chances of winning a reward increase. In contrast, maltreated children fail to show sensitivity to important environmental cues, such as changing rewards (Guyer et al., 2006; Mueller et al., 2012; Weller & Fisher, 2013). Reports of primate behavior also suggest that maltreated monkeys display less interest in rewards relative to control monkeys (Pryce, Dettling, Spengler, Schnell, & Feldon, 2004). While these findings emphasize the importance of attention in learning processes, a greater understanding of the brain regions associated with learning reward or punishment is likely to help account for the effects of the environment on these children's interpersonal behavior. Indeed, a few candidate brain systems have emerged as potentially underlying these phenomena and provide clues about the development of psychopathology.

Child Maltreatment and the Development of Neural Systems Underlying Learning

Potential brain circuits that might be affected by child maltreatment include the prefrontal cortex (a likely candidate because of its protracted period of postnatal development, as well as ties to behavioral regulation abilities such as impulse control and executive functions), the amygdala (because of ties to emotional regulation), and the basal ganglion (BG), and orbitofrontal cortex (OFC)—which, together, seem to represent the outcomes of situations that the organism has experienced (for a review, see McCrory, De Brito, & Viding, 2010).

Much current research activity has been focused on the role of maltreatment on children's cognitive abilities, specifically executive functioning dependent on the prefrontal cortex (PFC). For example, childhood maltreatment is associated with weakened connectivity between the ventral PFC and subcortical regions such as the amygdala and hippocampus, which may play a role in fear regulation and the development of post-traumatic stress disorder (Birn, Partriat, Phillips, Germain, & Herringa, 2014). Similarly, children reared in deprived environments, such as institutions for the care of orphaned or abandoned children, are at increased risk for attention and behavior regulation difficulties often associated with development of the PFC. Behavioral measures of sustained attention indicate that these children have difficulty with attentional functioning, and event-related potential (ERP) findings have revealed differences in inhibitory control and error monitoring, as post-institutionalized children had smaller N2 amplitudes on a Go/NoGo task as well as smaller error-related negativity on a flanker task (Loman et al., 2012). This pattern of results raises questions regarding the nature of attention difficulties for these children. The behavioral errors likely reflect difficulties in overall sustained attention, whereas the ERP results are consistent with deficits in inhibitory control and error monitoring. However, recent research with children who have experienced severe abuse found increased activation in the dorsomedial frontal cortex during a tracking stop-signal task suggesting greater sensitivity in error monitoring (Lim et al., 2015). To clarify the nature of these effects, further research is needed to explore whether factors such as the severity, chronicity, or type of abuse may differentially influence cognitive functioning. Additionally, greater consistency in tasks and measurements across studies may help in generalizing and reconciling conflicting findings.

The anterior cingulate cortex (ACC) is an area of the frontal cortex implicated in associative learning. Neuronal loss and smaller volumes in the ACC have been reported in children who have suffered physical abuse compared to non-maltreated children (Carrion et al., 2009; De Bellis, Keshavan, Spencer, & Hall, 2000; Teicher, Anderson, Ohashi, & Polcari, 2014; Thomaes, Dorrepaal, & Draijer, 2010). Hanson and colleagues (Hanson et al., 2012) found that children who experienced high levels of early life stress had smaller volumes in the ACC and also more errors during an executive functioning task. In that study, individual differences in ACC volumes accounted for the association between levels of early life stress and the number of errors children made during the task. Research in non-human animals has also noted structural differences in the ACC, with lower dendritic branching in this area in rodents exposed to early stress (Gos, Bock, Poeggel, & Braun, 2008). Functional brain imaging has also revealed lower brain activity in ACC during a cognitive control task in adolescents who suffered abuse (Mueller et al., 2010). Similarly, resting-state functional connectivity points to effects of child maltreatment in the circuit-level dynamics of the ACC related to abuse (Herringa, Birn, & Ruttle, 2013). Computational models, single-unit recording in non-human animals, studies of human patients with brain damage, and basic cognitive neuroscience studies in typically developing humans all cohere in suggesting that the ACC plays a central role in how organisms make predictions and improve those predictions by processing prediction errors (Botvinick, Cohen, & Carter, 2004; Ridderinkhof, 2004; Schultz & Dickinson, 2000). Prediction errors are engines of learning because detecting differences in outcomes guides subsequent actions. Taken together, these findings are consistent with the possibility that children who have suffered physical abuse experience problems related to associative learning processes.

Such processes may lead to a cascade of developmental challenges because they are a major component of adaptive social learning. In this manner, learning difficulties may undermine children's attempts to develop effective strategies to cope with changing environmental contingencies.

The BG is a diverse network of subcortical structures that work in concert to orchestrate and execute planned, motivated behaviors that require integration of movement, thinking, and feeling (Haber, 2003). The OFC is a rapidly flexible associative learning area that is crucial for signaling outcome expectancies such as reward/punishment and the regulation of flexible behavior (Kringelbach & Rolls, 2004). Current thinking is that the BG guides learning based on assessments of the probability of a positive outcome, while the OFC represents gain–loss information and, together, these systems provide a robust way for the organism to learn from and adapt to the environment (Frank & Claus, 2006). As expected, impairments in these systems are associated with poor learning from environmental cues. It is especially interesting that OFC neurons do not stop firing in response to the reward after learning, suggesting that these neurons support predictions on the basis of afferent input and anticipation prior to other emotion-processing regions such as the amygdala (Schoenbaum, Roesch, Stalnaker, & Takahashi, 2009).

Supporting the role of the OFC in associative learning, damage to the OFC causes deficits in reversal learning, reduces the speed of reward learning, and is activated in humans during processes such as regret and counterfactual reasoning (Honey, Kötter, & Breakspear, 2007; Passingham, Stephan, & Kötter, 2002). Common to these examples is the need to signal, in real time, information about outcomes predicted by circumstances in the environment. Some emerging evidence suggests functional changes in the OFC and BG during reward processing in adolescents. This further suggests that these systems are a source of developmental changes in social behavior (Galvan et al., 2006).

There is also some evidence that functioning of these systems may account, in part, for how child maltreatment confers pervasive lifetime risks for children. Many kinds of early life stressors (maternal separation, social defeat, chronic stress exposure, and abuse) appear to alter neurotransmitters and receptors in the BG that are subsequently associated with impairments in learning (DeSteno & Schmauss, 2009). In this regard, child maltreatment has been associated with lower BG recruitment during a reward task (Mehta et al., 2010), and children who experienced early life stress have smaller brain volumes in the OFC (Hanson et al., 2010).

There is less consistency in the literature regarding the effects of physical abuse on the structure and function of the orbitofrontal cortex (OFC). The OFC plays a central role in flexibly adapting behavior in response to changing contingencies (Murray, O'Doherty, & Schoenbaum, 2007). There have been reports of both smaller volumes (Hanson et al., 2010; Holz et al., 2015; McCrory, De Brito, & Viding, 2012) and larger volumes (Carrion et al., 2009) in the OFC for children and adolescents who have suffered physical abuse. No clear explanation exists to date regarding these opposing findings, as researchers have examined similar age participants and with similar types of early life stress. Inconsistencies have also been found in non-human animals, with both dendritic expansion (Liston et al., 2006) and retraction (Helmeke et al., 2009) reported in the OFC after chronic stress exposure. Functional brain imaging may help in clarifying the role of frontal lobe circuitry in developmental problems associated with maltreatment. However, a major limitation of structural imaging is that brain structure and a region's function may not always be in concordance. For example, brain areas may be smaller in volume but exhibit greater activity for specific tasks; brain regions may be larger in volume, but no differences in brain activity may actually be present after controlling for these factors.

There has also been much research attention, as well as inconsistency in findings, regarding the amygdala and its role in emotional dysregulation. The divergence in findings may stem from methodological factors, heterogeneous samples of at-risk children, nonlinear effects of life stress, or a combination of all three. To address some of these issues, Hanson et al. (2015) completed rigorous hand tracing of the amygdala in samples of children who experienced different forms of early stress including physical abuse, early neglect, or extreme family poverty. They found smaller amygdala volumes for children exposed to these different forms of stress, with brain development associated with both greater cumulative stress exposure and the emergence of child behavioral problems (Hanson et al., 2015). These data suggest that early and severe life stress may be associated with increased excitation and cell death, reflected in reductions in brain volume. However, as mentioned previously, brain structure and function are not always concordant. For example, while Hanson et al.'s study found smaller amygdala volume among children who have experienced early life stress, child maltreatment is also associated with a heightened response in the amygdala when viewing negative emotional images (McLaughlin, Peverill, Gold, Alves, & Sheridan, 2015). Caution must be used when inferring developmental patterns from cross-sectional studies; only longitudinal research can truly validate such a model of amygdala development after early stress exposure. Structural and functional alterations in the amygdala may help us understand individual differences in risk and resilience to behavioral problems as related to toxic stress.

What developmental processes might link the above-mentioned components of neural circuitry? One well-understood system is the hypothalamic–pituitary–adrenal (HPA) axis, which is central for understanding the negative effects of stress and trauma on children. When an individual encounters a stressor, corticotropin-releasing hormone (CRH) is secreted from the hypothalamus. This hormone acts on the pituitary gland, causing it to release adrenocorticotropic hormone (ACTH). ACTH then acts upon the adrenal gland, resulting in the production of cortisol. Cortisol binds with glucocorticoid (GR) receptors in the hippocampus to regulate the HPA axis and inhibit further release of CRH. Similarly, cortisol released in response to stress binds with GR receptors at the cellular level to regulate the immune system (Lupien, McEwen, Gunnar, & Heim, 2009). This system promotes adaptation in response to normative stressors. In this manner, toxic or extreme levels of early life stress exposure may impair this system (Koss, Hostinar, Donzella, & Gunnar, 2014).

Other hormone systems also hold potential for understanding how early life adversity affects subsequent social behavior. For example, a recent study examined functioning of the neuropeptide oxytocin (OT) in children aged 8–11 years following a social stressor. Girls with histories of physical abuse showed higher levels of urinary OT and lower levels of salivary cortisol following the stressor when compared to controls (Seltzer, Ziegler, Connolly, Prososki, & Pollak, 2013). Abused and control boys, however, did not differ in their hormonal responses. These data suggest that early adversity may disrupt the development of the stress regulation system in girls by middle childhood, and disruptions of this system have implications for not only children's successful regulation of emotion, but also aspects of comforting behaviors such as the establishment of stable and secure interpersonal relationships. A related study examined the role of the oxytocin receptor gene as a moderator between social support and psychological symptoms among abused children. The polymorphism of the oxytocin receptor gene (rs53576) differentiated outcomes between children with low social support in terms of internalizing symptoms. This is striking in that these groups of children did not differ on objective measures of maltreatment such as type, duration, or severity or abuse (Hostinar, Cicchetti, & Rogosch, 2014). The authors speculated that, unlike maltreated A-carriers, individuals with G/G homozygotes might be more attuned to negative social experiences.

From a developmental perspective, it is important to emphasize that enhanced threat detection (as well as the myriad systems that children use to promote self-regulation and comforting) is critical for children living in contexts that do not provide adequate protection. Thus, neuropeptide systems such as glucocorticoids and oxytocin that play a role in coordinating these responses (Hostinar & Gunnar, 2013) may be important targets for interventions aimed at improving children's adjustment. Additionally, other biological approaches such as epigenetics may further inform our understanding of the influence of child maltreatment on development as well as help in designing effective treatments.

Child Maltreatment and Epigenetic Changes

The use of epigenetic approaches (i.e., regulatory interactants, such as DNA methylation and histone modifications, that determine gene expression) to understand emotion regulatory processes holds tremendous promise for advancing new treatments for children who have experienced maltreatment. Epigenetics may well provide new traction in understanding etiological processes in a range of psychological disorders. While in the past, inheritance was conceptualized in terms of structured base sequences of the DNA code passed from parents' egg and sperm, we now know that the functional expression (or lack of expression) of DNA is inheritable via non-genetic markers arising from parental experiences. Parental behavior can write information onto DNA completely bypassing egg and sperm, adding a level of flexibility that extends the DNA code. This biological flexibility seems quite logical: Through experience, individuals use information about the world they are growing up in, changing DNA to adapt to the environment.

Of particular importance for understanding developmental processes affected by child maltreatment, there appear to be many ways to trigger epigenetic changes. One avenue is the actual characteristics of the environment that might affect gene functioning—such as violence, threat, or instability. But it is also possible that children's interpretations and subjective perceptions of their experience may be enough to trigger epigenetic changes (Slavich & Cole, 2013). As reviewed above, there have been many studies indicating that maltreated children overly attend to threat/hostility in their environments. For example, children who suffered physical abuse are more likely to view others as hostile and the world as generally unsafe (Gibb, 2002; Keil & Price, 2009). These biases influence information processing, with physically abused children incorrectly encoding social cues and exhibiting hostile attributional biases (Teisl & Cicchetti, 2007). Such attentional processes may reflect short-term adaptation to hostile environments, but carry long-term risk for health and behavior, especially given that the behavioral problems of maltreated children are largely accounted for by experiential rather than genetic risk factors (Jaffee, Caspi, Moffitt, & Taylor, 2004).

Although the mechanisms of these effects likely involve diverse cellular and molecular pathways, there is emerging evidence supporting the hypothesis that certain epigenetic changes mediate the effects of early life variations on social interactions (see also Mulder, Rijlaarsdam, & Van IJzendoorn, Chap. 7). Moreover, there may be plasticity within these epigenetic pathways at later developmental time points, such that the social experiences of juveniles and adults may also induce epigenetic change (for review, see Champagne & Curley, 2011). These findings have implications for understanding the emergence of behavior problems—both in early childhood (such as emotion regulation problems) as well as distal problems in adulthood (such as cancer and cardiovascular disease). These data also highlight the dynamic bidirectional interactions occurring between genes and environments during the course of development.

Recently, epigenetic changes in the glucocorticoid receptor gene were examined in whole blood from children aged 11–14 years (Romens, McDonald, Svaren, & Pollak, 2014). The promotor region of the gene is the sequence needed to turn the gene on and off. It is usually found near the beginning of a gene and has binding sites for enzymes that make RNA. In Romens et al.'s study, abused children had more methylation on several sites within exon 1F of the promotor region of the NR3C1 gene, especially CpG site 3, which may have important implications for brain development given that it is the binding site for nerve growth factor (NGF; Weaver et al., 2014). In simple terms, increased methylation of this DNA region in maltreated children functionally depletes the formation of stress receptors, compromising the development of a healthy stress response system. These results have been found in several samples of children who have experienced various forms of early life adversity (for a review, see Palma-Gudiel, Córdova -Palomera, Leza, & Fañanás, 2015). This pattern of results highlights molecular mechanisms linking childhood stress with biological changes that may lead to mental and physical disorders. Indeed, epigenetic changes in several genes (ID3, GRIN1, TPPP) in combination with the experience of maltreatment are associated with an increased risk of depression (Weder et al., 2014). Consistent findings across both rodent and human studies suggest that better parental care and less parental stress decrease methylation of the GR promoter, increasing GR expression. Increased GR expression in the hippocampus reduces stress responsiveness. Though this is an oversimplified explanation (other factors are involved, such as chromatin and histones), the general idea is that methylation inhibits gene transcription and can be thought of as a useful framework for understanding the complexities of gene expression.

But translation of findings across species is difficult. The current GR epigenetic data are consistent with the view that genes can be turned on and off, yet such studies in humans do not imply causality and are limited in terms of specificity of the cellular processes occurring in the brains of living children. They also do not reflect gene expression but rather influence it. What the animal studies can do is to control for confounding variables that are not possible to account for in studies of humans, where we need to be opportunistic in our research. One clear link between controlled animal studies and peripheral measurement of epigenetic changes in humans concerns effects of early stress on immune system competence. Indeed, consistent with peripheral changes in methylation of the glucocorticoid receptor gene, children with early stress exposure show deficits in immune functions (Danese, 2014; Shirtcliff et al., 2009). Such deficits are believed to be a result of poor caregiving experiences, persist into adulthood, and contribute to the development of numerous mental and physical health concerns (Shirtcliff et al., 2009). As such, interventions for at-risk children would benefit from a focus on not only problematic behaviors but also parenting practice.

Clinical Implications

An understanding of developmental processes includes understanding adaptation as well as maladaptation. Therefore, a key aspect of developmentally appropriate interventions requires contextualizing a child's behavior in terms of how it may have been useful to the child in the past. It appears that some cognitive, affective, and behavioral patterns that emerge in stress-exposed children may have allowed children to cope with aberrant life circumstances. As an example, in a psychiatric context, we construe anxiety as a disadvantage. Indeed, anxiety is problematic for individuals living in low-danger, highly consistent environments. But if danger or uncertainty is high, then keeping a low profile and responding quickly to possible threat may be useful. For this reason, it is important to view symptoms within the child's life context rather than solely within their present circumstances. If a child is continuing to live in family context that is unstable, where threat is high, it may well be harmful to reduce the child's anxiety or vigilance to threat. Even at high cost, children need the supports to cope with the realities of their lives.

There is hope for effective interventions. Although data suggest that social experiences can alter human physiology, these changes are not necessarily permanent. For example, there is some evidence for epigenetic reversibility from rodents within the glucocorticoid receptor system (Weaver, 2005). Such advances will require not only that we discover ways to target and change biobehavioral processes, but that we are able to personalize or individualize treatments based on the nature and timing of a child's experience and the individual child's sensitivity/reactivity to those experiences.

Given the considerable effects of the timing and chronicity of early life stress on behavior and neurocognitive functioning (Cowell, Cicchetti, Rogosch, & Toth, 2015), early identification of children who have experienced trauma is crucial. As less than a quarter of adults identified as maltreated during childhood or adolescence have been found to access outpatient mental health services (Ringeisen, Casanueva, Urato, & Stambaugh, 2009), schools and primary care providers are often the first and only contact with the healthcare system. This places school and medical professionals in a critical role to both identify high-risk children and provide appropriate interventions. Research documenting deficits in executive functioning, speech and language, motor skills, memory, attention, and intelligence among maltreated children suggest ways to aid in early identification through administering neuropsychological assessments in schools that target these areas of concern (Davis, Moss, Nogin, & Webb, 2015).

These deficits may also hold promise as targets for intervention. One example is the proliferation of attention bias modification paradigms that have been used to alter emotional attention biases associated with psychopathology (Shechner et al., 2011). Effective behavioral methods have been developed to ameliorate symptoms in a range of mental health problems including anxiety (Amir, Beard, Burns, & Bomyea, 2009), depression (Beevers, Clasen, Enoch, & Schnyer, 2015), phobias (Amir, Taylor, & Donohue, 2011), disordered eating (Renwick, Campbell, & Schmidt, 2013), and substance abuse (Field, Duke, Tyler, & Schoenmakers, 2009). These advances suggest that similar types of approaches—if appropriately tailored—may also help address the threat biases and concomitant behavioral problems among maltreated children.

Evidence-based treatments for victims of maltreatment are also becoming available (Cohen, Scheid, & Gerson, 2014). For example, trauma-focused cognitive behavior therapy is a treatment for traumatized children that provides individual and family therapy and includes parental or caregiver participation as a critical component (Cohen & Mannarino, 2015). Trauma-focused cognitive behavior therapy provides psychoeducation, targets emotion regulation and cognitive processing, and has strong empirical support for improving symptoms of anxiety, depression, and PTSD in addition to behavioral, cognitive, and relationship problems for both children and parents. Greater education in trauma-informed care for professionals in all childcare services will be important in implementing these types of interventions. Beyond the need for more education, successful intervention is going to require collaboration and integrated systems of care to ensure access to appropriate treatments and the provision of community supports and resources for high-risk children in any setting. Such integration will also allow for interventions aimed at preventing child maltreatment.

While treatment for victims of maltreatment may help improve health and behavior outcomes, preventing the occurrence of maltreatment before it occurs remains the most desirable intervention. Given the massive lifetime economic burden of maltreatment (Fang et al., 2012), prevention is also a more cost-effective intervention. To this end, prevention strategies are being developed and implemented in a variety of settings. One example is the Chicago-based Child-Parent Centers (CPC; Reynolds & Robertson, 2003). CPCs provide education for preschool and school-aged children and support services for families in high-poverty areas. The goal of CPCs is to provide environmental support during the transition to school to assist parents in meeting the educational and social needs of their children. A longitudinal examination of the Chicago-based CPCs found that program participants had nearly 50% lower rates of reported maltreatment through age 17 than those who participated in an alternative preschool intervention (Reynolds & Robertson, 2003). Such interventions hold promise for reducing the prevalence and consequences of child maltreatment (see also Havighurst & Kehoe, Chap. 12).

As clinicians and researchers begin to develop new and effective treatments for children, a challenge will involve learning how to tailor interventions for given individuals given those individuals' specific biological and environmental circumstances. At present, many treatments for children remain somewhat generic, with popular approaches such as cognitive behavioral, mindfulness, or attachment-oriented therapies being applied similarly across a range of mental health conditions, ages, and individual differences. In addition, intervention studies tend to focus on very broad, non-specific behavioral outcome measures, such as ratings or interviews of overt symptomatology, school achievement, or observed ratings of behavior. But our behavioral constructs have not yet evolved to have the same level of mechanistic specificity as newer biological measures. As described above, great efforts have been made to provide treatment and prevention for high-risk children; however, more sensitive and specific behavioral measures will be necessary to truly discern the processes underlying mental health issues.

Implications for Understanding Parenting

A critical component of these types of interventions is addressing the parent–child relationship. Research on parenting stress, as outlined in this book, demonstrates the profound impact of individuals' environments and mental and physical health on various domains of parenting. This includes the impact of children's own behavior and functioning on their parents as a source of stress. As research focuses on the impact of aberrant parenting on children's development, the role of parents themselves has often been overlooked. While it may be true that some parents lack the ability to appropriately care for children, it is more likely the case that parents' caregiving is impacted by environmental circumstances (Neece, Green, & Baker, 2012; Whipple & Webster-Stratton, 1991; see also Finegood & Blair, Chap. 8; Neece & Chan, Chap. 5). As economic and familial stressors mount, caregiving quality is likely to decline. In this way, as poor parenting influences children's behavior, so too does children's compromised behavior (e.g., poor self-regulation) impact parents' burden of stress. Indeed, some of the behaviors identified as possible consequences of child maltreatment described above may result in increased stress and problems for parents. It may be that highly stressed and overburdened parents are less likely to model appropriate behaviors and mood regulation that may contribute to the exacerbation of externalizing behaviors and dysregulation found in maltreated children (see Bernard, Zwerling, & Dozier, 2015; Heleniak et al. 2015). This transactional relationship outlines the reciprocal nature of parenting and children's behaviors and emphasizes the need to target both the parent and child for intervention.

Research examining the mechanisms linking children's early social environments and later functioning has helped inform the timing and means of intervention for at-risk youth. Similarly, elucidating the role of child development and behavior on parental stress may help guide the development of appropriate interventions for parents. Fortunately, as mentioned above, some of the interventions designed to target children's behaviors that may manifest as a result of adverse experiences incorporate parenting as a key component. Such treatments aim to improve children's environments and reduce problematic behaviors but do so acknowledging the important role of parents in dictating their children's environment. In this way, treating and educating parents and children alike may help improve both child and parent health.

Conclusion

As illustrated in this chapter, successful social adaptation reflects children's ability to learn from complex and varied interpersonal experiences. Children need to discern factors including cues for approach versus withdrawal, actions that lead to punishments versus rewards, and which behaviors lead to success in having needs and desires met. These processes become increasingly intricate and fine-tuned as relevant neuroanatomical systems develop, and as the range, complexity, and amount of social information increase for the developing child. A focus on developmental processes across levels of analysis allows us to formulate questions about which neural mechanisms humans use to process socio-emotional information, how these mechanisms are themselves shaped by social context, why adverse social environments confer risk for children, and, perhaps, what sorts of neurally informed interventions might remediate deficits in self-regulation.

References

Amir, N., Beard, C., Burns, M., & Bomyea, J. (2009). Attention modification program in individuals with generalized anxiety disorder. *Journal of Abnormal Psychology, 118*(1), 28–33. doi:10.1037/a0012589

Amir, N., Taylor, C. T., & Donohue, M. C. (2011). Predictors of response to an attention modification program in generalized social phobia. *Journal of Consulting and Clinical Psychology, 79*(4), 533–541. doi:10.1037/a0023808

Ardizzi, M., Martini, F., Umiltà, M. A., Evangelista, V., Ravera, R., & Gallese, V. (2015). Impact of childhood maltreatment on the recognition of facial expressions of emotions. *PloS One, 10* (10), e0141732–19. doi:10.1371/journal.pone.0141732

Bakermans-Kranenburg, M. J., & Van IJzendoorn, M. H. (2011). Differential susceptibility to rearing environment depending on dopamine-related genes: New evidence and a meta-analysis. *Development and Psychopathology, 23*(01), 39–52. doi:10.1017/S0954579410000635

Beevers, C. G., Clasen, P. C., Enoch, P. M., & Schnyer, D. M. (2015). Attention bias modification for major depressive disorder: Effects on attention bias, resting state connectivity, and symptom change. *Journal of Abnormal Psychology, 124*(3), 463–475. doi:10.1037/abn0000049

Bernard, K., Zwerling, J., & Dozier, M. (2015). Effects of early adversity on young children's diurnal cortisol rhythms and externalizing behavior. *Developmental Psychobiology, 57*(8), 935–947. doi:10.1002/dev.21324

Bigelow, A. E., & DeCoste, C. (2003). Sensitivity to social contingency from mothers and strangers in 2-, 4-, and 6-month-old infants. *Infancy, 4*(1), 111–140. doi:10.1207/S15327078IN0401_6

Birn, R. M., Patriat, R., Phillips, M. L., Germain, A., & Herringa, R. J. (2014). Childhood maltreatment and combat posttraumatic stress differentially predict fear-related fronto-subcortical connectivity. *Depression and Anxiety, 31*(10), 880–892. doi:10.1002/da.22291

Botvinick, M. M., Cohen, J. D., & Carter, C. S. (2004). Conflict monitoring and anterior cingulate cortex: An update. *Trends in Cognitive Sciences, 8*(12), 539–546. doi:10.1016/j.tics.2004.10.003

Bousha, D. M., & Twentyman, C. T. (1984). Mother–child interactional style in abuse, neglect, and control groups: Naturalistic observations in the home. *Journal of Abnormal Psychology*. doi:10.1037/0021-843X.93.1.106

Briggs-Gowan, M. J., Pollak, S. D., Grasso, D., Voss, J., Mian, N. D., Zobel, E., … & Pine, D.S. (2015). Attention bias and anxiety in young children exposed to family violence. *Journal of Child Psychology and Psychiatry, 56*(11), 1194–1201. doi:10.1111/jcpp.12397

Burgess, K. B., Wojslawowicz, J. C., Rubin, K. H., Rose-Krasnor, L., & Booth-LaForce, C. (2006). Social information processing and coping strategies of shy/withdrawn and aggressive children: Does friendship matter? *Child Development, 77*(2), 371–383. doi:10.1111/j.1467-8624.2006.00876.x

Call, J. (2001). Chimpanzee social cognition. *Trends in Cognitive Sciences, 5*(9), 388–393. doi:10.1016/S1364-6613(00)01728-9

Capitanio, J. P. (1984). Early experience and social processes in Rhesus macaques (Macaca Mulatta): I. Dyadic social interaction. *Journal of Comparative Psychology, 98*(1), 35. doi:10.1037/0735-7036.98.1.35

Carrion, V. G., Weems, C. F., Watson, C., Eliez, S., Menon, V., & Reiss, A. L. (2009). Converging evidence for abnormalities of the prefrontal cortex and evaluation of midsagittal structures in pediatric posttraumatic stress disorder: An MRI study. *Psychiatry Research: Neuroimaging, 172*(3), 226–234. doi:10.1016/j.pscychresns.2008.07.008

Champagne, F. A., & Curley, J. P. (2011). Epigenetic influence of the social environment. In *Brain, Behavior and Epigenetics* (pp. 185–208). Berlin Heidelberg: Springer. doi:10.1007/978-3-642-17426-1_10

Cicchetti, D., & Curtis, W. (2005). An event-related potential study of the processing of affective facial expressions in young children who experienced maltreatment during the first year of life. *Development and Psychopathology, 17*(03), 641–677. doi:10.1017/S0954579405050315

Cohen, J. A., & Mannarino, A. P. (2015). Trauma-focused cognitive behavior therapy for traumatized children and families. *Child Adolescent Psychiatric Clinics of North America, 24* (3), 557–570. doi:10.1016/j.chc.2015.02.005

Cohen, J. A., Scheid, J., & Gerson, R. (2014). Transforming trajectories for traumatized children. *Journal of the American Academy of Child and Adolescent Psychiatry, 53*(1), 9–13. doi:10.1016/j.jaac.2013.10.004

Cowell, R. A., Cicchetti, D., Rogosch, F. A., & Toth, S. L. (2015). Childhood maltreatment and its effect on neurocognitive functioning: Timing and chronicity matter. *Development and Psychopathology, 27*(02), 521–533. doi:10.1017/S0954579415000139

Curtis, W. J., & Cicchetti, D. (2011). Affective facial expression processing in young children who have experienced maltreatment during the first year of life: An event-related potential study. *Development and Psychopathology, 23*(02), 373–395. doi:10.1017/S0954579411000125

da Silva Ferreira, G. C., Crippa, J. A. S., & de Lima Osório, F. (2014). Facial emotion processing and recognition among maltreated children: A systematic literature review. *Frontiers in Psychology, 5*. doi:10.3389/fpsyg.2014.01460/abstract

Danese, A. (2014). Developmental psychoneuroimmunology: From bench to bedside. *Brain Behavior and Immunity, 36*(C), 27–28. doi:10.1016/j.bbi.2013.11.001

Danese, A., Moffitt, T. E., Harrington, H., Milne, B. J., Polanczyk, G., Pariante, C. M., … & Caspi, A. (2009). Adverse childhood experiences and adult risk factors for age-related disease. *Archives of Pediatrics & Adolescent Medicine, 163*(12), 1–17. doi:10.1001/archpediatrics.2009.214

Davis, J. S., Fani, N., Ressler, K., Jovanovic, T., Tone, E. B., & Bradley, B. (2014). Attachment anxiety moderates the relationship between childhood maltreatment and attention bias for emotion in adults. *Psychiatry Research, 217*(1–2), 79–85. doi:10.1016/j.psychres.2014.03.010

Davis, A. S., Moss, L. E., Nogin, M. M., & Webb, N. E. (2015). Neuropsychology of child maltreatment and implications for school psychologists. *Psychology in the Schools, 52*(1), 77–91. doi:10.1002/pits.21806

De Bellis, M. D., Keshavan, M. S., Spencer, S., & Hall, J. (2000). N-Acetylaspartate concentration in the anterior cingulate of maltreated children and adolescents with PTSD. *American Journal of Psychiatry, 157*(7), 1175–1177. doi:10.1176/appi.ajp.157.7.1175

DeCasper, A. J., & Carstens, A. A. (1981). Contingencies of stimulation: Effects on learning and emotion in neonates. *Infant Behavior & Development, 4(1)*, 19–35. doi:10.1016/S0163-6383(81)80004-5

DeSteno, D. A., & Schmauss, C. (2009). A role for dopamine D2 receptors in reversal learning. *Neuroscience, 162*(1), 118–127. doi:10.1016/j.neuroscience.2009.04.052

Fang, X., Brown, D. S., Florence, C. S., & Mercy, J. A. (2012). The economic burden of child maltreatment in the United States and implications for prevention. *Child Abuse and Neglect, 36* (2), 156–165. doi:10.1016/j.chiabu.2011.10.006

Fang, X., & Corso, P. S. (2007). Child maltreatment, youth violence, and intimate partner violence. *American Journal of Preventive Medicine, 33*(4), 281–290. doi:10.1016/j.amepre.2007.06.003

Felitti, M. D., Vincent, J., Anda, M. D., & Robert, F. (1998). Relationship of childhood abuse and household dysfunction to many of the leading causes of death in adults: The adverse childhood experiences (ACE) study. *American Journal of Preventative Medicine, 14*(4), 245–258. doi:10.1016/S0749-3797(98)00017-8

Field, M., Duka, T., Tyler, E., & Schoenmakers, T. (2009). Attentional bias modification in tobacco smokers. *Nicotine & Tobacco Research, 11*(7), 812–822. doi:10.1093/ntr/ntp067

Frank, M. J., & Claus, E. D. (2006). Anatomy of a decision: Striato-orbitofrontal interactions in reinforcement learning, decision making, and reversal. *Psychological Review, 113*(2), 300–326. doi:10.1037/0033-295X.113.2.300

Fraser, M. W., Galinsky, M. J., Smokowski, P. R., Day, S. H., Terzian, M. A., Rose, R. A., et al. (2005). Social information-processing skills training to promote social competence and prevent aggressive behavior in the third grades. *Journal of Consulting and Clinical Psychology, 73*(6), 1045–1055. doi:10.1037/0022-006X.73.6.1045

Galvan, A., Hare, T. A., Parra, C. E., Penn, J., Voss, H., Glover, G., et al. (2006). Earlier development of the accumbens relative to orbitofrontal cortex might underlie risk-taking behavior in adolescents. *The Journal of Neuroscience, 26*(25), 6885–6892. doi:10.1523/JNEUROSCI.1062-06.2006

Gibb, B. E. (2002). Childhood maltreatment and negative cognitive styles. *Clinical Psychology Review, 22*(2), 223–246. doi:10.1016/S0272-7358(01)00088-5

Gibb, B. E., McGeary, J. E., & Beevers, C. G. (2015). Attentional biases to emotional stimuli: Key components of the RDoC constructs of sustained threat and loss. *American Journal of Medical Genetics Part B: Neuropsychiatric Genetics, 171*(1), 65–80. doi:10.1002/ajmg.b.32383

Gilbert, R., Widom, C. S., Browne, K., Fergusson, D., Webb, E., & Johnson, S. (2009). Burden and consequences of child maltreatment in high-income countries. *The Lancet, 373*(9657), 68–81. doi:10.1016/S0140-6736(08)61706-7

Gos, T., Bock, J., Poeggel, G., & Braun, K. (2008). Stress-induced synaptic changes in the rat anterior cingulate cortex are dependent on endocrine developmental time windows. *Synapse, 62*(3), 229–232. doi:10.1002/syn.20477

Gottfried, J. A., O'Doherty, J., & Dolan, R. J. (2003). Encoding predictive reward value in human amygdala and orbitofrontal cortex. *Science, 301*(5636), 1104–1107. doi:10.1126/science.1087919

Guyer, A. E., Kaufman, J., Hodgdon, H. B., Masten, C. L., Jazbec, S., Pine, D. S., et al. (2006). Behavioral alterations in reward system function. *Journal of the American Academy of Child and Adolescent Psychiatry, 45*(9), 1059–1067. doi:10.1097/01.chi.0000227882.50404.11

Haber, S. N. (2003). The primate basal ganglia: Parallel and integrative networks. *Journal of Chemical Neuroanatomy, 26*(4), 317–330. doi:10.1016/j.jchemneu.2003.10.003

Hanson, J. L., Adluru, N., Chung, M. K., Alexander, A. L., Davidson, R. J., & Pollak, S. D. (2013a). Early neglect is associated with alterations in white matter integrity and cognitive functioning. *Child Development, 84*(5), 1566–1578. doi:10.1111/cdev.12069

Hanson, J. L., Chung, M. K., Avants, B. B., Rudolph, K. D., Shirtcliff, E. A., Gee, J. C., … & Pollak, S. D. (2012). Structural variations in prefrontal cortex mediate the relationship between early childhood stress and spatial working memory. *The Journal of Neuroscience, 32*(23), 7917–7925. doi:10.1523/JNEUROSCI.0307-12.2012

Hanson, J. L., Chung, M. K., Avants, B. B., Shirtcliff, E. A., Gee, J. C., Davidson, R. J., et al. (2010). Early stress is associated with alterations in the orbitofrontal cortex: A tensor-based morphometry investigation of brain structure and behavioral risk. *The Journal of Neuroscience, 30*(22), 7466–7472. doi:10.1523/JNEUROSCI.0859-10.2010

Hanson, J. L., Hair, N., Shen, D. G., Shi, F., Gilmore, J. H., Wolfe, B. L., & Pollak, S. D. (2013b). Family poverty affects the rate of human infant brain growth. *PloS One, 8*(12), e80954–9. doi:10.1371/journal.pone.0080954

Hanson, J. L., Nacewicz, B. M., Sutterer, M. J., Cayo, A. A., Schaefer, S. M., Rudolph, K. D., … Davidson, R. J. (2015). Behavioral problems after early life stress: Contributions of the hippocampus and amygdala. *Biological Psychiatry, 77*(4), 314–323. doi:10.1016/j.biopsych.2014.04.020

Heleniak, C., Jenness, J. L., Vander Stoep, A., McCauley, E., & McLaughlin, K. A. (2015). Childhood maltreatment exposure and disruptions in emotion regulation: A transdiagnostic pathway to adolescent internalizing and externalizing psychopathology. *Cognitive Therapy and Research*, 1–22. doi:10.1007/s10608-015-9735-z

Helmeke, C., Seidel, K., Poeggel, G., Bredy, T. W., Abraham, A., & Braun, K. (2009). Paternal deprivation during infancy results in dendrite- and time-specific changes of dendritic development and spine formation in the orbitofrontal cortex of the biparental rodent Octodon Degus. *Neuroscience, 163*(3), 790–798. doi:10.1016/j.neuroscience.2009.07.008

Herringa, R. J., Birn, R. M., & Ruttle, P. L. (2013). Childhood maltreatment is associated with altered fear circuitry and increased internalizing symptoms by late adolescence. *Proceedings of the National Academy of Science, 110*(47), 19119–19124. doi:10.1073/pnas.1310766110/-/DCSupplemental

Hilt, L. M., Leitzke, B. T., & Pollak, S. D. (2014). Cognitive control and rumination in youth: The importance of emotion. *Journal of Experimental Psychopathology, 5*(3), 302–313. doi:10.5127/jep.038113

Hilt, L. M., & Pollak, S. D. (2012). Getting out of rumination: Comparison of three brief interventions in a sample of youth. *Journal of Abnormal Child Psychology, 40*(7), 1157–1165. doi:10.1007/s10802-012-9638-3

Hilt, L. M., & Pollak, S. D. (2013). Characterizing the ruminative process in young adolescents. *Journal of Clinical Child and Adolescent Psychology, 42*(4), 519–530. doi:10.1080/15374416.2013.764825

Holz, N. E., Boecker, R., Hohm, E., Zohsel, K., Buchmann, A. F., Blomeyer, D., … & Laucht, M. (2015). The long-term impact of early life poverty on orbitofrontal cortex volume in adulthood: Results from a prospective study over 25 years. *Neuropsychopharmacology, 40*(4), 996–1004. doi:10.1038/npp.2014.277

Honey, C. J., Kötter, R., & Breakspear, M. (2007). Network structure of cerebral cortex shapes functional connectivity on multiple time scales. *Proceedings of the National Academy of Sciences, 104*(24), 10240–10245. doi:10.1073/pnas.0701519104

Hostinar, C. E., Cicchetti, D., & Rogosch, F. A. (2014). Oxytocin receptor gene polymorphism, perceived social support, and psychological symptoms in maltreated adolescents. *Development and Psychopathology, 26*(02), 465–477. doi:10.1017/S0954579414000066

Hostinar, C. E., & Gunnar, M. R. (2013). The developmental effects of early life stress: An overview of current theoretical frameworks. *Current Directions in Psychological Science, 22* (5), 400–406. doi:10.1177/0963721413488889

Jaffee, S. R., Caspi, A., Moffitt, T. E., & Taylor, A. (2004). Physical maltreatment victim to antisocial child: Evidence of an environmentally mediated process. *Journal of Abnormal Psychology, 113*(1), 44–55. doi:10.1037/0021-843X.113.1.44

Keil, V., & Price, J. M. (2009). Social information-processing patterns of maltreated children in two social domains. *Journal of Applied Developmental Psychology, 30*(1), 43–52. doi:10.1016/j.appdev.2008.10.003

Kiecolt-Glaser, J. K., Gouin, J. P., Weng, N. P., Malarkey, W. B., Beversdorf, D. Q., & Glaser, R. (2011). Childhood adversity heightens the impact of later-life caregiving stress on telomere length and inflammation. *Psychosomatic Medicine, 73,* 16–22. doi:10.1097/PSY.0b013e31820573b6

Koenen, K. C., Moffitt, T. E., Poulton, R., Martin, J., & Caspi, A. (2007). Early childhood factors associated with the development of post-traumatic stress disorder: Results from a longitudinal birth cohort. *Psychological Medicine, 37*(02), 181–192. doi:10.1017/S0033291706009019

Koss, K. J., Hostinar, C. E., Donzella, B., & Gunnar, M. R. (2014). Social deprivation and the HPA axis in early development. *Psychoneuroendocrinology, 50,* 1–13. doi:10.1016/j.psyneuen.2014.07.028

Kringelbach, M., & Rolls, E. (2004). The functional neuroanatomy of the human orbitofrontal cortex: Evidence from neuroimaging and neuropsychology. *Progress in Neurobiology, 72*(5), 341–372. doi:10.1016/j.pneurobio.2004.03.006

Lauterbach, D., & Armour, C. (2015). Symptom trajectories among child survivors of maltreatment: Findings from the longitudinal studies of child abuse and neglect (LONGSCAN). *Journal of Abnormal Child Psychology*, 1–11. doi:10.1007/s10802-015-9998-6

Leeb, R.T., Paulozzi, L., Melanson, C., Simon, T., & Arias, I. (2008). *Child maltreatment surveillance: Uniform definitions for public health and recommended data elements.* Centers for Disease Control and Prevention, National Center for Injury Prevention and Control.

Lemerise, E. A., & Arsenio, W. F. (2000). An integrated model of emotion processes and cognition in social information processing. *Child Development, 71*(1), 107–118. doi:10.1111/1467-8624.00124

Lim, L., Hart, H., Mehta, M. A., Simmons, A., Mirza, K., & Rubia, K. (2015). Neural correlates of error processing in young people with a history of severe childhood abuse: An fMRI study. *American Journal of Psychiatry, 172*(9), 892–900. doi:10.1176/appi.ajp.2015.14081042

Liston, C., Miller, M. M., Goldwater, D. S., Radley, J. J., Rocher, A. B., Hof, P. R., … & McEwen, B. S. (2006). Stress-induced alterations in prefrontal cortical dendritic morphology predict selective impairments in perceptual attentional set-shifting. *The Journal of Neuroscience, 26*(30), 7870–7874. doi:10.1523/JNEUROSCI.1184-06.2006

Loman, M. M., Johnson, A. E., Westerlund, A., Pollak, S. D., Nelson, C. A., & Gunnar, M. R. (2012). The effect of early deprivation on executive attention in middle childhood. *Journal of Child Psychology and Psychiatry, 54*(1), 37–45. doi:10.1111/j.1469-7610.2012.02602.x

Lupien, S. J., McEwen, B. S., Gunnar, M. R., & Heim, C. (2009). Effects of stress throughout the lifespan on the brain, behaviour and cognition. *Nature Reviews Neuroscience, 10*(6), 434–445. doi:10.1038/nrn2639

Lyons-Ruth, K., & Block, D. (1996). The disturbed caregiving system: Relations among childhood trauma, maternal caregiving, and infant affect and attachment. *Infant Mental Health Journal, 17*(3), 257–275. doi:10.1002/(SICI)1097-0355(199623)17:3<257:AID-IMHJ5>3.0.CO;2-L

Mason, W. A., & Capitanio, J. P. (1988). Formation and expression of filial attachment in Rhesus monkeys raised with living and inanimate mother substitutes. *Developmental Psychobiology*. doi:10.1002/dev.420210502/pdf

Mason, W. A., & Kenney, M. D. (1974). Redirection of filial attachments in Rhesus monkeys: dogs as mother surrogates. *Science, 183*(4130), 1209–1211. doi:10.1126/science.183.4130.1209

Matthews, K., & Robbins, T. W. (2003). Early experience as a determinant of adult behavioural responses to reward: The effects of repeated maternal separation in the rat. *Neuroscience and Biobehavioral Reviews, 27*(1–2), 45–55. doi:10.1016/S0149-7634(03)00008-3

McCrory, E., De Brito, S. A., & Viding, E. (2010). Research Review: The neurobiology and genetics of maltreatment and adversity. *Journal of Child Psychology and Psychiatry, 51*(10), 1079–1095. doi:10.1111/j.1469-7610.2010.02271.x

McCrory, E., De Brito, S. A., & Viding, E. (2012). The link between child abuse and psychopathology: A review of neurobiological and genetic research. *Journal of the Royal Society of Medicine, 105*(4), 151–156. doi:10.1258/jrsm.2011.110222

McLaughlin, K. A., Peverill, M., Gold, A. L., Alves, S., & Sheridan, M. A. (2015). Child maltreatment and neural systems underlying emotion regulation. *Journal of the American Academy of Child and Adolescent Psychiatry, 54*(9), 753–762. doi:10.1016/j.jaac.2015.06.010

Mehta, M. A., Gore-Langton, E., Golembo, N., Colvert, E., Williams, S. C., & Sonuga-Barke, E. (2010). Hyporesponsive reward anticipation in the basal ganglia following severe institutional deprivation early in life. *Journal of Cognitive Neuroscience, 22*(10), 2316–2325. doi:10.1162/jocn.2009.21394

Miller, G. E., Chen, E., & Parker, K. J. (2011). Psychological stress in childhood and susceptibility to the chronic diseases of aging: Moving toward a model of behavioral and biological mechanisms. *Psychological Bulletin, 137*(6), 959–997. doi:10.1037/a0024768

Moles, A., Kieffer, B. L., & D'Amato, F. R. (2004). Deficit in attachment behavior in mice lacking the μ-opioid receptor gene. *Science, 304*(5679), 1983–1986. doi:10.1126/science.1095943

Mueller, S. C., Hardin, M. G., Korelitz, K., Daniele, T., Bemis, J., Dozier, M., … & Ernst, M. (2012). Incentive effect on inhibitory control in adolescents with early-life stress: An antisaccade study. *Child Abuse & Neglect, 36*(3), 217–225. doi:10.1016/j.chiabu.2011.10.010

Mueller, S. C., Maheu, F. S., Dozier, M., Peloso, E., Mandell, D., Leibenluft, E., … & Ernst, M. (2010). Early-life stress is associated with impairment in cognitive control in adolescence: An fMRI study. *Neuropsychologia, 48*(10), 3037–3044. doi:10.1016/j.neuropsychologia.2010.06.013

Murray, E. A., O'Doherty, J. P., & Schoenbaum, G. (2007). What we know and do not know about the functions of the orbitofrontal cortex after 20 years of cross-species studies. *The Journal of Neuroscience, 27*(31), 8166–8169. doi:10.1523/JNEUROSCI.1556-07.2007

Nanni, V., Uher, R., & Danese, A. (2014). Childhood maltreatment predicts unfavorable course of illness and treatment outcome in depression: A meta-analysis. *American Journal of Psychiatry*. doi:10.1176/appi.ajp.2011.11020335

Neece, L. C., Green, S. A., & Baker, B. L. (2012). Parenting stress and child behavior problems: A transactional relationship across time. *American Journal of Intellectual Developmental Disabilities, 117,* 48–66. doi:10.1352/1944-7558-117.1.48

Nolen-Hoeksema, S., Wisco, B. E., & Lyubomirsky, S. (2008). Rethinking rumination. *Perspectives on Psychological Science, 3*(5), 400–424. doi:10.1111/j.1745-6924.2008.00088.x

Oldershaw, L., Walters, G. C., & Hall, D. K. (1986). Control strategies and noncompliance in abusive mother-child dyads: An observational study. *Child Development*. 722–732. doi:10.2307/1130349

Palma-Gudiel, H., Córdova-Palomera, A., Leza, J. C., & Fañanás, L. (2015). Glucocorticoid receptor gene (NR3C1) methylation processes as mediators of early adversity in stress-related disorders causality: A critical review. *Neuroscience and Biobehavioral Reviews, 55,* 520–535. doi:10.1016/j.neubiorev.2015.05.016

Papoušek, H., & Papoušek, M. (2008). Cognitive aspects of preverbal social interaction between human infants and adults. In *Ciba Foundation Symposium 33—Parent-Infant Interaction* (pp. 241–269). Chichester, UK: John Wiley. doi:10.1002/9780470720158.ch14

Passingham, R. E., Stephan, K. E., & Kötter, R. (2002). The anatomical basis of functional localization in the cortex. *Nature Reviews Neuroscience, 3*(8), 606–616. doi:10.1038/nrn893

Paul, E., & Eckenrode, J. (2015). Childhood psychological maltreatment subtypes and adolescent depressive symptoms. *Child Abuse and Neglect, 47,* 38–47. doi:10.1016/j.chiabu.2015.05.018

Perlman, S. B., Kalish, C. W., & Pollak, S. D. (2008). The role of maltreatment experience in children's understanding of the antecedents of emotion. *Cognition and Emotion, 22*(4), 651–670. doi:10.1080/02699930701461154

Pollak, S. D., Cicchetti, D., Hornung, K., & Reed, A. (2000). Recognizing emotion in faces: Developmental effects of child abuse and neglect. *Developmental Psychology, 36*(5), 679–688. doi:10.1037//0012-1649.36.5.679

Pollak, S. D., Nelson, C. A., Schlaak, M. F., Roeber, B. J., Wewerka, S. S., Wiik, K. L., ... & Gunnar, M. R. (2010). Neurodevelopmental effects of early deprivation in postinstitutionalized children. *Child Development, 81*(1), 224–236. doi:10.1111/j.1467-8624.2009.01391.x

Pollak, S. D., Vardi, S., Putzer Bechner, A. M., & Curtin, J. J. (2005). Physically abused children's regulation of attention in response to hostility. *Child Development, 76*(5), 968–977. doi:10.1111/j.1467-8624.2005.00890.x

Poulton, R., Moffitt, T. E., & Silva, P. A. (2015). The Dunedin multidisciplinary health and development study: Overview of the first 40 years, with an eye to the future. *Social Psychiatry and Psychiatric Epidemiology, 50*(5), 679–693. doi:10.1007/s00127-015-1048-8

Pryce, C. R., Dettling, A. C., Spengler, M., Schnell, C. R., & Feldon, J. (2004). Deprivation of parenting disrupts development of homeostatic and reward systems in Marmoset monkey offspring. *Biological Psychiatry, 56*(2), 72–79. doi:10.1016/j.biopsych.2004.05.002

Quiggle, N. L., Garber, J., & Panak, W. F. (1992). Social information processing in aggressive and depressed children. *Child Development, 63*(6), 1305–1320. doi:10.1111/j.1467-8624.1992.tb01696.x/full

Ramrakha, S., Bell, M. L., Paul, C., & Dickson, N. (2007). Childhood behavior problems linked to sexual risk taking in young adulthood: A birth cohort study. *Journal of the American Academy of Child and Adolescent Psychiatry, 46*(10), 1272–1279. doi:10.1097/chi.0b013e3180f6340e

Renwick, B., Campbell, I. C., & Schmidt, U. (2013). Attention bias modification: A new approach to the treatment of eating disorders? *International Journal of Eating Disorders, 46*(5), 496–500. doi:10.1002/eat.22107

Reynolds, A. J., & Robertson, D. L. (2003). School-based early intervention and later child maltreatment in the Chicago longitudinal study. *Child Development, 74*(1), 3–26. doi:10.1111/1467-8624.00518

Ridderinkhof, K. R. (2004). The role of the medial frontal cortex in cognitive control. *Science, 306* (5695), 443–447. doi:10.1126/science.1100301

Ringeisen, H., Casanueva, C. E., Urato, M., & Stambaugh, L. F. (2009). Mental health service use during the transition to adulthood for adolescents reported to the child welfare system. *Psychiatric Services, 60,* 1084–1091.

Rohrbeck, C. A., & Twentyman, C. T. (1986). Multimodal assessment of impulsiveness in abusing, neglecting, and nonmaltreating mothers and their preschool children. *Journal of Consulting and Clinical Psychology, 54*(2), 231. doi:10.1037/0022-006X.54.2.231

Romens, S. E., McDonald, J., Svaren, J., & Pollak, S. D. (2014). Associations between early life stress and gene methylation in children. *Child Development, 86*(1), 303–309. doi:10.1111/cdev.12270

Romens, S. E., & Pollak, S. D. (2011). Emotion regulation predicts attention bias in maltreated children At-risk for depression. *Journal of Child Psychology and Psychiatry, 53*(2), 120–127. doi:10.1111/j.1469-7610.2011.02474.x

Schoenbaum, G., Roesch, M. R., Stalnaker, T. A., & Takahashi, Y. K. (2009). A new perspective on the role of the orbitofrontal cortex in adaptive behaviour. *Nature Reviews Neuroscience, 10* (12), 885–892. doi:10.1038/nrn2753

Schultz, W., Dayan, P., & Montague, P. R. (1997). A neural substrate of prediction and reward. *Science, 275*(5306), 1593–1599. doi:10.1126/science.275.5306.1593

Schultz, W., & Dickinson, A. (2000). Neuronal coding of prediction errors. *Annual Review of Neuroscience, 23*(1), 473–500. doi:10.1146/annurev.neuro.23.1.473

Seltzer, L. J., Ziegler, T., Connolly, M. J., Prososki, A. R., & Pollak, S. D. (2013). Stress-induced elevation of oxytocin in maltreated children: Evolution, neurodevelopment, and social behavior. *Child Development, 85*(2), 501–512. doi:10.1111/cdev.12136

Shackman, J. E., Fatani, S., Camras, L. A., Berkowitz, M. J., Bachorowski, J.-A., & Pollak, S. D. (2010). Emotion expression among abusive mothers is associated with their children's emotion processing and problem behaviours. *Cognition and Emotion, 24*(8), 1421–1430. doi:10.1080/02699930903399376

Shackman, J. E., & Pollak, S. D. (2014). Impact of physical maltreatment on the regulation of negative affect and aggression. *Development and Psychopathology*, 1–13. doi:10.1017/S0954579414000546

Shackman, J. E., Shackman, A. J., & Pollak, S. D. (2007). Physical abuse amplifies attention to threat and increases anxiety in children. *Emotion, 7*(4), 838–852. doi:10.1037/1528-3542.7.4.838

Shechner, T., Britton, J. C., Pérez-Edgar, K., Bar-Haim, Y., Ernst, M., Fox, N. A., … & Pine, D. S. (2011). Attention biases, anxiety, and development: Toward or away from threats or rewards? *Depression and Anxiety, 29*(4), 282–294. doi:10.1002/da.20914

Sheridan, M. A., Fox, N. A., & Zeanah, C. H. (2012). Variation in neural development as a result of exposure to institutionalization early in childhood. *Proceedings of the National Academy of Sciences, 109*(32), 12927–12932. doi:10.1073/pnas.1200041109/-/DCSupplemental

Shipman, K. L., Schneider, R., Fitzgerald, M. M., Sims, C., Swisher, L., & Edwards, A. (2007). Maternal emotion socialization in maltreating and non-maltreating families: Implications for children's emotion regulation. *Social Development, 16*(2), 268–285. doi:10.1111/j.1467-9507.2007.00384.x

Shirtcliff, E. A., Coe, C. L., & Pollak, S. D. (2009). Early childhood stress is associated with elevated antibody levels to herpes simplex virus type 1. *Proceedings of the National Academy of Sciences, 106*(8), 2963–2967. doi:10.1073/pnas.0806660106

Shonkoff, J. P., Garner, A. S., & The Committee on Psychosocial, Developmental, and Behavioral Pediatrics (2012). The lifelong effects of early childhood adversity and toxic stress. *Pediatrics, 129*(1), e232–e246. doi:10.1542/peds.2011-2663

Slavich, G. M., & Cole, S. W. (2013). The emerging field of human social genomics. *Clinical Psychological Science, 1*(3), 331–348. doi:10.1177/2167702613478594
Taylor, S. E., Way, B. M., & Seeman, T. E. (2011). Early adversity and adult health outcomes. *Development and Psychopathology, 23*(3), 939–954. doi:10.1017/S0954579411000411
Teicher, M. H., Anderson, C. M., Ohashi, K., & Polcari, A. (2014). Childhood maltreatment: altered network centrality of cingulate, precuneus, temporal pole and insula. *Biological Psychiatry, 76*(4), 297–305. doi:10.1016/j.biopsych.2013.09.016
Teisl, M., & Cicchetti, D. (2007). Physical abuse, cognitive and emotional processes, and aggressive/disruptive behavior problems. *Social Development, 17*(1), 1–23. doi:10.1111/j.1467-9507.2007.00412.x
Thomaes, K., Dorrepaal, E., & Draijer, N. (2010). Reduced anterior cingulate and orbitofrontal volumes in child abuse-related complex PTSD. *Journal of Clinical Psychiatry, 71*(12), 1636. doi:10.4088/JCP.08m04754blu
Thornberry, T. P., Henry, K. L., Ireland, T. O., & Smith, C. A. (2010). The causal impact of childhood-limited maltreatment and adolescent maltreatment on early adult adjustment. *Journal of Adolescent Health, 46*(4), 359–365. doi:10.1016/j.jadohealth.2009.09.011
Timmons, A. C., & Margolin, G. (2014). Family conflict, mood, and adolescents' daily achool problems: Moderating roles of internalizing and externalizing symptoms. *Child Development, 86*(1), 241–258. doi:10.1111/cdev.12300
Vachon, D. D., Krueger, R. F., Rogosch, F. A., & Cicchetti, D. (2015). Assessment of the harmful psychiatric and behavioral effects of different forms of child maltreatment. *JAMA Psychiatry, 72*(11), 1135–1138. doi:10.1001/jamapsychiatry.2015.1792
Wasserman, E. A., & Miller, R. R. (1997). What's elementary about associative learning? *Annual Review of Psychology, 48*(1), 573–607. doi:10.1146/annurev.psych.48.1.573
Weaver, I. C. (2005). Reversal of maternal programming of stress responses in adult offspring through methyl supplementation: Altering epigenetic marking later in life. *The Journal of Neuroscience, 25*(47), 11045–11054. doi:10.1523/JNEUROSCI.3652-05.2005
Weaver, I. C., Hellstrom, I. C., Brown, S. E., Andrews, S. D., Dymov, S., Diorio, J., … & Meaney, M. J. (2014). The methylated-DNA binding protein MBD2 enhances NGFI-A (egr-1)-mediated transcriptional activation of the glucocorticoid receptor. *Philosophical Transactions of the Royal Society B: Biological Sciences, 369*(1652), 20130513. doi:10.1098/rstb.2013.0513
Weder, N., Zhang, H., Jensen, K., Yang, B. Z., Simen, A., Jackowski, A., … & O'Loughlin, K. (2014). Child Abuse, Depression, and Methylation in Genes involved with Stress, Neural Plasticity, and Brain Circuitry. *Journal of the American Academy of Child & Adolescent Psychiatry, 53*(4), 417–424. doi:10.1016/j.jaac.2013.12.025
Weller, J. A., & Fisher, P. A. (2013). Decision-making Deficits among Maltreated Children. *Child Maltreatment, 18*(3), 184–194. doi:10.1177/1077559512467846
Whipple, E. E., & Webster-Stratton, C. (1991). The role of parental stress in physically abusive families. *Child Abuse and Neglect, 15,* 279–291. doi:10.1016/0145-2134(91)90072-L
Widom, C. S., & Maxfield, M. G. (2001). An Update on the" Cycle of Violence". *Research in Brief.* doi:10.1037/e528142006-001

Chapter 10
How Being Mothered Affects the Development of Mothering

Viara R. Mileva-Seitz and Alison S. Fleming

For better or for worse, parents draw on past experiences, sometimes repeating the behaviour of their own parents. Yet how precisely do they do so? What aspects of their early 'experience' become influential to new parents, and by what mechanisms? As with any complex behaviour, the transmission of parenting from one generation to another is unlikely to follow a single pathway or mechanism. Social and biological processes are intertwined. Advances in genetic and epigenetic techniques allow us to probe mechanisms underlying this transmission across generations. Such research also bears a responsibility. It must ultimately answer the following questions: What dimensions of parenting tend to be transmitted across generations? Are these dimensions at the mercy of biological and environmental programming? How flexible is the intergenerational transmission of parenting? Here we will review some major aspects of intergenerational transmission of mothering.

Parenting is a hugely complex and potentially stressful time of life. Sometimes parental stress leads to less-than-optimal parental behaviours, which can be strongly influential for subsequent generations. The identification of mechanisms of transmission of parental behaviour across generations will help to eventually shape interventions and policies aimed at reducing parental stress and abuse and neglect of the offspring. One potential such mechanism which we discuss below is the following: maternal stress can alter aspects of psychobiological function in offspring such that daughters grow up to mother in the same way (e.g. low-licking moms produce daughters who grow up to be low-licking moms). The focus on mothering—versus other types of caregiving—is due to the overall lack of research into fathers, grandparents, and other caregivers.

V.R. Mileva-Seitz (✉) · A.S. Fleming
Department of Psychology, University of Toronto, Toronto, Canada
e-mail: viara.mileva@gmail.com

A.S. Fleming
e-mail: Alison.fleming@utoronto.ca

K. Deater-Deckard and R. Panneton (eds.), *Parental Stress and Early Child Development*, DOI 10.1007/978-3-319-55376-4_10

Variations in Mothering

Animals (including humans) exhibit natural variations in the types and quantities of species-specific maternal care they exhibit. Studying animals in the laboratory is useful to untangle some of the underlying influences on maternal behaviour and on the transmission of behaviour across generations. One of the most widely studied animal models of parenting is the rat. Rats exhibit stereotyped maternal behaviours: they nurse, lick, and groom their pups, build a nest, and retrieve the pups back to the nest. The mother and the nest provide nutrition, warmth, and protection. They also provide social and other stimuli that affect pups' neural and endocrine development and later behaviour (Lonstein, Lévy, & Fleming, 2015). Moreover, the young learn to prefer their mother's odour over time, which guides subsequent social interactions and even their responses to their own offspring later on (Abel, Ronca, & Alberts, 1998; Hofer & Sullivan, 2001; Shah, Oxley, Lovic, & Fleming, 2002; Wilson & Sullivan, 1994). Maternal licking has a particularly pronounced effect on offspring development. The somatosensory stimulation has long-term effects on the quality of mothering pups adopt towards their own young. The most effective period for transmission of licking effects seems to be in the first post-partum week when the rat brain is still rapidly developing (Champagne, Francis, Mar, & Meaney, 2003; Gonzalez, Lovic, Ward, Wainwright, & Fleming, 2001). Licking and grooming during early life thus have a non-genetic influence on the next generations and are therefore crucial for optimal development. The absence or disruption of licking and grooming, such as during maternal separation or deprivation, has documented developmental consequences as well.

In humans, as in other mammals, there also occurs a continuity of parenting styles (subtypes of parental behaviours) across generations (Bailey, Hill, Oesterle, & Hawkins, 2009; Belsky, Jaffee, Sligo, Woodward, & Silva, 2005; Conger, Neppl, Kim, & Scaramella, 2003; Neppl, Conger, Scaramella, & Ontai, 2009; Scaramella, Neppl, Ontai, & Conger, 2008). For instance, a large prospective study with direct parent–child behavioural observations during a puzzle task showed continuity in both positive parenting (supportive, warm, helpful, and involved parenting during the task) and negative/harsh parenting (critical, aggressive, unkind, irritable, and 'pressureful' parenting during the task) (Scaramella et al., 2008). Moreover, human studies suggest a bi-directional role for parent–child interactions in the developmental process. On the one hand, early parenting might influence developmental trajectories. On the other hand, children's own behaviours might elicit specific types of parenting through evocative effects and—given shared genetic factors—through evocative gene–environment correlations (Ge et al., 1996; Jaffee & Price, 2008; Maccoby, 2000).

In addition to normal variations in parenting affecting the parental behaviour of the next generation, there is ample evidence both in non-human animals and in humans that manipulated extremes in parenting affects the offspring and their subsequent parental behaviour. This has been well demonstrated in rats (Fleming et al., 2002; Hofer, 2002). The most severe rat deprivation paradigm involves raising pups without a mother in an artificial rearing variant on Hall's 'pup-in-a-cup' environment, and then comparing these pups to mother-reared sibling controls (Hall, Wilkinson, Humby, & Robbins, 1999; Thoman & Arnold, 1968). This animal model is reminiscent of the environment provided by human institutionalization and produces many of the same effects on young (Brett, Humphreys, Fleming, Kraemer, & Drury, 2015). Unlike the limited deprivation during short-term daily separations and reunions (short-term stress), the 'pup-in-the-cup' procedure is a continuous isolation, where pups never know their mothers and siblings but are raised alone, with some human contact. As adults, these pups show deficits in maternal licking and crouching over their pups, consistent with the extent of the adversity or separations experienced in early life (Gonzalez et al., 2001; Lovic & Fleming, 2004; Lovic, Gonzalez, & Fleming, 2001; Rees & Fleming, 2001). Short-term deprivations produce the least deficits, whereas artificially reared pups produce the greatest reductions in pup body licking, genital licking, and crouching subsequently as adults (Fleming et al., 2002; Gonzalez et al., 2001; Liu et al., 1997). Yet when artificially reared pups are given additional licking-like stimulation by 5–8 daily strokes with a paintbrush, or if they are reared more socially with another single sibling, the isolation effects on subsequent behaviour are considerably reduced (Lomanowska & Melo, 2016).

Hence a deficit experienced by isolated pups resides in how much somatosensory, vestibular, and tactile stimulation (and possibly contingent interactions) they receive in their pre-weaning life (Hofer & Sullivan, 2001). Most relevant to the current discussion is that the effect of artificial rearing *persists across generations*. Offspring of isolated pups who were not themselves isolated or maternally deprived, also show disrupted mothering as adults (Champagne et al., 2003; Fleming et al., 2002; Gonzalez et al., 2001; Hofer & Sullivan, 2001; Kraemer, 1992; Lévy, Melo, Galef, Madden, & Fleming, 2003; Lomanowska & Melo, 2016; Lovic & Fleming, 2004; Melo et al., 2006; Numan, Fleming, & Levy, 2006; Palombo, Nowoslawski, & Fleming, 2010; Wilson & Sullivan, 1994). Similar effects are seen in non-human primates (Champoux et al., 2002; Fleming et al., 2002; Maestripieri, 2005; Maestripieri et al., 2006; Maestripieri, Lindell, & Higley, 2007; Suomi, 1999).

In humans as well, extreme parental abuse, neglect, or deprivation and social isolation have serious consequences that affect the behaviour of subsequent generations. About 30% of women abused as children go on to abuse their own children, a rate of abuse substantially higher than that in the general population of 5% (Kaufman & Zigler, 1987; Knutson, 1995). Some of the associated outcomes of early abuse or neglect include more aggressive, intrusive, or generally 'poor' parenting (Moehler, Biringen, & Poustka, 2007; Newcomb & Locke, 2001), a decreased female interest in becoming a mother, higher levels of child neglect, diminished parental confidence and self-appraisal, greater use of physical punishment, and a lack of emotional control in parenting situations (Roberts, O'Connor, Dunn, & Golding, 2004). Less severe negative early experiences (e.g. harsh parenting and high levels of family discord) are also transmitted intergenerationally (Capaldi, Pears, Patterson, & Owen, 2003). For instance, mothers who experienced early parental rejection show more negative affect towards their children (Belsky, Youngblade, & Pensky, 1989).

Positive early experiences also influence later maternal behaviour (Belsky et al., 2005; Chen & Kaplan, 2001; Chen, Liu, & Kaplan, 2008). Mothers who had positive childhood relationships with their own parents are more responsive towards their children (Gara, Rosenberg, & Herzog, 1996). Less authoritarianism, more positive family 'climate', and a positive attachment in childhood are predictive of warm, sensitive, and stimulating maternal behaviour in adulthood (Belsky et al., 2005). Early life experiences are thus part of a spectrum, from very negative to very positive (Belsky et al., 2009), and both the 'good' and the 'bad' can be transmitted cross-generationally. The most evident question arising from this intergenerational research is the question of *how* parental behaviour is transmitted, particularly when it appears to happen sometimes in the absence of the very same environment that triggered particular parental behaviours in previous generations.

Is Parenting Stable Over Time?

The quest for finding mechanisms of intergenerational transmission of parenting begins with the assumption that parenting practices are, to a degree, stable over time for a given parent. The evidence only partially corroborates this view, however. For instance, some studies indicate maternal sensitivity is stable over time (Behrens, Hart, & Parker, 2012; Vereijken & Marianne Ri, 1997), whereas others report the opposite (Lohaus, Keller, Ball, Voelker, & Elben, 2004). Therefore, single snapshots of mother–infant interactions may not be optimal for assessing the true nature of maternal sensitivity (Lindhiem, Bernard, & Dozier, 2011).

Mothers may get more comfortable over time and repeated assessments, or they may gradually fall into more stable patterns of interactions with their infants over the first year (Pauli-Pott, 2008). As well, mothers clearly respond differently to different children within the family, and family effects at one time can feed back and affect mothers' relationship with different children at later times (Jenkins, McGowan, & Knafo-Noam, 2016). Furthermore, individual susceptibility to parenting effects might also be only moderately stable. That is, there might be different sensitivity periods (Windhorst et al., 2015), so that the interactions between parenting and the child's susceptibility alleles might change over time. This has not been well explored, and nothing is known about the stability of gene–environment interactions in mothers lives as they acquire experience with their own children.

Mechanisms for the Intergenerational Transmission of Parenting

The effects of early rearing experiences on later parenting might be mediated by shared genetics, shared environment, physiology, brain development, and epigenetic modifications. We will briefly review evidence for each of these multiple mechanisms. New rat mothers who themselves experienced adequate early parenting in infancy, when compared to mothers who experienced varying periods of separation from mother, show a good balance in approach-withdrawal behaviours when in both novel environments and when with their pups; they show reduced fearfulness and enhanced attentiveness, and they are better able to respond to positive features of their young (Barrett & Fleming, 2011; Fleming & Li, 2002; Lomanowska, Boivin, Hertzman, & Fleming, 2016; Lonstein et al., 2015). In contrast, early adversity and isolation results in changes in the animals' fearfulness in an elevated plus maze (Lomanowska & Melo, 2016; Lomanowska, Rana, McCutcheon, Parker, & Wainwright, 2006), produces hyperactivity in an open field and in activity boxes (Gonzalez et al., 2001), increases overall impulsivity assessed in a DRL paradigm (Lovic & Fleming, 2015), enhances inattention in a set shifting task (Lovic & Fleming, 2004), and alters the hedonic value of pups in the new mother (Afonso, King, Chatterjee, & Fleming, 2009). Paradoxically, early deprivation also enhances an animal's responsiveness to natural or conditioned cues associated with a primary reward (Lomanowska et al., 2011; Lomanowska & Kraemer, 2014). Thus, early experiences affect reward processing and executive functioning in animals. These cognitive processes are important to mothering, and therefore offer an indirect neural mechanism by which early experiences affect subsequent maternal behaviour in rats.

We believe a similar set of relations applies to human mothers. After giving birth, mothers are more attracted to infant odours and more sympathetic to infant cries than are non-mothers, and the extent of sympathy or attraction is associated with mothers' expressed maternal behaviour and their heart-rate and cortisol responses to those cues (Fleming et al., 1993; Fleming, Steiner, & Corter, 1997; Giardino, Gonzalez, Steiner, & Fleming, 2008; Porter, Cernoch, & McLaughlin, 1983; Porter, Makin, Davis, & Christensen, 1991; Stallings, Fleming, Corter, Worthman, & Steiner, 2001). Infant sensory cues are inherently rewarding to human mothers (Lonstein et al., 2015). They activate regions of the adult brain that are associated with reward and pleasure [e.g. (Kringelbach, 2008)]. Moreover, infant cues can grab and/or disrupt adult attention (Dudek, Faress, Bornstein, & Haley, 2016), depending on the valence of these cues.

Moreover, experience with salient infant cues enhances maternal attention to these cues, as illustrated in studies that examined attentional capture or bias by infant and adult faces in women during late pregnancy (Pearson, Lightman, & Evans, 2011). Mothers were much less able to disengage from a distressed infant face than from a non-distressed infant face, in order to attend to a neutral stimulus in the periphery. This differential maternal attention to distressed faces was related to later maternal self-reported postpartum bonding with the infant. Also, a study of event-related potential (ERP) responses to infant cues (Proverbio, Brignone, Matarazzo, Del Zotto, & Zani, 2006) indicated that parents find infant cues more salient and better discriminate between different infant emotional expressions, suggesting heightened attention to infant features.

While too little attention bias to infant cues is clearly problematic for parenting, too much attention bias to infant cues can also interfere with parenting. Mothers who were overly distractible to infant cues and unable to selectively attend to a target task and ignore infant cries have greater insecure maternal attachment history (Haley & Ryan, personal communication, 2016) and less emotion regulation as indexed by reduced control of their autonomic activity (Haley & Jabrayan, personal communication, 2016). Finally, non-parents have been shown to display greater heart-rate reactivity than parents in response to hearing infant cries (Out, Pieper, Bakermans-Kranenburg, & van IJzendoorn, 2010). This, as Pedersen, Huffman, del Carmen, and Bryan (1996) suggested, might be due to the fact that parents perceive infant cries more accurately and can better select an appropriate response to infant cries (Pedersen et al., 1996). In general, parents have had more experience with infant cries than have non-parents and hence may simply be habituated to their effects. Taken together, mothers showing moderate attention biases to infant cues—rather than too little or too much—exercise greater cognitive flexibility and selective attention, which may enhance parenting experiences and parenting adequacy. Both experience and underlying biological factors are likely to shape individual differences in these attention biases.

Early experiences of adversity likely affects human mothers' attraction to infants and their reinforcing value, although this has not been specifically addressed (summarized in Afonso, Grella, Chatterjee, & Fleming, 2008; Barrett & Fleming, 2011). Correlational behavioural and imaging studies suggest that early adversity affects reward processing (Boecker et al., 2014; Pechtel & Pizzagalli, 2011). Furthermore, indirect evidence is mounting that early experiences with parenting influence brain development and behaviour in the child. For instance, child neglect and institutionalized rearing is associated with later-life difficulties of inhibitory control that may reflect altered attribution of salience to external stimuli (Brett et al., 2015). Even less severe early negative experiences, such as harsh parenting and low maternal sensitivity, have been associated with decreased inhibitory control in children (Lucassen et al., 2015).

Early neglect or adversity also appears to have neurological consequences for children. For instance, early maltreatment is associated with reductions in hippocampal volume (Riem, Alink, Out, Van IJzendoorn, & Bakermans-Kranenburg, 2015), whereas more sensitive parenting is associated with larger grey matter volume (i.e. neuronal density), and total brain volume (Kok et al., 2015). Positive maternal behaviour in early childhood is also associated with an attenuated growth of the amygdala of adolescents (Whittle et al., 2014). Such attenuation (e.g. reduced hippocampal volume) might relate to decreased emotional reactivity, though further research is needed to implicate this in a cross-generational effect on subsequent parenting. In general, however, if early experience-associated changes in brain morphology and executive functioning persist into adulthood, they are likely to have effects on parenting.

Genetic and Physiological Mediators of Mothering

Early experiences and environmental influences affect the quality of exhibited mothering, and yet not all mothers respond in the same way to these environmental influences. Mothers vary in their susceptibility to environmental effects, possibly owing at least in part to mothers' genetic profiles. Some genetic variants might make individuals more susceptible to specific types of environmental input, and there is a growing literature on this topic. A caveat to this research is that studies have been mostly correlational and associations between a genetic variant and an environmental susceptibility are modest at best. Since human maternal responsiveness is a highly complex phenotype, it is unlikely scientists will find individual genetic variants with large influences on such phenotypes. Effects are likely to be small, polygenic, and involve numerous, ongoing, interactions with environmental factors. The search for candidate genes associated with human parenting has centred on three key neurotransmitter/neuropeptide systems (Mileva-Seitz, Bakermans-Kranenburg, & van IJzendoorn, 2015): dopamine, oxytocin, and serotonin. Because of their clear involvement regulating animal parental responsiveness and processing of infant cues, the following discussion focuses on the first two: dopamine and oxytocin.

Dopamine and Mothering

Dopamine is a major catecholaminergic neurotransmitter implicated in reward, mood, attention, and mothering, at least in non-humans. Dopamine reflects and enhances the rewarding properties or salience of stimuli. Depending on an animal's 'motivational' state, relevant stimuli are food (to the hungry animal), a sexually experienced male (for an oestrous female), or pups (for a new mother) (Afonso et al., 2008, 2009; Afonso, King, Novakov, Burton, & Fleming, 2011; Berridge & Robinson, 1998). In the new mother rat, progesterone and oestrogen suppress baseline activity of the dopamine system in the nucleus accumbens (NA); in hormonally primed non-mother rats, subsequent pup stimulation produces an increase in dopamine over baseline, which is proportionally greater than it would be if the baseline were high (Afonso et al., 2011). Therefore, the hormonal effect acts to tune the dopamine system by enhancing the ratio of dopamine signal to baseline noise when pups are presented (Afonso et al., 2011).

Rat dams exhibit individual differences in levels of dopamine release into the nucleus accumbens (e.g. high-lickers and groomers have greater dopamine release than low-lickers and groomers; Champagne et al., 2004). Postpartum females have naturally suppressed dopamine baseline levels, but these levels increase significantly when they are exposed to pups (Afonso et al., 2009), or following reunion with pups after a separation (Hansen, Bergvall, & Nyiredi, 1993). Pups are so rewarding that new rat mothers prefer pups to cocaine until about day eight postpartum (Mattson, Williams, Rosenblatt, & Morrell, 2001). Even cycling (non-postpartum) females, who normally avoid pups, when exposed to pups show dopamine increases proportional to their prior pup exposure (Afonso et al., 2008).

In addition to looking at dopamine levels associated with mothering, there is substantial evidence that dopamine receptors which determine the sensitivity of the brain to the dopamine that is released also change in the new mother, and that in different sites different receptors are activated. For instance, the expression of dopamine receptor genes D1 and D2 (DRD1 and DRD2, respectively) is up-regulated during pregnancy in the rat (Mann, 2014), and dopamine receptor D4 (DRD4) and dopamine transporter (DAT1) mRNA increase in the medial pre-optic area following pup exposure, regardless of maternal parity (Akbari et al., 2013). This evidence implies that dopamine, known to be implicated in stimulus salience and 'reward', is one of the major neurotransmitters involved in rat maternal regulation.

Rat pups might be partially responsible for the onset and ongoing maintenance of maternal behaviour (Rosenblatt, 1967), via stimulation of gene expression in the mother. Natural bursts of dopamine-firing neurons in the mammalian striatum are said to be key for the pup-regulated aspects of maternal care (i.e. maternal care in response to pup-cues) (Robinson, Zitzman, & Williams, 2011). Other rodent models provide additional evidence for the dopamine-mothering link. In hypodopaminergic mice (genetically engineered to express less dopamine), striatal dopamine is key for 'active' maternal behaviours such as pup-retrieval and liking/grooming of pups, but not for 'passive' behaviours such as nursing (Henschen, Palmiter, & Darvas, 2013). In voles, the dopamine antagonist haloperidol has similar effects on parenting behaviour as in rats, reducing 'active' components of maternal behaviour (e.g. duration of licking), although species-specific differences in the effects can be seen (Lonstein, 2002).

Much of these natural variations in rodent dopamine levels are not clearly associated with underlying genotypes, suggesting that genetic association studies may not be useful. However, in humans, genetic association studies offer one of the only ways to study natural variation in dopamine levels. This is because the invasive procedures used in animal research (e.g. extraction of region-specific brain tissue for genetic expression analyses) are not possible in humans. Human studies rely mostly on the genotyping of specifics genes or gene loci to determine whether genetic variation is associated with differences in behavioural phenotypes.

Other ways to study possible relationships between genetic factors and parental behaviour in humans are by using brain imaging studies. Functional magnetic resonance imaging (fMRI) studies in which mothers were exposed to infant vocalizations (Lorberbaum et al., 2002; Sander, Frome, & Scheich, 2007; Seifritz et al., 2003), pictures (Barrett et al., 2011; Bartels & Zeki, 2004; Leibenluft, Gobbini, Harrison, & Haxby, 2004; Nitschke et al., 2004; Strathearn, Li, Fonagy, &

Montague, 2008), or video fragments (Noriuchi, Kikuchi, & Senoo, 2008; Ranote et al., 2004), report activation of either dopaminergic regions, or regions that directly interact with dopaminergic regions (Georges & Aston-Jones, 2002). Candidate gene studies have explored dopamine genetic polymorphisms in association with human parenting. Genetic polymorphisms in DRD1, DRD2, DRD4, COMT (coding for catechol-*O*-methyltransferase, a dopamine deactivating enzyme), and DAT1 have all been associated with differences in maternal behaviours, including sensitivity and vocalizing (Lee et al., 2008; Mileva-Seitz, Fleming, et al., 2012; van IJzendoorn, Bakermans-Kranenburg, & Mesman, 2008). Not all studies find significant associations, however. Mills-Koonce et al. (2007) reported no significant association between maternal genotype at a dopamine-related polymorphism on the gene ANKK1 and observed maternal sensitivity. These studies used observed measures of parenting, which is a significant strength because they represent a more objective and unbiased assessment of parental behaviour than can be obtained by parental self-report questionnaires (the alternate method for assessing parenting differences). Yet further replication is crucial before the role of dopamine gene polymorphisms in human maternal behaviour is clear.

A central limitation to the molecular genetic studies of parenting is the indirect way in which genotype is used as a proxy of actual gene expression in the brain, and this is particularly so for genotypes that have no known functional significance (i.e. genotypes that are not readily linked with up- or down-regulation of gene expression). Another limitation is that genetic variants interact with non-genetic factors (e.g. early rearing history) in ways that are not yet fully understood. This limits the ability to detect main effects of genotype alone. Furthermore, there is ongoing discussion whether main effects of higher order interactive effects are, in fact, more plausible. Given relatively small sample sizes, particularly when it comes to human behavioural studies, it is an added challenge to find these interactive effects in the first place. The future of parenting research will likely see small strides towards elucidating these important but complex mechanisms.

Oxytocin/Vasopressin and Mothering

In many non-primate mammalian species, the nine-amino-acid peptide oxytocin is key to regulating the onset of maternal behaviour (Fahrbach, Morrell, & Pfaff, 1985; Kendrick, 2000; Numan, 2015; Pedersen, Caldwell, Walker, Ayers, & Mason, 1994). Individual differences in centrally inducible oxytocin receptors predict rat maternal behaviour (Champagne, Diorio, Sharma, & Meaney, 2001). Oxytocin might also mediate maternal behaviour in rat dams indirectly by modulating anxiety levels, which in turn affect maternal behaviour (Bosch, 2010). In sheep, oxytocin administration results in maternal behaviour towards foreign lambs (Keverne & Kendrick, 1992) and decreases aggression and aversion to newborn lambs (Insel & Young, 2001). In oxytocin receptor knockout mice, maternal behaviour is impaired (Takayanagi et al., 2005).

In primates, oxytocin is not essential for the establishment of maternal care, but is associated with post-parturition bonding and maternal behaviour (Broad, Curley, & Keverne, 2006; Saltzman & Maestripieri, 2010). Pregnancy hormones prime the mesolimbic dopamine projections to the NA and up-regulate oxytocin receptors in the brain. These modulations of the reward system facilitate mother–infant bonds at birth (Broad et al., 2006). Additionally, peripheral administration of an oxytocin receptor blocker in rhesus macaques reduces interest in the infant (e.g. lip-smacking, approaching, touching) (Boccia, Goursaud, Bachevalier, Anderson, & Pedersen, 2007). Whereas cerebrospinal (hence, 'central') levels of oxytocin in multiparous rhesus macaque females do not correlate with mother–infant interaction (Cooke et al., 1997), *plasma* (hence, peripheral) levels of oxytocin are highly correlated with 'maternal warmth' (Maestripieri, Hoffman, Anderson, Carter, & Higley, 2009).

The evidence in primates points to the numerous functions of oxytocin, and the complex regulation mechanisms that peripheral versus central oxytocin might be involved in. However, as is true of many of the other maternal hormones, oxytocin enhances responsiveness but it does not cause it, and in many instances maternal behaviour will be exhibited in the absence of the polypeptide. If virgin female rats are administered progesterone followed by oestrogen in a series of silastic capsules, they will exhibit maternal behaviour to foster pups without the addition of oxytocin—and in the rat, oxytocin will not affect maternal behaviour onset without prior oestrogen priming (see reviews by Bridges, 2016; Lonstein et al., 2015).

Turning to humans, increased plasma oxytocin from early to mid-late pregnancy correlates with higher scores on ratings of attachment to the foetus (Levine, Zagoory-Sharon, Feldman, & Weller, 2007), indicating the important role of oxytocin for bonding even before birth. Maternal and infant salivary oxytocin levels are correlated with each other and with mother–infant affect synchrony (Feldman, Gordon, & Zagoory-Sharon, 2010), and high levels of plasma oxytocin predict high levels of affectionate touch towards infants (Feldman, Gordon, Schneiderman, Weisman, & Zagoory-Sharon, 2010). Increased oxytocin levels are found in mothers who recently touched or interacted with their infants (Light et al., 2000). Oxytocin is thus important in human parenting (Galbally, Lewis, van IJzendoorn, & Permezel, 2011), not purely during parturition and breastfeeding but during the expression of behavioural and attachment responses to infants. However, oxytocin has a multiple-site release, many functions, and a diurnal rhythm in the cerebrospinal fluid but not peripherally (Amico, Tenicela, Johnston, & Robinson, 1983), making it difficult to accurately measure. Since it does not cross the blood–brain barrier in adults (Saltzman & Maestripieri, 2010), plasma and cerebrospinal fluid levels may not be identical, although they are highly correlated (Carson et al., 2014). Again, this makes research with oxytocin genotypes challenging, as a simple DNA sequence along oxytocin-related genes does not necessarily indicate whether central or peripheral gene expression is associated with this genotype, and how this might relate to parenting.

Candidate gene studies of oxytocin in humans have shown significant association between polymorphic variants and parental behaviour. For instance, the rs53576 polymorphism on the oxytocin receptor gene (OXTR) is associated with parental sensitive responsiveness (Bakermans-Kranenburg & van IJzendoorn, 2008), maternal warmth (Klahr, Klump, & Burt, 2014), positive parenting, and neural activation of brain regions previously associated with positive parenting (Michalska et al., 2014). This polymorphism is also associated with differences in maternal cardiac reactivity to infant cries, moderated by maternal depressive symptoms (Riem, Pieper, Out, Bakermans-Kranenburg, & van IJzendoorn, 2011). However, although this polymorphism might influence oxytocin function (Meyer-Lindenberg, Domes, Kirsch, & Heinrichs, 2011) and to represent an important direction in parenting research (Taylor, 2008), a meta-analysis of 48 studies ($N = 17{,}559$) found no significant effect for five domains of outcomes (biology, personality, social behaviour, psychopathology, and autism) (Bakermans-Kranenburg & van IJzendoorn, 2014). This further emphasizes the limitation of using genetic polymorphisms with unclear functional significance in human candidate gene studies.

Other single nucleotide polymorphisms (SNPs) in OXTR-related genes have also been explored in relation to differences in human parenting. For instance, parents with the CD38 CC genotype and the OXTR rs1042778 TT genotype touched their infants less frequently than parents with other genotypes (Feldman et al., 2012). CD38 regulates oxytocin release and is related to autism spectrum disorders (Munesue et al., 2010). Mice-knockouts for the CD38 gene exhibit reduced oxytocin levels and deficits in social and maternal behaviour (Jin et al., 2007), suggesting some possible function for these in human parenting. Another study showed that two SNPs in the oxytocin peptide-coding gene (OXT rs2740210 and OXT rs4813627) were significantly associated with differences in maternal vocalizing to the infant, but not maternal 'sensitivity' (Mileva-Seitz et al., 2013). That SNPs associate with some but not other maternal behaviour outcomes could indicate that the multiple dimensions of parental behaviour have differential genetic regulation. It also highlights the measurement issues inherent in complex behavioural research (such as parenting). 'Parenting' can be sliced in multiple ways, but the discriminant validity of specific parenting dimensions is often less than clear.

Finally, polymorphic variation in the vasopressin receptor 1A gene associates with differences in maternal sensitivity (Bisceglia et al., 2012) and maternal structuring and support (Avinun, Ebstein, & Knafo, 2012). Vasopressin has structural similarity to oxytocin and evidence suggests it is involved in the regulation of social behaviour (Ebstein, Knafo, Mankuta, Chew, & Lai, 2012; Heinrichs & Domes, 2008; Meyer-Lindenberg et al., 2011), so it is another potential system for candidate gene studies. However, the lack of knowledge about the function of many of these SNPs limits the conclusions that can be drawn. Replications and functional studies of oxytocin and vasopressin genes are necessary. One approach is to use candidate genes/alleles only if their function in cell or cellular networks is known. However, this too, has the potential to bias our genetic research to specific known genetic polymorphisms. Thus, a combination approach would be most productive. For instance, a hypothesis-generating genome-wide association (GWA) approach might first be used to identify genetic loci that have not been obvious candidates from a functional perspective alone. Later, these regions could be more carefully probed in observational studies of parenting.

Furthermore, some of these studies provide suggestive evidence for a moderating role of the environment (e.g. Mileva-Seitz et al., 2011; van IJzendoorn et al., 2008). Gene–environment interplay is likely to involve multiple genes and multiple environmental conditions, and we are only beginning to understanding these complex effects. Gene–environment interactions and correlations may explain why parents are differentially affected by their experiences, by their early life, and by their current stressors. Studies of gene–environment interplay have grown substantially in number over recent years (Fortuna et al., 2011), increasingly supporting the *for better and for worse* paradigm of differential susceptibility. For instance, in a large cohort of American children (Lee, Brooks-Gunn, McLanahan, Notterman, & Garfinkel, 2013), mothers with one genetic variant on the ANKK1 gene—related to DRD2 function—exhibited differential susceptibility: for them, harsh parenting increased as macroeconomic conditions worsened but decreased as conditions improved. For mothers with the alternate genetic variant, harsh parenting was not related to changes in macroeconomic conditions.

A working hypothesis emerging from these studies is that under conditions of stress, parents carrying differential susceptibility alleles are among the less parentally sensitive parents (i.e. exhibiting less optimal parental behaviours), whereas under conditions of no stress, they are among the more sensitive parents (i.e. exhibiting more optimal parental behaviours). Additional support for this comes from studies indicating that the short allele on the serotonin transporter polymorphism (5HTTLPR) is associated with greater maternal sensitivity (Cents et al., 2014; Mileva-Seitz et al., 2011). This is an allele that unpublished work of ours suggests is also related to greater rates of depressive symptoms in these same, more sensitive mothers. Thus, mothers with this allele might not only be more likely to be influenced by more adverse experiences, but also might generally be more responsive to ongoing environmental input, of which the new infant forms a large proportion in the early postpartum period. In other words, a mother who is more emotionally labile or susceptible might also be *able,* under optimal conditions, to respond better to their infants.

From an evolutionary perspective, maintaining a diverse gene pool has allowed for some phenotypes that are able to cope with greater stress (the less susceptible parents) and whose behaviour is not greatly affected by the environment, and for other phenotypes that are highly reactive to ongoing environmental stimuli and whose behaviour might suffer as a result of high stress, but benefit as a result of low stress. With historical fluctuations in the levels of environmental stress (e.g. famines, war, drought), the maintenance of a full range of genotypes might have been facilitated. At any given slice in history, however, some phenotypes might be more advantageous than others. Of course, this thinking is highly simplified and speculative. Much more work is required in this domain.

Epigenetic Effects on Mothering

If environmental interactions with genetic polymorphisms are codified, and they are passed across generations as well, how does this occur? Current theoretical and empirical evidence implicates 'epigenetic' mechanisms, an umbrella term covering processes by which the environment interfaces with, and changes the influence of, underlying genetic variants without altering those variants.

Complex epigenetic processes regulate gene expression in response to environmental input (Brookes & Shi, 2014; Kundakovic & Champagne, 2014; Meaney, 2010). In rats, licking/grooming and arch-back nursing can alter pup methylation patterns and gene expression and can be passed on to the pup's pups (e.g. Meaney, 2010; Szyf, Weaver, Champagne, Diorio, & Meaney, 2005). Thus, epigenetic changes can be acquired through experience and/or inherited (Meaney, 2010). Differential methylation of the glucocorticoid receptor (GR) gene as a result of early experience induces long-term changes in response to stress that span into the next generation (Weaver et al., 2004; Zhang & Meaney, 2010; Zhang, Labonté, Wen, Turecki, & Meaney, 2013). The first epigenetic study on human behavioural development showed GR gene expression in the hippocampus of suicide victims was decreased only in the group who had experienced child abuse (McGowan, Sasaki, & D'Alessio, 2009). Similar epigenetic changes have been found as a result of child maltreatment (Perroud et al., 2014) or structural neglect in orphanages (Naumova et al., 2012).

Aside from the involvement of direct DNA information carried by gametes, there are multiple suggested transmission mechanisms, including for example hormones, cytokines, and microorganisms (Toth, 2015). Mileva-Seitz et al. (2015) outlined a mediated moderation model of intergenerational transmission of parental behaviour. In this model, abusive grandparental behaviour might alter methylation patterns of multiple candidate genes of interest in the offspring, leading to altered parental behaviour set-points, and this behavioural system might be further moderated by existing genotypes in parental susceptibility genes, and existing environments, to affect the third generation.

The fact that there might be potential effects on several generations arising as a result of environmental or behavioural exposures in the first generation, presents a set of interesting challenges for the study of intergenerational transmission of parental behaviour. Moreover, it has consequences for interventions and policy-building. We feel that we are yet at too early of a stage to directly apply this epigenetic research and reasoning towards clinical implementations, but it is an exciting area of research that is rapidly gaining momentum. Large-scale human behavioural studies are beginning to examine epigenome-wide methylation differences and patterns within populations, with the potential to identify previously unknown loci of interest that can in turn regulate the genetic variants we have been studying for years, and other, new genetic variants that genome-wide association studies are providing. There has arguably never been a more exciting time to be in parenting research.

Future Directions

'Human parenting' is in fact clusters of behaviours with underlying motivational, physiological, genetic, epigenetic, and environmental interactants. Parenting behaviours exhibit variation over time and place and culture (see Cassells & Evans, Chap. 2 this volume; Nomaguchi & Milkie, Chap. 3 this volume; Mileva-Seitz, Afonso, & Fleming, 2012; Mileva-Seitz & Fleming, 2011). To study the underlying mechanisms of transmission of such behaviours, we suggest it would be best to adopt a multi-pronged approach. On the one hand, we should continue to explore how broad parenting concepts (e.g. maternal 'sensitivity') are shaped by experience and biology. On the other hand, we ought to also dissect the broader phenotypes of parenting into smaller, discrete behavioural components. In animal research, this approach has been fruitful: the use of micro-behavioural analysis, quantifying exact behaviours and their durations, frequencies, and contingencies, has helped untangle some of the complexity. The smaller components of parenting might have more direct biological or environmental underpinnings.

Future research should also analyze interactions *between* multiple levels of influence: genetic, epigenetic, and environmental. Individuals with more environmentally 'susceptible' genotypes might have different epigenetic profiles, and we are only scratching the surface of these interactions to peek into the shaping of parental behaviour over time and place. Prenatal effects—which have been argued to constitute a form of early parenting (Mileva-Seitz et al., 2015)—must also be explored. The choices mothers make and behaviours they perform while pregnant might be just as important to the growing foetus, as the behaviours following birth. We recently showed that there are no large effects of prenatal maternal stress exposure on neonatal DNA methylation profiles (Rijlaarsdam et al., 2016), but these efforts require replication before we can dismiss prenatal stress as inconsequential.

Finally, it would be highly beneficial to peer into the parental brain. The field so far has used brain imaging and molecular genetics studies of genes thought to be expressed in the brain. Future techniques which allow a more direct view of the human parental brain—and genes expressed in different neural regions—would be the ultimate approach to understanding parental behaviour. Animal studies have a lot to offer, as they permit the use of invasive techniques to map and monitor gene expression in the brain. However, there are limits to the amount of extrapolation we can and ought to do from non-human to human parenting, imparted by the greater complexity of human parenting behaviour and cortical organization (Lonstein et al., 2015).[1]

The many changes that new parenthood entails often bring about a large amount of stress. Parental ability to cope with stress is likely codified at multiple levels, from the genetic to the epigenetic. The expression of parental behaviour during stressful times is a hugely important predictor for children's well-being. Parenting scientists are only beginning to explore the mechanisms by which stress interacts with the biology of the parent to shape their behaviour (see Neuenschwander & Oberlander, Chap. 6 this volume; Crnic & Ross, Chap. 11 this volume). As far as impactful implications, we ought to focus on research that can give rise to predictable and replicable intervention strategies for those most at risk. From a research perspective, we are a long way from understanding the complexities of the systems that help shape parental behaviour, but we have made great strides by considering both animal and human research and tackling them both at multiple levels of influence, from the genetic to the behavioural.

References

Abel, R. A., Ronca, A. E., & Alberts, J. R. (1998). Perinatal stimulation facilitates suckling onset in newborn rats. *Developmental Psychobiology*, *32*(2), 91–99. Retrieved from http://www.ncbi.nlm.nih.gov/pubmed/9526684

Afonso, V. M., Grella, S. L., Chatterjee, D., & Fleming, A. S. (2008). Previous maternal experience affects accumbal dopaminergic responses to pup-stimuli. *Brain Research, 1198,* 115–123.

Afonso, V. M., King, S., Chatterjee, D., & Fleming, A. S. (2009). Hormones that increase maternal responsiveness affect accumbal dopaminergic responses to pup- and food-stimuli in the female rat. *Hormones and Behavior*, *56*(1), 11–23. doi:10.1016/j.yhbeh.2009.02.003

Afonso, V. M., King, S. J., Novakov, M., Burton, C. L., & Fleming, A. S. (2011). Accumbal dopamine function in postpartum rats that were raised without their mothers. *Hormones and Behavior*, *60*(5), 632–643. doi:10.1016/j.yhbeh.2011.08.016

Akbari, E. M., Shams, S., Belay, H. T., Kaiguo, M., Razak, Z., Kent, C. F., … Fleming, A. S. (2013). The effects of parity and maternal behavior on gene expression in the medial preoptic area and the medial amygdala in postpartum and virgin female rats: A microarray study. *Behavioral Neuroscience*, *127*(6), 913–922. doi:10.1037/a0034884

Amico, J. A., Tenicela, R., Johnston, J., & Robinson, A. G. (1983). A time-dependent peak of oxytocin exists in cerebrospinal fluid but not in plasma of humans. *The Journal of Clinical Endocrinology and Metabolism*, *57*(5), 947–951. Retrieved from http://www.ncbi.nlm.nih.gov/pubmed/6619269

Avinun, R., Ebstein, R. P., & Knafo, A. (2012). Human maternal behaviour is associated with arginine vasopressin receptor 1A gene. *Biology Letters*, *8*(5), 894–896. doi:10.1098/rsbl.2012.0492

[1]Sections of the present chapter are based on Lonstein et al. (2015) and on Lomanowska et al. (2016), in which neural and molecular (non-genetic) mechanisms of early adversity and maternal behaviour are further explored.

Bailey, J. A., Hill, K. G., Oesterle, S., & Hawkins, J. D. (2009). Parenting practices and problem behavior across three generations: Monitoring, harsh discipline, and drug use in the intergenerational transmission of externalizing behavior. *Developmental Psychology*, *45*(5), 1214–1226. doi:10.1037/a0016129

Bakermans-Kranenburg, M. J., & van IJzendoorn, M. H. (2008). Oxytocin receptor (OXTR) and serotonin transporter (5-HTT) genes associated with observed parenting. *Social Cognitive and Affective Neuroscience*, *3*(2), 128–134. doi:10.1093/scan/nsn004

Bakermans-Kranenburg, M. J., & van IJzendoorn, M. H. (2014). A sociability gene? Meta-analysis of oxytocin receptor genotype effects in humans. *Psychiatric Genetics*, *24*(2), 45–51. doi:10.1097/YPG.0b013e3283643684

Barrett, J., & Fleming, A. S. (2011). All mothers are not created equal: neural and psychobiological perspectives on mothering and the importance of individual differences. *Journal of Child Psychology and Psychiatry, and Allied Disciplines*, *52*(4), 368–397. doi:10.1111/j.1469-7610.2010.02306.x

Barrett, J., Wonch, K. E., Gonzalez, A., Ali, N., Steiner, M., Hall, G. B., et al. (2011). Maternal affect and quality of parenting experiences are related to amygdala response to infant faces. *Social Neuroscience*, (February 2012), 37–41. doi:10.1080/17470919.2011.609907

Bartels, A., & Zeki, S. (2004). The neural correlates of maternal and romantic love. *NeuroImage*, *21*(3), 1155–1166. doi:10.1016/j.neuroimage.2003.11.003

Behrens, K. Y., Hart, S. L., & Parker, A. C. (2012). Maternal Sensitivity: Evidence of stability across time, contexts, and measurement instruments. *Infant and Child Development*. doi:10.1002/icd

Belsky, J., Jaffee, S. R., Sligo, J., Woodward, L., & Silva, P. A. (2005). Intergenerational transmission of warm-sensitive-stimulating parenting: A prospective study of mothers and fathers of 3-year-olds. *Child Development*, *76*(2), 384–396. doi:10.1111/j.1467-8624.2005.00852.x

Belsky, J., Jonassaint, C., Pluess, M., Stanton, M., Brummett, B. H., & Williams, R. (2009). Vulnerability genes or plasticity genes? *Molecular Psychiatry*, *14*(8), 746–754. doi:10.1038/mp.2009.44

Belsky, J., Youngblade, L., & Pensky, E. (1989). Childrearing history, marital quality, and maternal affect: Intergenerational transmission in a low-risk sample. *Development and Psychopathology*, *1*, 291–304. Retrieved from http://journals.cambridge.org/abstract_S0954579400000481

Berridge, K. C., & Robinson, T. E. (1998). What is the role of dopamine in reward: hedonic impact, reward learning, or incentive salience? *Brain Research. Brain Research Reviews*, *28*(3), 309–369. Retrieved from http://www.ncbi.nlm.nih.gov/pubmed/9858756

Bisceglia, R., Jenkins, J. M., Wigg, K. G., O'Connor, T. G., Moran, G., & Barr, C. L. (2012). Arginine vasopressin 1a receptor gene and maternal behavior: evidence of association and moderation. *Genes, Brain, and Behavior*, *11*(3), 262–268. doi:10.1111/j.1601-183X.2012.00769.x

Boccia, M. L., Goursaud, A. P. S., Bachevalier, J., Anderson, K. D., & Pedersen, C. A. (2007). Peripherally administered non-peptide oxytocin antagonist, L368, 899®, accumulates in limbic brain areas: A new pharmacological tool for the study of social motivation in non-human primates. *Hormones and Behavior*, *52*(3), 344–351. doi:10.1016/j.yhbeh.2007.05.009

Boecker, R., Holz, N. E., Buchmann, A. F., Blomeyer, D., Plichta, M. M., Wolf, I., … Laucht, M. (2014). Impact of early life adversity on reward processing in young adults: EEG-fMRI results from a prospective study over 25 years. *PloS One*, *9*(8), e104185. doi:10.1371/journal.pone.0104185

Bosch, O. J. (2010). Maternal nurturing is dependent on her innate anxiety: The behavioral roles of brain oxytocin and vasopressin. *Hormones and Behavior*, *59*(2), 202–212. doi:10.1016/j.yhbeh.2010.11.012

Brett, Z. H., Humphreys, K. L., Fleming, A. S., Kraemer, G. W., & Drury, S. S. (2015). Using cross-species comparisons and a neurobiological framework to understand early social deprivation effects on behavioral development. *Development and Psychopathology*, *27*(2), 347–367. doi:10.1017/S0954579415000036

Bridges, R. S. (2016). Long-term alterations in neural and endocrine processes induced by motherhood in mammals. *Hormones and Behavior*, *77*, 193–203. doi:10.1016/j.yhbeh.2015.09.001

Broad, K. D., Curley, J. P., & Keverne, E. B. (2006). Mother-infant bonding and the evolution of mammalian social relationships. *Philosophical Transactions of the Royal Society of London. Series B, Biological Sciences*, *361*(1476), 2199–2214. doi:10.1098/rstb.2006.1940

Brookes, E., & Shi, Y. (2014). Diverse epigenetic mechanisms of human disease. *Annual Review of Genetics*, *48*, 237–268. doi:10.1146/annurev-genet-120213-092518

Capaldi, D. M., Pears, K. C., Patterson, G. R., & Owen, L. D. (2003). Continuity of parenting practices across generations in an at-risk sample: A prospective comparison of direct and mediated associations. *Journal of Abnormal Child Psychology*, *31*(2), 127–142. Retrieved from http://www.ncbi.nlm.nih.gov/pubmed/12735396

Carson, D. S., Berquist, S. W., Trujillo, T. H., Garner, J. P., Hannah, S. L., Hyde, S. A, … Parker, K. J. (2014). Cerebrospinal fluid and plasma oxytocin concentrations are positively correlated and negatively predict anxiety in children. *Molecular Psychiatry*, (August), 1–6. doi:10.1038/mp.2014.132

Cents, R. A. M., Kok, R., Tiemeier, H., Lucassen, N., Székely, E., Bakermans-Kranenburg, M. J., … Lambregtse-van den Berg, M. P. (2014). Variations in maternal 5-HTTLPR affect observed sensitive parenting. *Journal of Child Psychology and Psychiatry, and Allied Disciplines*, *55*(9), 1025–1032. doi:10.1111/jcpp.12205

Champagne, F., Chretien, P., Stevenson, C. W., Zhang, T. Y., Gratton, A., & Meaney, M. J. (2004). Variations in nucleus accumbens dopamine associated with individual differences in maternal behavior in the rat. *The Journal of Neuroscience : The Official Journal of the Society for Neuroscience*, *24*(17), 4113–4123. doi:10.1523/JNEUROSCI.5322-03.2004

Champagne, F., Diorio, J., Sharma, S., & Meaney, M. J. (2001). Naturally occurring variations in maternal behavior in the rat are associated with differences in estrogen-inducible central oxytocin receptors. *Proceedings of the National Academy of Sciences of the United States of America*, *98*(22), 12736–12741. Retrieved from http://www.pubmedcentral.nih.gov/articlerender.fcgi?artid=60123&tool=pmcentrez&rendertype=abstract

Champagne, F., Francis, D. D., Mar, A., & Meaney, M. J. (2003). Variations in maternal care in the rat as a mediating influence for the effects of environment on development. *Physiology & Behavior*, *79*, 359–371. doi:10.1016/S0031-9384(03)00149-5

Champoux, M., Bennett, A. J., Shannon, C., Higley, J. D., Lesch, K.-P., & Suomi, S. J. (2002). Serotonin transporter gene polymorphism, differential early rearing, and behavior in rhesus monkey neonates. *Molecular Psychiatry*, *7*(10), 1058–1063. doi:10.1038/sj.mp.4001157

Chen, Z., & Kaplan, H. B. (2001). Intergenerational transmission of constructive parenting. *Journal of Marriage and Family, 63*(February), 17–31.

Chen, Z., Liu, R. X., & Kaplan, H. B. (2008). Mediating mechanisms for the intergenerational transmission of constructive parenting. *Journal of Family Issues*, *29*(12), 1574. doi:10.1177/0192513X08318968

Conger, R. D., Neppl, T., Kim, K. J., & Scaramella, L. (2003). Angry and aggressive behavior across three generations: A prospective, longitudinal study of parents and children. *Journal of Abnormal Child Psychology*, *31*(2), 143–160. Retrieved from http://www.ncbi.nlm.nih.gov/pubmed/12735397

Cooke, B., Higley, J. D., Shannon, C., Lindell, S. G., Higley, H., Suomi, S. J., et al. (1997). Rearing history and CSF Oxytocin as predictors of maternal competency in rhesus macaques. *American Journal of Primatology*, *42*(2), 102.

Dudek, J., Faress, A., Bornstein, M. H., & Haley, D. W. (2016). Infant cries rattle adult cognition. *PloS One*, *11*(5), e0154283. doi:10.1371/journal.pone.0154283

Ebstein, R. P., Knafo, A., Mankuta, D., Chew, S. H., & Lai, P. S. (2012). The contributions of oxytocin and vasopressin pathway genes to human behavior. *Hormones and Behavior*, *61*(3), 359–379. doi:10.1016/j.yhbeh.2011.12.014

Fahrbach, S. E., Morrell, J., & Pfaff, D. W. (1985). Possible role for endogenous oxytocin in estrogen-facilitated maternal behavior in rats. *Neuroendocrinology*, *40*(6), 526–532. Retrieved from http://www.ncbi.nlm.nih.gov/pubmed/4010891

Feldman, R., Gordon, I., Schneiderman, I., Weisman, O., & Zagoory-Sharon, O. (2010). Natural variations in maternal and paternal care are associated with systematic changes in oxytocin following parent-infant contact. *Psychoneuroendocrinology*, *35*(8), 1133–1141. doi:10.1016/j.psyneuen.2010.01.013

Feldman, R., Gordon, I., & Zagoory-Sharon, O. (2010). The cross-generation transmission of oxytocin in humans. *Hormones and Behavior*, *58*(4), 669–676. doi:10.1016/j.yhbeh.2010.06.005

Feldman, R., Zagoory-Sharon, O., Weisman, O., Schneiderman, I., Gordon, I., Maoz, R., … Ebstein, R. P. (2012). Sensitive parenting is associated with plasma oxytocin and polymorphisms in the OXTR and CD38 genes. *Biological Psychiatry*, *72*(3), 175–181. doi:10.1016/j.biopsych.2011.12.025

Fleming, A. S., Corter, C., Franks, P., Surbey, M., Schneider, B., & Steiner, M. (1993). Postpartum factors related to mother's attraction to newborn infant odors. *Developmental Psychobiology*, *26*(2), 115–132. doi:10.1002/dev.420260204

Fleming, A. S., Kraemer, G. W., Gonzalez, A., Lovic, V., Rees, S., & Melo, A. (2002). Mothering begets mothering: the transmission of behavior and its neurobiology across generations. *Pharmacology, Biochemistry, and Behavior*, *73*(1), 61–75. Retrieved from http://www.ncbi.nlm.nih.gov/pubmed/12076725

Fleming, A. S., & Li, M. (2002). Psychobiology of maternal behavior and its early determinants in nonhuman mammals. *Handbook of Parenting*, *2*, 61–97. Retrieved from https://judzrun-children.googlecode.com/files/Handbook%20of%20Parenting%202nd%20vol%202,%20Biology%20and%20Ecology%20of%20Pare.pdf#page=94

Fleming, A. S., Steiner, M., & Corter, C. (1997). Cortisol, hedonics, and maternal responsiveness in human mothers. *Hormones and Behavior*, *32*(2), 85–98. doi:10.1006/hbeh.1997.1407

Fortuna, K., van IJzendoorn, M. H., Mankuta, D., Kaitz, M., Avinun, R., Ebstein, R. P., et al. (2011). Differential genetic susceptibility to child risk at birth in predicting observed maternal behavior. *PloS One*, *6*(5), e19765. doi:10.1371/journal.pone.0019765

Galbally, M., Lewis, A. J., van IJzendoorn, M. H., & Permezel, M. (2011). The role of oxytocin in mother-infant relations: A systematic review of human studies. *Harvard Review of Psychiatry*, *19*(1), 1–14. doi:10.3109/10673229.2011.549771

Gara, M., Rosenberg, S., & Herzog, E. P. (1996). The abused child as parent. *Child Abuse and Neglect, 20*(9), 797–807.

Ge, X., Conger, R. D., Cadoret, R. J., Neiderhiser, J. M., Yates, W., Troughton, E., et al. (1996). The developmental interface between nature and nurture: A mutual influence model of child antisocial behavior and parent behaviors. *Developmental Psychology*, *32*(4), 574–589. doi:10.1037/0012-1649.32.4.574

Georges, F., & Aston-Jones, G. (2002). Activation of ventral tegmental area cells by the bed nucleus of the stria terminalis: A novel excitatory amino acid input to midbrain dopamine neurons. *The Journal of Neuroscience : The Official Journal of the Society for Neuroscience*, *22*(12), 5173–5187. Retrieved from http://www.jneurosci.org/content/22/12/5173.full

Giardino, J., Gonzalez, A., Steiner, M., & Fleming, A. S. (2008). Effects of motherhood on physiological and subjective responses to infant cries in teenage mothers: a comparison with non-mothers and adult mothers. *Hormones and Behavior*, *53*(1), 149–158. doi:10.1016/j.yhbeh.2007.09.010

Gonzalez, A., Lovic, V., Ward, G. R., Wainwright, P. E., & Fleming, A. S. (2001). Intergenerational effects of complete maternal deprivation and replacement stimulation on maternal behavior and emotionality in female rats. *Developmental Psychobiology*, *38*(1), 11–32. Retrieved from http://www.ncbi.nlm.nih.gov/pubmed/11150058

Hall, F. S., Wilkinson, L. S., Humby, T., & Robbins, T. W. (1999). Maternal deprivation of neonatal rats produces enduring changes in dopamine function. *Synapse (New York, N.Y.)*, *32* (1), 37–43. doi:10.1002/(SICI)1098-2396(199904)32:1<37::AID-SYN5>3.0.CO;2-4

Hansen, S., Bergvall, A. H., & Nyiredi, S. (1993). Interaction with pups enhances dopamine release in the ventral striatum of maternal rats: A microdialysis study. *Pharmacology, Biochemistry, and Behavior, 45*(3), 673–676. Retrieved from http://linkinghub.elsevier.com/retrieve/pii/009130579390523V

Heinrichs, M., & Domes, G. (2008). Neuropeptides and social behaviour: Effects of oxytocin and vasopressin in humans. *Progress in Brain Research, 170*(8), 337–350. doi:10.1016/S0079-6123(08)00428-7

Henschen, C. W., Palmiter, R. D., & Darvas, M. (2013). Restoration of dopamine signaling to the dorsal striatum is sufficient for aspects of active maternal behavior in female mice. *Endocrinology, 154*(11), 4316–4327. doi:10.1210/en.2013-1257

Hofer, M. A. (2002). Unexplained infant crying: An evolutionary perspective. *Acta Paediatrica (Oslo, Norway : 1992), 91*(5), 491–496. Retrieved from http://www.ncbi.nlm.nih.gov/pubmed/12113311

Hofer, M. A., & Sullivan, R. (2001). Toward a neurobiology of attachment. In C. Nelson & M. Luciana (Eds.), *Handbook of Developmental Cognitive Neuroscience* (pp. 599–616). Cambridge.

Insel, T. R., & Young, L. J. (2001). The neurobiology of attachment. *Nature Reviews Neuroscience, 2*(2), 129–136. doi:10.1038/35053579

Jaffee, S. R., & Price, T. S. (2008). Genotype-environment correlations: Implications for determining the relationship between environmental exposures and psychiatric illness. *Psychiatry, 7*(12), 496–499. doi:10.1016/j.mppsy.2008.10.002

Jenkins, J. M., McGowan, P., & Knafo-Noam, A. (2016). Parent–offspring transaction: Mechanisms and the value of within family designs. *Hormones and Behavior, 77*, 53–61. doi:10.1016/j.yhbeh.2015.06.018

Jin, D., Liu, H.-X., Hirai, H., Torashima, T., Nagai, T., Lopatina, O., … Higashida, H. (2007). CD38 is critical for social behaviour by regulating oxytocin secretion. *Nature, 446*(7131), 41–45. doi:10.1038/nature05526

Kaufman, J., & Zigler, E. (1987). Do abused children become abusive parents? *The American Journal of Orthopsychiatry, 57*(2), 186–192. Retrieved from http://www.ncbi.nlm.nih.gov/pubmed/3296775

Kendrick, K. M. (2000). Oxytocin, motherhood and bonding. *Experimental Physiology, 85S*, 111S–124S. Retrieved from http://onlinelibrary.wiley.com/doi/10.1111/j.1469-445X.2000.tb00014.x/abstract

Keverne, E. B., & Kendrick, K. M. (1992). Oxytocin facilitation of maternal-behavior in sheep. *Annals of the New York Academy of Sciences, 652,* 83–101.

Klahr, A. M., Klump, K., & Burt, S. A. (2014). A constructive replication of the association between the oxytocin receptor genotype and parenting. *Journal of Family Psychology : JFP : Journal of the Division of Family Psychology of the American Psychological Association (Division 43).* doi:10.1037/fam0000034

Knutson, J. F. (1995). Psychological characteristics of maltreated children: Putative risk factors and consequences. *Annual Review of Psychology, 46*, 401–431. doi:10.1146/annurev.ps.46.020195.002153

Kok, R., Thijssen, S., Bakermans-Kranenburg, M. J., Jaddoe, V. W. V, Verhulst, F. C., White, T., … Tiemeier, H. (2015). Normal variation in early parental sensitivity predicts child structural brain development. *Journal of the American Academy of Child and Adolescent Psychiatry, 54* (10), 824–831.e1. doi:10.1016/j.jaac.2015.07.009

Kraemer, G. W. (1992). A psychobiological theory of attachment. Retrieved from http://philpapers.org/rec/KRAAPT-2

Kringelbach, M. (2008). The hedonic brain: A functional neuroanatomy of human pleasure. In M. Kringelbach & K. Berridge (Eds.), *Pleasures of the brain*. Oxford, UK: Oxford University Press.

Kundakovic, M., & Champagne, F. A. (2014). Early-life experience, epigenetics, and the developing brain. *Neuropsychopharmacology : Official Publication of the American College of Neuropsychopharmacology, 40*(1), 140–152. doi:10.1038/npp.2014.140

Lee, D., Brooks-Gunn, J., McLanahan, S. S., Notterman, D., & Garfinkel, I. (2013). The Great Recession, genetic sensitivity, and maternal harsh parenting. *Proceedings of the National Academy of Sciences of the United States of America*, *110*(34), 13780–13784. doi:10.1073/pnas.1312398110

Lee, S. S., Chronis-Tuscano, A., Keenan, K., Pelham, W. E., Loney, J., Van Hulle, C. A, … Lahey, B. B. (2008). Association of maternal dopamine transporter genotype with negative parenting: Evidence for gene x environment interaction with child disruptive behavior. *Molecular Psychiatry*, *15*(5), 548–558. doi:10.1038/mp.2008.102

Leibenluft, E., Gobbini, M. I., Harrison, T., & Haxby, J. V. (2004). Mothers' neural activation in response to pictures of their children and other children. *Biological Psychiatry*, *56*(4), 225–232. doi:10.1016/j.biopsych.2004.05.017

Levine, A., Zagoory-Sharon, O., Feldman, R., & Weller, A. (2007). Oxytocin during pregnancy and early postpartum: individual patterns and maternal-fetal attachment. *Peptides*, *28*(6), 1162–1169. doi:10.1016/j.peptides.2007.04.016

Lévy, F., Melo, A. I., Galef, B. G., Madden, M., & Fleming, A. S. (2003). Complete maternal deprivation affects social, but not spatial, learning in adult rats. *Developmental Psychobiology*, *43*(3), 177–191. doi:10.1002/dev.10131

Light, K. C., Smith, T. E., Johns, J. M., Brownley, K. A., Hofheimer, J. A., & Amico, J. A. (2000). Oxytocin responsivity in mothers of infants: A preliminary study of relationships with blood pressure during laboratory stress and normal ambulatory activity. *Health Psychology*, *19*(6), 560. Retrieved from http://psycnet.apa.org/journals/hea/19/6/560/

Lindhiem, O., Bernard, K., & Dozier, M. (2011). Maternal sensitivity: Within-person variability and the utility of multiple assessments. *Child Maltreatment*, *16*(1), 41–50. doi:10.1177/1077559510387662

Liu, D., Diorio, J., Tannenbaum, B., Caldji, C., Francis, D. D., Freedman, A., … Meaney, M. J. (1997). Maternal care, hippocampal glucocorticoid receptors, and hypothalamic-pituitary-adrenal responses to stress. *Science (New York, N.Y.)*, *277*(5332), 1659–1662. Retrieved from http://www.ncbi.nlm.nih.gov/pubmed/9287218

Lohaus, A., Keller, H., Ball, J., Voelker, S., & Elben, C. (2004). Maternal sensitivity in interactions with three-and 12-month-old infants: Stability, structural composition, and developmental consequences. *Infant and Child Development*, *13*(3), 235–252. doi:10.1002/icd.

Lomanowska, A. M., Boivin, M., Hertzman, C., & Fleming, A. S. (2016). Parenting begets parenting: A neurobiological perspective on early adversity and the transmission of parenting styles across generations. *Neuroscience*. doi:10.1016/j.neuroscience.2015.09.029

Lomanowska, A. M., & Kraemer, G. W. (2014). Increased behavioral output but intact goal-directed and habitual responding for food reward following early-life social deprivation in rats. *Behavioural Brain Research*, *271*, 94–105. doi:10.1016/j.bbr.2014.05.062

Lomanowska, A. M., Lovic, V., Rankine, M. J., Mooney, S. J., Robinson, T. E., & Kraemer, G. W. (2011). Inadequate early social experience increases the incentive salience of reward-related cues in adulthood. *Behavioural Brain Research*, *220*(1), 91–99. doi:10.1016/j.bbr.2011.01.033

Lomanowska, A. M., & Melo, A. I. (2016). Deconstructing the Function of Maternal Stimulation in Offspring Development: Insights from the Artificial Rearing Model in Rats. *Hormones and Behavior*, *77*(October), 224–236. doi:10.1016/j.yhbeh.2015.05.017

Lomanowska, A. M., Rana, S., McCutcheon, D., Parker, L., & Wainwright, P. E. (2006). Artificial rearing alters the response of rats to natural and drug-mediated rewards. *Developmental Psychobiology*, *48*, 301–314. doi:10.1002/dev

Lonstein, J. S. (2002). Effects of dopamine receptor antagonism with haloperidol on nurturing behavior in the biparental prairie vole. *Pharmacology, Biochemistry, and Behavior*, *74*(1), 11–19. Retrieved from http://www.ncbi.nlm.nih.gov/pubmed/12376148

Lonstein, J. S., Lévy, F., & Fleming, A. S. (2015). Common and divergent psychobiological mechanisms underlying maternal behaviors in non-human and human mammals. *Hormones and Behavior*, *73*, 156–85. doi:10.1016/j.yhbeh.2015.06.011

Lorberbaum, J. P., Newman, J. D., Horwitz, A. R., Dubno, J. R. J. R. J. R., Lydiard, R. B. B., Hamner, M. B., … George, M. S. M. S. (2002). A potential role for thalamocingulate circuitry in human maternal behavior. *Biological Psychiatry*, *51*(6), 431–445. doi:10.1016/S0006-3223(01)01284-7

Lovic, V., & Fleming, A. S. (2004). Artificially-reared female rats show reduced prepulse inhibition and deficits in the attentional set shifting task—reversal of effects with maternal-like licking stimulation. *Behavioural Brain Research*, *148*(1–2), 209–219. doi:10.1016/S0166-4328(03)00206-7

Lovic, V., & Fleming, A. S. (2015). Propagation of maternal behavior across generations is associated with changes in non-maternal cognitive and behavioral processes. *Behavioural Processes*, *117*, 42–47. doi:10.1016/j.beproc.2015.02.016

Lovic, V., Gonzalez, A., & Fleming, A. S. (2001). Maternally separated rats show deficits in maternal care in adulthood. *Developmental Psychobiology*, *39*(1), 19–33. Retrieved from http://www.ncbi.nlm.nih.gov/pubmed/11507706

Lucassen, N., Kok, R., Bakermans-Kranenburg, M. J., Van IJzendoorn, M. H., Jaddoe, V. W. V, Hofman, A., … Tiemeier, H. (2015). Executive functions in early childhood: the role of maternal and paternal parenting practices. *The British Journal of Developmental Psychology*, *33*(4), 489–505. doi:10.1111/bjdp.12112

Maccoby, E. E. (2000). Parenting and its effects on children: on reading and misreading behavior genetics. *Annual Review of Psychology*, *51*, 1–27. doi:10.1146/annurev.psych.51.1.1

Maestripieri, D. (2005). Early experience affects the intergenerational transmission of infant abuse in rhesus monkeys. *Proceedings of the National Academy of Sciences of the United States of America*, *102*(27), 9726–9729. Retrieved from http://www.pubmedcentral.nih.gov/articlerender.fcgi?artid=1172276&tool=pmcentrez&rendertype=abstract

Maestripieri, D., Higley, J. D., Lindell, S. G., Newman, T. K., McCormack, K., & Sanchez, M. M. (2006). Early maternal rejection affects the development of monoaminergic systems and adult abusive parenting in rhesus macaques (*Macaca mulatta*). *Behavioral Neuroscience*, *120*(5), 1017–1024. doi:10.1037/0735-7044.120.5.1017

Maestripieri, D., Hoffman, C. L., Anderson, G. M., Carter, C. S., & Higley, J. D. (2009). Mother-infant interactions in free-ranging rhesus macaques: relationships between physiological and behavioral variables. *Physiology & Behavior*, *96*(4–5), 613–619. doi:10.1016/j.physbeh.2008.12.016

Maestripieri, D., Lindell, S. G., & Higley, J. D. D. (2007). Intergenerational transmission of maternal behavior in rhesus macaques and its underlying mechanisms. *Developmental Psychobiology*, *49*(2), 165–171. doi:10.1002/dev

Mann, P. E. (2014). Gene expression profiling during pregnancy in rat brain tissue. *Brain Sciences*, *4*(1), 125–135. doi:10.3390/brainsci4010125

Mattson, B., Williams, S., Rosenblatt, J., & Morrell, J. (2001). Comparison of two positive reinforcing stimuli: Pups and cocaine throughout the postpartum period. *Behavioral Neuroscience*, *115*(3), 683. Retrieved from http://psycnet.apa.org/journals/bne/115/3/683/

McGowan, P., Sasaki, A., & D'Alessio, A. (2009). Epigenetic regulation of the glucocorticoid receptor in human brain associates with childhood abuse. *Nature Neuroscience*, *12*(3), 342–348. doi:10.1038/nn.2270

Meaney, M. J. (2010). Epigenetics and the biological definition of gene x environment interactions. *Child Development*, *81*(1), 41–79. doi:10.1111/j.1467-8624.2009.01381.x

Melo, A. I., Lovic, V., Gonzalez, A., Madden, M., Sinopoli, K., & Fleming, A. S. (2006). Maternal and littermate deprivation disrupts maternal behavior and social-learning of food preference in adulthood: Tactile stimulation, nest odor, and social rearing prevent these effects. *Developmental Psychobiology*, *48*(3), 209–219. doi:10.1002/dev

Meyer-Lindenberg, A., Domes, G., Kirsch, P., & Heinrichs, M. (2011). Oxytocin and vasopressin in the human brain: Social neuropeptides for translational medicine. *Nature Reviews Neuroscience*, *12*(9), 524–538. doi:10.1038/nrn3044

Michalska, K. J., Decety, J., Liu, C., Chen, Q., Martz, M. E., Jacob, S., … Lahey, B. B. (2014). Genetic imaging of the association of oxytocin receptor gene (OXTR) polymorphisms with positive maternal parenting. *Frontiers in Behavioral Neuroscience*, *8*(February), 21. doi:10.3389/fnbeh.2014.00021

Mileva-Seitz, V. R., Afonso, V. M., & Fleming, A. S. (2012). Dopamine: Another "Magic Bullet" for caregiver responsiveness? In T. R. Gleason, D. Narvaez, J. Panksepp, & Allan N. Schore (Eds.), *Evolution, early experience and human development: from research to practice and policy* (pp. 152–178). Oxford Scholarship Online.

Mileva-Seitz, V. R., Bakermans-Kranenburg, M. J., & van IJzendoorn, M. H. (2015). Genetic mechanisms of parenting. *Hormones and Behavior*, *77*, 211–223. doi:10.1016/j.yhbeh.2015.06.003

Mileva-Seitz, V. R., & Fleming, A. S. (2011). How mothers are born: A psychobiological analysis of mothering. In A. Booth, S. M. McHale, & N. S. Landale (Eds.), *Biosocial foundations of family processes* (pp. 3–34). New York, NY: Springer.

Mileva-Seitz, V. R., Fleming, A. S., Meaney, M. J., Mastroianni, A., Sinnwell, J. P., Steiner, M., … Sokolowski, M. B. (2012). Dopamine receptors D1 and D2 are related to observed maternal behavior. *Genes, Brain, and Behavior*, *11*(6), 684–694. doi:10.1111/j.1601-183X.2012.00804.x

Mileva-Seitz, V. R., Kennedy, J., Atkinson, L., Steiner, M., Levitan, R., Matthews, S. G., … Fleming, A. S. (2011). Serotonin transporter allelic variation in mothers predicts maternal sensitivity, behavior and attitudes toward 6-month-old infants. *Genes, Brain, and Behavior*, *10* (3), 325–333. doi:10.1111/j.1601-183X.2010.00671.x

Mileva-Seitz, V. R., Steiner, M., Atkinson, L., Meaney, M. J., Levitan, R., Kennedy, J. L., … Fleming, A. S. (2013). Interaction between oxytocin genotypes and early experience predicts quality of mothering and postpartum mood. *PloS One*, *8*(4), e61443. doi:10.1371/journal.pone.0061443

Mills-Koonce, W. R., Propper, C. B., Gariepy, J.-L., Blair, C., Garrett-Peters, P., & Cox, M. J. (2007). Bidirectional genetic and environmental influences on mother and child behavior: the family system as the unit of analyses. *Development and Psychopathology*, *19*(4), 1073–1087. doi:10.1017/S0954579407000545

Moehler, E., Biringen, Z., & Poustka, L. (2007). Emotional availability in a sample of mothers with a history of abuse. *The American Journal of Orthopsychiatry*, *77*(4), 624–628. doi:10.1037/0002-9432.77.4.624

Munesue, T., Yokoyama, S., Nakamura, K., Anitha, A., Yamada, K., Hayashi, K., … Higashida, H. (2010). Two genetic variants of CD38 in subjects with autism spectrum disorder and controls. *Neuroscience Research*, *67*(2), 181–191. doi:10.1016/j.neures.2010.03.004

Naumova, O. Y., Lee, M., Koposov, R., Szyf, M., Dozier, M., & Grigorenko, E. L. (2012). Differential patterns of whole-genome DNA methylation in institutionalized children and children raised by their biological parents. *Development and Psychopathology*, *24*(1), 143–155. doi:10.1017/S0954579411000605

Neppl, T. K., Conger, R. D., Scaramella, L. V, & Ontai, L. L. (2009). Intergenerational continuity in parenting behavior: mediating pathways and child effects. *Developmental Psychology*, *45*(5), 1241–1256. doi:10.1037/a0014850

Newcomb, M. D., & Locke, T. F. (2001). Intergenerational cycle of maltreatment: a popular concept obscured by methodological limitations. *Child Abuse & Neglect*, *25*(9), 1219–1240. Retrieved from http://www.ncbi.nlm.nih.gov/pubmed/11700694

Nitschke, J. B., Nelson, E. E., Rusch, B. D., Fox, A. S., Oakes, T. R., & Davidson, R. J. (2004). Orbitofrontal cortex tracks positive mood in mothers viewing pictures of their newborn infants. *NeuroImage*, *21*(2), 583–592. doi:10.1016/j.neuroimage.2003.10.005

Noriuchi, M., Kikuchi, Y., & Senoo, A. (2008). The functional neuroanatomy of maternal love: mother's response to infant's attachment behaviors. *Biological Psychiatry*, *63*(4), 415–423. doi:10.1016/j.biopsych.2007.05.018

Numan, M. (2015). *Neurobiology of social behavior: Toward an understanding of the prosocial and antisocial brain*. London, UK: Academic Press.

Numan, M., Fleming, A. S., & Levy, F. (2006). Maternal behavior. In J. D. Neill (Ed.), *Knobil & Neill's physiology of reproduction* (pp. 1921–1993). New York: Elsevier Inc.

Out, D., Pieper, S., Bakermans-Kranenburg, M. J., & van IJzendoorn, M. H. (2010). Physiological reactivity to infant crying: A behavioral genetic study. *Genes, Brain, and Behavior*, *9*(8), 868–876. doi:10.1111/j.1601-183X.2010.00624.x

Palombo, D. J., Nowoslawski, M., & Fleming, A. S. (2010). Motherless rats show deficits in maternal behavior towards fostered pups. *Developmental Psychobiology*, *52*(2), 142–148. doi:10.1002/dev.20422

Pauli-Pott, U. (2008). Mothers with depressive symptoms: cross-situational consistency and temporal stability of their parenting behavior. *Infant Behavior & Development*, *31*(4), 679–687. doi:10.1016/j.infbeh.2008.04.010

Pearson, R. M., Lightman, S. L., & Evans, J. (2011). Attentional processing of infant emotion during late pregnancy and mother-infant relations after birth. *Archives of Women's Mental Health*, *14*(1), 23–31. doi:10.1007/s00737-010-0180-4

Pechtel, P., & Pizzagalli, D. A. (2011). Effects of early life stress on cognitive and affective function: an integrated review of human literature. *Psychopharmacology*, *214*(1), 55–70. doi:10.1007/s00213-010-2009-2

Pedersen, C. A., Caldwell, J. D., Walker, C., Ayers, G., & Mason, G. A. (1994). Oxytocin activates the postpartum onset of rat maternal behavior in the ventral tegmental and medial preoptic areas. *Behavioral Neuroscience, 108*(6), 1163.

Pedersen, F. A., Huffman, L. C., del Carmen, R., & Bryan, Y. E. (1996). Prenatal maternal reactivity to infant cries predicts postnatal perceptions of infant temperament and marriage appraisal. *Child Development*, *67*(5), 2541–2552. Retrieved from http://www.ncbi.nlm.nih.gov/pubmed/9022255

Perroud, N., Dayer, A., Piguet, C., Nallet, A., Favre, S., Malafosse, A., & Aubry, J.-M. (2014). Childhood maltreatment and methylation of the glucocorticoid receptor gene NR3C1 in bipolar disorder. *The British Journal of Psychiatry : The Journal of Mental Science*, *204*(1), 30–35. doi:10.1192/bjp.bp.112.120055

Porter, R. H., Cernoch, J. M., & McLaughlin, F. J. (1983). Maternal recognition of neonates through olfactory cues. *Physiology & Behavior*, *30*(1), 151–154. Retrieved from http://www.ncbi.nlm.nih.gov/pubmed/6836038

Porter, R. H., Makin, J. W., Davis, L. B., & Christensen, K. M. (1991). An assessment of the salient olfactory environment of formula-fed infants. *Physiology & Behavior*, *50*(5), 907–911. Retrieved from http://www.ncbi.nlm.nih.gov/pubmed/1805280

Proverbio, A. M., Brignone, V., Matarazzo, S., Del Zotto, M., & Zani, A. (2006). Gender and parental status affect the visual cortical response to infant facial expression. *Neuropsychologia*, *44*(14), 2987–2999. doi:10.1016/j.neuropsychologia.2006.06.015

Ranote, S., Elliott, R., Abel, K. M., Mitchell, R., Deakin, J. F. W., & Appleby, L. (2004). The neural basis of maternal responsiveness to infants: an fMRI study. *NeuroReport*, *15*(11), 1825–1829. doi:10.1097/01.wnr.0000137078.64128.6a

Rees, S. L., & Fleming, A. S. (2001). How early maternal separation and juvenile experience with pups affect maternal behavior and emotionality in adult postpartum rats. *Animal Learning & Behavior*, *29*(3), 221–233. doi:10.3758/BF03192889

Riem, M. M. E., Alink, L. R. A., Out, D., Van IJzendoorn, M. H., & Bakermans-Kranenburg, M. J. (2015). Beating the brain about abuse: Empirical and meta-analytic studies of the association between maltreatment and hippocampal volume across childhood and adolescence. *Development and Psychopathology*, *27*(2), 507–520. doi:10.1017/S0954579415000127

Riem, M. M. E., Pieper, S., Out, D., Bakermans-Kranenburg, M. J., & van IJzendoorn, M. H. (2011). Oxytocin receptor gene and depressive symptoms associated with physiological reactivity to infant crying. *Social Cognitive and Affective Neuroscience*, *6*(3), 294–300. doi:10.1093/scan/nsq035

Rijlaarsdam, J., Pappa, I., Walton, E., Bakermans-Kranenburg, M. J., Mileva-Seitz, V. R., Rippe, R. C. A., … van IJzendoorn, M. H. (2016). An epigenome-wide association meta-analysis of prenatal maternal stress in neonates: A model approach for replication. *Epigenetics*, 1–10. doi:10.1080/15592294.2016.1145329

Roberts, R., O'Connor, T., Dunn, J., & Golding, J. (2004). The effects of child sexual abuse in later family life; mental health, parenting and adjustment of offspring. *Child Abuse & Neglect, 28*(5), 525–545. doi:10.1016/j.chiabu.2003.07.006

Robinson, D. L., Zitzman, D. L., & Williams, S. K. (2011). Mesolimbic dopamine transients in motivated behaviors: focus on maternal behavior. *Frontiers in Psychiatry, 2*, 23. doi:10.3389/fpsyt.2011.00023

Rosenblatt, J. (1967). Nonhormonal basis of maternal behavior in the rat. *Science, 156*, 1512–1513.

Saltzman, W., & Maestripieri, D. (2010). The neuroendocrinology of primate maternal behavior. *Progress in Neuro-psychopharmacology & Biological Psychiatry, 35*(5), 1192–1204. doi:10.1016/j.pnpbp.2010.09.017

Sander, K., Frome, Y., & Scheich, H. (2007). FMRI activations of amygdala, cingulate cortex, and auditory cortex by infant laughing and crying. *Human Brain Mapping, 28*(10), 1007–1022. doi:10.1002/hbm.20333

Scaramella, L. V, Neppl, T. K., Ontai, L. L., & Conger, R. D. (2008). Consequences of socioeconomic disadvantage across three generations: parenting behavior and child externalizing problems. *Journal of Family Psychology (JFP) : Journal of the Division of Family Psychology of the American Psychological Association (Division 43), 22*(5), 725–733. doi:10.1037/a0013190

Seifritz, E., Esposito, F., Neuhoff, J. G., Lüthi, A., Mustovic, H., Dammann, G., … Tedeschi, G. (2003). Differential sex-independent amygdala response to infant crying and laughing in parents versus nonparents. *Biological Psychiatry, 54*(12), 1367–1375. doi:10.1016/S0006-3223(03)00697-8

Shah, A., Oxley, G., Lovic, V., & Fleming, A. S. (2002). Effects of preweaning exposure to novel maternal odors on maternal responsiveness and selectivity in adulthood. *Developmental Psychobiology, 41*(3), 187–196. doi:10.1002/dev.10064

Stallings, J., Fleming, A. S., Corter, C., Worthman, C., & Steiner, M. (2001). The effects of infant cries and odors on sympathy, cortisol, and autonomic responses in new mothers and nonpostpartum women. *Parenting, 1*(1), 71–100. doi:10.1207/S15327922PAR011&2_5

Strathearn, L., Li, J., Fonagy, P., & Montague, P. R. (2008). What's in a smile? Maternal brain responses to infant facial cues. *Pediatrics, 122*(1), 40–51. doi:10.1542/peds.2007-1566

Suomi, S. J. (1999). Attachment in rhesus monkeys. In J. Cassidy & P. R. Shaver (Eds.), *Handbook of attachment: Theory, research, and clinical applications* (pp. 181–197). New York: Guilford Press.

Szyf, M., Weaver, I. C. G., Champagne, F. A., Diorio, J., & Meaney, M. J. (2005). Maternal programming of steroid receptor expression and phenotype through DNA methylation in the rat. *Frontiers in Neuroendocrinology, 26*(3–4), 139–162. doi:10.1016/j.yfrne.2005.10.002

Takayanagi, Y., Yoshida, M., Bielsky, I. F., Ross, H. E., Kawamata, M., Onaka, T., … Nishimori, K. (2005). Pervasive social deficits, but normal parturition, in oxytocin receptor-deficient mice. *Proceedings of the National Academy of Sciences of the United States of America, 102*(44), 16096–16101. doi:10.1073/pnas.0505312102

Taylor, S. E. (2008). Genetic contributions to sensitive parenting. *Social Cognitive and Affective Neuroscience, 3*(2), 89–90. doi:10.1093/scan/nsn015

Thoman, E. B., & Arnold, W. J. (1968). Effects of incubator rearing with social deprivation on maternal behavior in rats. *Journal of Comparative and Physiological Psychology, 65*(3), 441–446. Retrieved from http://www.ncbi.nlm.nih.gov/pubmed/5667385

Toth, M. (2015). Mechanisms of Non-Genetic Inheritance and Psychiatric Disorders. *Neuropsychopharmacology : Official Publication of the American College of Neuropsychopharmacology, 40*(1), 129–140. doi:10.1038/npp.2014.127

van IJzendoorn, M. H., Bakermans-Kranenburg, M. J., & Mesman, J. (2008). Dopamine system genes associated with parenting in the context of daily hassles. *Genes, Brain, and Behavior, 7*(4), 403–410. doi:10.1111/j.1601-183X.2007.00362.x

Vereijken, C. M. J. L., Riksen-Walraven J. M., & Kondo-Ikemura, K. (1997). Maternal sensitivity and infant attachment security in Japan: A longitudinal study. *International Journal of Behavioral Development*, *21*(1), 35–50. doi:10.1080/016502597384974

Weaver, I. C. G., Cervoni, N., Champagne, F., D'Alessio, A. C., Sharma, S., Seckl, J. R., … Meaney, M. J. (2004). Epigenetic programming by maternal behavior. *Nature Neuroscience*, *7* (8), 847–854. doi:10.1038/nn1276

Whittle, S., Simmons, J. G., Dennison, M., Vijayakumar, N., Schwartz, O., Yap, M. B. H., … Allen, N. B. (2014). Positive parenting predicts the development of adolescent brain structure: A longitudinal study. *Developmental Cognitive Neuroscience*, *8*, 7–17. doi:10.1016/j.dcn.2013.10.006

Wilson, D. A., & Sullivan, R. M. (1994). Neurobiology of associative learning in the neonate: Early olfactory learning. *Behavioral and Neural Biology*, *61*(1), 1–18. doi:10.1016/S0163-1047(05)80039-1

Windhorst, D. A., Mileva-Seitz, V. R., Linting, M., Hofman, A., Jaddoe, V. W. V, Verhulst, F. C., … Bakermans-Kranenburg, M. J. (2015). Differential susceptibility in a developmental perspective: DRD4 and maternal sensitivity predicting externalizing behavior. *Developmental Psychobiology*, *57*(1), 35–49. doi:10.1002/dev.21257

Zhang, T. Y., Labonté, B., Wen, X. L., Turecki, G., & Meaney, M. J. (2013). Epigenetic mechanisms for the early environmental regulation of hippocampal glucocorticoid receptor gene expression in rodents and humans. *Neuropsychopharmacology : Official Publication of the American College of Neuropsychopharmacology*, *38*(1), 111–123. doi:10.1038/npp.2012.149

Zhang, T.-Y., & Meaney, M. J. (2010). Epigenetics and the environmental regulation of the genome and its function. *Annual Review of Psychology*, *61*, 439–466, C1-3. doi:10.1146/annurev.psych.60.110707.163625

Part III
Pathways to Managing Parental Stress

Chapter 11
Parenting Stress and Parental Efficacy

Keith Crnic and Emily Ross

Among determinants of parenting, few constructs have engendered the kind of attention as has stress. Since Belsky's seminal determinants paper in 1984, and to some degree even before, stress has had a prominent place in understanding why parents parent the way that they do. The effect of stress on parenting, especially the adverse influences on aspects of parental efficacy, has been studied extensively across the last several decades. Indeed, it has become almost typical that studies of the determinants of parenting, especially if any risk condition is present, include some measurement of reported stress.

Several conceptual frameworks for understanding parenting stress currently exist and influence the nature of the research that has been done to explicate the construct. Despite differences in conceptualizations, the defining characteristics of parenting stress are similar and are well captured by Deater-Deckard's (2004) description of parenting stress as "a set of processes that lead to aversive psychological and physiological reactions arising from attempts to adapt to the demands of parenthood" (p.6). Given these defining qualities, it is reasonable to expect that parenting stress would present a significant challenge to parents' self-efficacy and sense of competence or well-being.

It is nevertheless important to recognize here that parenting stress cannot be simply viewed as an attribute or response of an individual mother or father at any one point in time. A mother's or father's perception of parenting stress and the implications of that experience reflect systemic processes within the family that are transactional, reciprocal, bidirectional, and developmental in their function. To date, a more systemic developmental perspective has not characterized the general approach to research on parenting stress. But in addressing the connections between

K. Crnic (✉) · E. Ross
Department of Psychology, Arizona State University, Tempe, AZ, USA
e-mail: keith.crnic@asu.edu

E. Ross
e-mail: EmilyRoss@asu.edu

K. Deater-Deckard and R. Panneton (eds.), *Parental Stress and Early Child Development*, DOI 10.1007/978-3-319-55376-4_11

parenting stress and parental self-efficacy, this chapter will promote approaches to understanding relations between parenting stress and parental functioning that encourage more systemic developmental perspectives.

Before delving more deeply into issues related to parenting stress, we first address conceptual perspectives on parental self-efficacy and the reasons why its links to parenting stress may be particularly important. Next, we address a number of critical issues in the conceptualization of parenting stress, with a particular eye toward its measurement, its developmental implications, and the transactional, systemic nature of the construct. From those perspectives, we then examine the evidence that links parenting stress to a variety of parenting processes, promoting a focus on reciprocal, transactional, and systemic perspectives. We conclude with a few recommendations for future research directions.

Parenting Self-efficacy

As O'Neil, Wilson, Shaw, and Dishion (2009) indicate, parental efficacy draws much from the basic concept of self-efficacy (Bandura, 1977), and parental self-efficacy (Glatz & Buchanan, 2015) addresses the extent to which parents believe they have the ability to influence their children's development and the contexts in which that development takes place. The expectation that one is efficacious as a parent is derived from multiple sources of input (O'Neil, Wilson, Shaw, & Dishion 2009), including parents' direct experience with their children and the nature of ecological contexts in which one's parenting experience occurs (Glatz & Buchanan, 2015). In this sense, parental self-efficacy emerges from the same experiential context as does parenting stress, giving rise to the likelihood that the two constructs might well align and that parenting stress may serve to change parental efficacy over time. There is some evidence that parental self-efficacy does change over time, increasing during early childhood (Weaver et al., 2008) only to decrease as children enter adolescence (Glatz & Buchanan, 2015). Whether such change can be tied to parenting stress is an important question for which the answer is not yet entirely known.

We have speculated before about whether parenting stress can serve as a change agent over time (Crnic & Low, 2002), essentially reducing parents' sense of their own efficacy as children develop and changing the nature or quality of parent–child relationships. The answer to whether such pathways of influence exist has not yet been fully explicated, but the effort to better understand the links between parenting stress and parent efficacy offers some important indications that there may be merit to such suggestions.

Nevertheless, when it comes to parenting, it seems clear that experience matters. There is a wealth of evidence that having the opportunities to develop mastery is an effective way to increase self-efficacy (Bandura, 1977), and indeed, parents with multiple children report higher parental self-efficacy than do parents of single children (Leahy-Warren & McCarthy, 2011). On the other hand, there is also evidence to suggest that parents with more children report higher parenting stress

(Crnic & Greenberg, 1990; Skreden et al., 2012; Spinelli, Poehlmann, & Bolt, 2013), balancing the effect of experience with the pressures of increased demand on parents.

Parents with high self-efficacy feel competent in the parenting role, have a sense that they can successfully accomplish parenting tasks, and believe that they can exert positive influence on a child's developmental competence. Parenting attitudes, parenting beliefs, and parenting behaviors are all relevant to this sense of self-efficacy, and each of these characteristics has some degree of impact on child development. Child characteristics, behavior, and relational qualities are also critical to parents' self-efficacy and may be more important than are the ecological contexts in which the parent–child relationship exists (see also McQuillian and Bates, Chap. 4 this volume; Glatz & Buchanan, 2015). Again, these attributes of parental self-efficacy share important features with parenting stress, which is also highly dependent on parental perspectives, children's developmental and behavioral qualities, and the quality of the parent–child relationship.

We are all likely to agree that parenting competence and self-efficacy (PSE) are important attributes of successful parenting (Shumow & Lomax, 2002; Teti & Gelfand, 1991) and are linked with a variety of positive and negative outcomes for parents and for children (Jones & Prinz, 2005). Identifying those factors that create risk for parenting competence is therefore important in constructing models for successful child development. The relations between parenting stress and parental self-efficacy are reciprocal, and the direction of effect can travel in either way. Further, there are likely to be critical pathways of influence at play. It may be that compromised parenting self-efficacy, in whatever form, can be a direct consequence of parenting stress. There is evidence to support such simple direct effects. On the other hand, it is likely that there are more complex pathways of influence in operation in which the links between parenting stress and parental self-efficacy are allied in mediated processes with implications for emerging parent and child well-being. Further, even more complex pathways that delineate moderated mediation processes (or vice versa) are also possible. For example, early parenting stress may predict later parental psychological distress (e.g., more depressive symptoms), but the effect may be indirectly affected (mediated) by parental self-efficacy. But, that mediated pathway may only be present under conditions where social support does not exist.

Conceptually, high parenting stress should have an adverse effect on parenting self-efficacy, creating doubt and hesitation or irritation and impulsive parental responding. On the other hand, low parent self-efficacy may well lead parents to perceive children's behavior and parenting processes as more stressful. Either direction is reasonable to assume and may in fact take place within the parent and parent–child dyad. Research models pursue both directions in an attempt to understand the complex interplay between parenting stress and parenting self-efficacy. But regardless of the directional conundrum, the relation between parenting stress and parenting self-efficacy is transactional; that is, the two factors affect one another across time. This renders the direction of effect issue as subject to the specific question at hand, and the timing of when that question is asked. Once a link is established between parenting stress and parenting self-efficacy, they become reciprocally influential to one another in ways that serve to perpetuate the connection. As the parent is stressed, she or he feels less efficacious. As efficacy becomes more compromised, parenting becomes more stressful, and the cycle is maintained between the two interdependent constructs.

Preliminary Considerations in Linking Parenting Stress and Parent Self-efficacy

In exploring the links between parenting stress and parenting efficacy, there are multiple issues to consider that help to define and explicate the nature of the connections that may exist. These issues are particularly germane to the synergy between parenting stress and parenting self-efficacy but are tied more specifically to parenting stress as an independent construct as well.

Conceptual Bases and Limitations

It is difficult to reach a full understanding of the implications of parenting stress on later competencies without addressing the ways in which it is has been both conceptualized and measured. Crnic and Low (2002) as well as Deater-Deckard (2004) have provided discussions of the issues and approaches, differentiating the more problem-focused parent–child-relationship (P-C-R) framework exemplified by Abidin's (1992) model, and the more normative, everyday experiential basis of parenting daily hassles (PDH) as indexed by the approach of Crnic and Greenberg (1990). By far, the majority of the research on parenting stress has utilized the P-C-R model and Abidin's (1995) Parenting Stress Index (PSI), and most often now its reliable and useful three-scale short form. As Deater-Deckard (2004) suggests, the PSI is most typically used with clinical or risk samples in which parenting stress is thought to be highly salient as a predictor of some adverse condition or a result of some problematic function. In contrast, the PDH targets more normative and adaptive everyday stresses that are typical of child behavior and parenting responsibilities, although it has important functions with risk groups as well (e.g. Gerstein, Crnic, Blacher, & Baker, 2009). Both approaches offer important perspectives on the parenting stress process, with some shared focus but divergent emphases. Beyond the American-focused approaches, the Swedish Parenthood Stress Questionnaire (SPSQ; Östberg, Hagekull, & Wettergren, 1997) was developed based on the model presented by Abidin's (1995) PSI but expanded on that framework to address broad elements of parenting along five scales (incompetence, role restriction, social isolation, spouse relationship problems, and health problems). There has been an emphasis on parenting stress research in Scandinavian countries, and the SPSQ has been used and validated in Sweden and Norway.

The fundamental difference between the P-C-R approach and that of the parenting daily hassles approach is the emphasis on existing problematic function. In many ways, the P-C-R model assumes that the presence of some problematic status (parental distress, child behavior problems, and parent–child relationship conflict) is stressful, which adversely affects the parenting context. Certainly, there is a wealth of evidence to support that conceptual connection. Nevertheless, it is not surprising that parenting stress measured within this framework would be associated with problematic functioning as the measure itself indexes existing problems in the family context.

The daily hassles approach, in contrast, identifies parenting tasks and child behaviors that reflect everyday experience that is essentially normative (sibling conflicts, child whining/complaining, repeatedly cleaning up messes, picky eating, etc.) but may be considered stressful, especially in the cumulative experience of the events over short periods of time. The measurement paradigm for parenting daily hassles (Crnic & Greenberg, 1990) judges parent response along two dimensions: the frequency with which parents experience each event (frequency scale) and the degree to which the event is judged to be stressful or irritating (intensity scale). Both frequency and intensity are rated separately along a 5-point scale for each item, providing indices that reflect how often parents experience these parenting events and how much they perceive them to be stressful. It is meant to capture normative rather than problematic experience but still discriminate between parents that are more and less stressed by the everyday parenting experience.

The P-C-R and parenting daily hassles approaches are not conflicting but are more complementary in what they offer current conceptualizations of parenting stress. Integrating the two may provide more robust perspectives on systemic family stress experience, capturing both the risk and normative processes through which most families evolve across the developmental periods that are characterized by caregiving.

Source of Stress

There is a need to distinguish between stressed parents and parenting stress. A stressed parent may result from any number of circumstances outside the context of the family or caregiving. Job stress, economic stress (see Cassells and Evans, Chap. 2 this volume), and interpersonal relationship stress may all contribute. There are large literatures on these stress contexts, and it is outside the scope of this chapter to detail those relations. Parenting stress, however, involves stressors that are tied specifically to the context of caregiving, parent–child relationships, and the broader parenting role (see Nomaguchi and Milkie, Chap. 3 this volume). This is not without its controversy (see *measurement issues* below). How we conceptualize and measure stress, and particularly how we measure *parenting* stress, is critical to understanding the various phenomena in which we are interested. Several studies that we have conducted that have included both measures of life stress and parenting stress indicate that parenting stress predicts parenting attitudes and behavior not only above and beyond the contribution of non-parenting related major life stresses, but also differentially (Crnic & Greenberg, 1990; Crnic, Gaze, & Hoffman, 2005).

Developmental Functions

One of the elements in the connection between parenting stress and parenting self-efficacy that has received far too little attention is the obvious developmental implications of this phenomenon. The literature has been woefully inadequate in considering the implication of child age and the likely differences across the developmental period that come into play in the connections between parenting stress and parenting processes. Parents of infants, toddlers, preschoolers, school-age children, and adolescents all face different developmental challenges with their children. Yet, there is a tendency to treat parenting stress as if it is a stable and coherent construct across the developmental period with little concern for the obvious developmental differences that may exist. There are exceptions, such as Spinelli et al. (2013) from four months to three years; Crnic and Booth (1991) across ages one, two, and three; Crnic et al. (2005) across ages three to five; Deater-Deckard, Pinkerton, and Scarr (1996) from preschool to early school age; and Putnick et al. (2010) across ages 10–14 years. Most of these studies that look across age spans, albeit relatively brief spans, find few differences in absolute amounts of parenting stress experienced by parents at differing ages or find strong stability across periods that are measured.

Although absolute stability and levels of stress may be similar when measured in the studies above, such analyses do not necessarily provide a full accounting. It could be that it is not the amount of stress that varies or changes, but the specific facets of parenting or child behavior that change across time. The parent of the preschooler and the parent of an adolescent may perceive the stressfulness of their parenting similarly on a general level, but the behaviors and childrearing responsibilities that create that stress are likely quite different and may have different implications for parent self-efficacy or other parenting attributes. The stability in parenting stress might also suggest that perceived parenting stress is more an underlying parent personality marker than an objective index of unique stressful experience, an explanation that has been raised by others as well (Deater-Deckard, 2004). Regardless, it is imperative that broader, more focused efforts be made to identify the underlying developmental processes that may differentiate the experience and effects of parenting stress from infancy through adolescence.

Systemic Considerations

One of the major shortcomings in parenting stress research to date is the fact that we do not tend to treat parenting stress as a systemic construct despite the fact that it truly reflects more multifaceted and multileveled influence than individual factors. Indeed, individual studies tend to focus on parenting stress related to a specific child at a particular age in families, as most studies are interested in targeted developmental phenomena. However, families often have children of other ages at home, even if those children are not the focus of the research of interest. Parents with multiple children are often asked to respond to parenting stress instruments in the context of the specific child of interest despite the fact that the stress of parenting comes from more than just the experiences related to a single child. That is, parenting stress is a dynamic construct that likely represents the cumulative and integrated influence of all children in the home or may differ for sibling children within the same home, as Deater-Deckard, Smith, Ivy, and Petrill (2005) have demonstrated. Further, there is evidence that the number of children in the home matters for parents' experience of stress (Crnic & Greenberg, 1990). The nature of such influence, however, may be dependent on the number and ages of the children and the specific research question at hand.

Another systemic factor involves the idea that mothers and fathers are not necessarily interchangeable in their perspectives on parenting stress. There is some evidence that there are similarities as well as differences between mothers and fathers with respect to parental self-efficacy (Jones & Prinz, 2005). Additionally, the differences in how mothers and fathers might perceive the stressfulness of parenting could present some interesting contrasts (Deater-Deckard, 2004) but have not really been studied in depth. How does mothers' stress affect fathers and fathers' stress affect mothers in the context of the family and individual parenting processes? These issues of influential crossover effects are addressed later in this chapter.

To address the systemic, dynamic nature of parenting stress, we offer a conceptual model that attempts to incorporate the salient elements that reflect the complex systemic nature of parenting stress as it might be related to parenting self-efficacy and beyond to any number of related parent and child competencies. The model (see Fig. 11.1) attempts to portray the complexity inherent in the reciprocal, bidirectional nature of the relations between parenting stress and parenting across time as well as indicates the possibility for crossover effects between caregivers that can be either direct or mediated. Further, child factors (e.g., developmental considerations and number of children) and family system attributes (e.g., marital functions and coparenting) both contribute to parenting stress processes and are affected by them over time. These complex transactional processes in turn have both immediate and longer term consequences for the well-being and competence of parents and children in the family.

Measurement Issues

Measuring stress, whether specific to parenting or not, is fraught with a number of methodological conundrums, and cautions are required regardless of the approach. These have been well detailed elsewhere (Crnic & Low, 2002; Deater-Deckard,

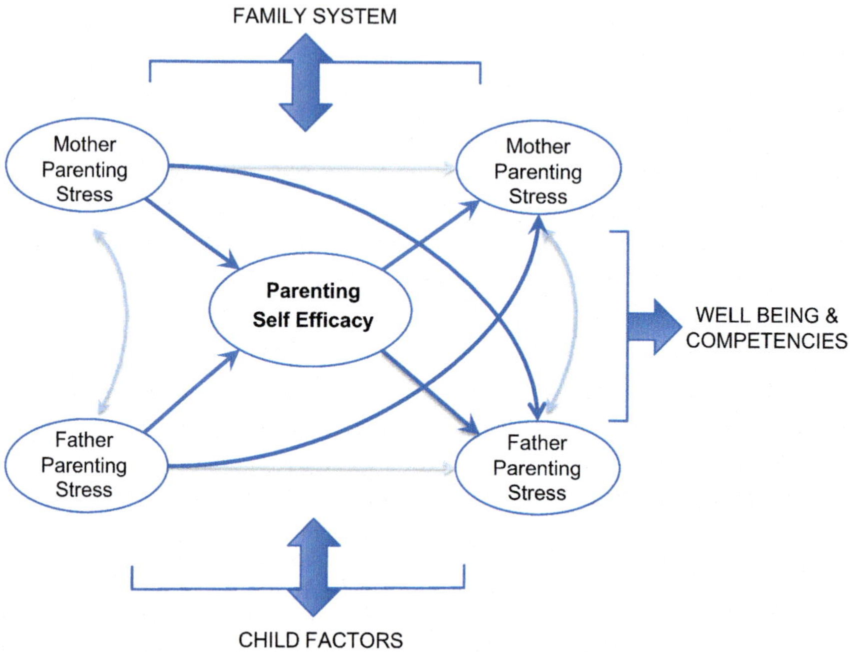

Fig. 11.1 Dynamic and systemic processes linking parenting stress and parenting processes within the family context

1998, 2004; Reitman, Currier, & Stickle, 2002) but involve concerns such as the objective versus more subjective appraisal of stressors and the extent to which stress indices may be contaminated by mood or affective wording, the latter which makes it difficult to differentiate between the stress predictor and psychological distress or other outcomes of interest. We are wise to be aware of the caution raised some time ago about the confound of "symptoms predicting symptoms" in the link between stress and psychological outcome (Dohrenwend & Shrout, 1985).

Evidence for Adverse Influence on Parenting Efficacy

In connecting parenting stress and parenting self-efficacy, research has taken a broad perspective with respect to what might reflect efficacy in the parenting role. Certainly, direct measures of parent beliefs about their own parenting self-efficacy are obvious targets, but there are multiple indirect markers that include a range of other parenting attitudes and beliefs, parenting styles, parent well-being or distress, parenting behaviors, and even more systemic family markers such as marital relationship quality and coparenting processes. We touch on each of these below.

Efficacy Beliefs

With an explicit focus of this chapter on the link between parenting stress and parental self-efficacy, it is worth exploring the central proposition that the experience of parenting stress is associated with direct makers of lower self-efficacy in parenting. Despite what must seem as a fairly intuitive relation to pursue, there is surprisingly little direct evidence that has accrued. Only a few studies have specifically assessed relations between parenting stress and parental self-efficacy, and the findings are consistent with expectations (e.g., Jones & Prinz, 2005). In a study of parents of clinically identified behavior problem preschoolers (Scheel & Rieckmann, 1998), parenting stress and parent self-efficacy were negatively related ($r = -.62$), and parenting stress predicted parental self-efficacy over and above the contribution of other indices of family functioning. Jackson and Huang (2000) likewise found that mothers of preschoolers who experienced more parenting stress reported less self-efficacy, and mothers' self-efficacy in turn mediated the relations between parenting stress and parenting behavior. In this case, parenting stress was indexed by a subset of seven items from the PSI, and parenting behavior was represented by a set of report and observational items from the HOME (Caldwell & Bradley, 1984). More recently, Dunninga and Giallo (2012) explored the connections between fatigue, parenting stress, and parent self-efficacy in mothers of infants, finding that parenting stress was negatively associated with parent efficacy, and in fact, mediated the relation between fatigue and maternal self-efficacy. This study supports the direct linkage not only between parenting stress and lower parent self-efficacy, but also between parental fatigue and parenting stress, which has important implications for emerging biopsychosocial models of parent health.

In all, the evidence supports the notion that parenting stress and parent efficacy are linked such that greater stress coincides with lower efficacy. Although direction of effect is indeterminant, or could certainly operate in either direction, it nevertheless follows that parental efficacy and its correlates might well be at risk under conditions in which parenting stress is high. Indeed, research not only tends to lead to such straightforward conclusions, but also suggests that there is a fair amount of nuance and specificity in the ways in which parenting stress is linked to broadly conceived markers of parental efficacy and competence.

Parent Psychopathology

We have all heard the classic parent refrain of "you kids are driving me crazy!" The extent to which that might literally be true has been the subject of a fair amount of research and not a small amount of interest. The connection between parenting stress and parent psychological distress is again one in which the pathways of influence are complex. It seems likely that parenting stress can lead to the experience of some psychological distress for mothers and fathers, and indeed, a wealth of evidence is available to support such connections. However, the evidence in support of a pathway from parenting stress to diagnosable disorder is less obvious. Although studies that connect parent depression and anxiety with parenting stress are apparent, it is often more typically dysphoria or anxious symptoms that are addressed as opposed to a specific diagnosed disorder. Thus, it is less clear that stresses associated with the parenting role are alone sufficiently robust to lead to clinical disorder. In contrast, the pathway from existing parental psychopathology to the experience of greater parenting stress is more conceptually robust, and existing research provides clear support for this linkage.

In the end, it may not matter whether there is a specific mental health diagnosis or not, as parental well-being is important in its own right and connects up well with other parenting processes to affect both parent and child functioning. Thus, understanding the ways in which parenting stress and various indices of parent well-being covary is an important goal. Consistent with stress research in almost any context, parenting stress and parental well-being are inextricably tied together such that higher stress is associated with less parental well-being (Cheah, Leung, Tahseen, & Schultz, 2009; Lamis, Wilson, Tarantino, Lansford, & Kaslow, 2014; Skreden et al., 2012). But again, the nature of these effects and the mechanisms that drive them are more complex than simple main effect models would suggest. The Skreden et al. (2012) study of Norwegian parents of preschoolers indicates that the processes by which mothers' and fathers' well-being is affected are differentially related to factors associated with parenting stress (e.g., social isolation and role restriction), and Cheah and colleagues (2009) present evidence to show the moderating influence of parenting stress on the connections between well-being and parenting styles.

Among indicators of parent distress, perhaps most frequently studied is parental depression, and especially maternal depression. Studies involving parental anxiety follow closely after that. In either case, the connections between symptoms and parenting stress are reliably strong and in the expected direction to indicate that greater parenting stress is linked to the endorsement of more symptoms (Delvecchio, Sciandra, Finos, Mazzeschi, & Di Riso, 2015; Gray et al., 2012; Nygren, Cartensen, Ludvigsson, & Frostell, 2012; Pripp, Skreden, Skari, Malt, & Emblem, 2010; Shea & Coyne, 2011; Skreden et al., 2012; Thomason et al., 2014). Further, parenting stress leads to decreased parental self-efficacy, and decreased parental efficacy has been found to be related to lower parental well-being and more depressive symptoms (Jones & Prinz, 2005; O'Neil et al., 2009). With respect to differences between mothers and fathers, the evidence does not clearly suggest that stress has differential effects on well-being for women and men. In some studies, mothers report more stress and more symptoms/less well-being than fathers (Skreden et al., 2012), whereas in others, such differences fail to emerge (Solmeyer & Feinberg, 2011).

The major issue with much of the research on parenting stress is that it relies on parent report to identify the extent of parent symptoms as well as the degree of parenting stress and is therefore subject to shared method variance biases. Much of it is also single point in time, cross-sectional research, which means that direction of effect cannot easily be discerned. Longitudinal studies that connect symptoms with parenting stress and offer the structural models necessary, or the cross-lagged analyses that are likely to help untangle the directionality issues, are simply too few. Nonetheless, Thomason et al. (2014) offer some compelling longitudinal findings that demonstrate the complexity of the connections that may exist, at least during infancy. Exploring overall parenting stress as well as the three short-form scales from the PSI, they demonstrated that overall parenting stress served to predict later maternal depressive symptoms in a cross-lagged analysis assessing parenting stress and depression across three-, seven-, and 14-months postpartum. However, when parenting stress components were examined individually, the findings became less consistent. For the parental distress scale, there were no cross-lagged effects to later depression. For the difficult child scale, depressive symptoms predicted stress rather than the other way around, and finally for the parent–child dysfunctional interaction scale, bidirectional cross-lagged relations emerged, but the model fit indices were poor. Other longitudinal research suggests that parent symptoms measured in infancy can lead to higher levels of reported parenting stress later (Pritchard et al., 2012). The high-risk nature of this sample may account at some level for the differences between these results and those of Thomason et al. (2014).

Whether the link between parenting stress and parental psychopathology is initiated by parental distress that leads to subsequent parenting stress or vice versa, it is likely that the process becomes transactional and cyclical, creating an ongoing feedback loop in which each factor facilitates the experience of the other across time. Depending upon child age and where in the cycle measurements are taken, one factor or the other may appear to be the precipitant. Minimally, we need to extend our research models beyond cross-sectional approaches as well as beyond the early childhood period to more fully understand the interplay between parenting stress and distress in parents.

Parenting Styles

One common focus of much of the research which has explored the connection between parenting stress and parenting processes has been on parenting styles, broadly conceived to represent parents' general approach to or attitudes about children and child rearing. In some early work, parent's perspectives about the complexity of child development showed some interesting relations to parenting stress (Crnic & Booth, 1991), such that the degree to which mothers were stressed depended on the complexity with which they viewed development. For mothers who viewed development as complex and dynamic, parenting younger children was perceived as more stressful. For parents who viewed development in more concrete or simple terms, preschoolers were perceived to be more stressful. This suggests the importance of developmental perspectives on parenting stress processes, as parents sense of the stresses associated with childrearing may depend to some extent on children's growing behavioral repertoires or skills and the goodness of fit with parental expectations about development.

More commonly, research on parenting stress has examined the connection to traditional parenting styles such as those identified by Baumrind (1991). Low parenting stress has been associated with more authoritative parenting styles, even when otherwise supportive contexts may be available to parents (Cheah et al., 2009). Likewise, parenting stress has been associated with inconsistent or more punitive parenting practices that are aligned with more authoritarian approaches (Shea & Coyne, 2011), as well as more demanding and less responsive parenting (Ponnet et al., 2013). Interestingly, even adolescents' reports about the parenting style of their parents (acceptance/rejection versus psychological autonomy/control) have been shown to connect to parent's report of parenting stress (Putnick et al., 2010), providing greater context for validation of the association.

Other attitudes and beliefs tend to confirm these same links, such that parenting stress connects in theoretically consistent ways with parents' perceptions of various parenting correlates. For example, parents who report high stress also report lower parenting satisfaction (Crnic & Greenberg, 1990), less perceived support (Cheah et al., 2009; Crnic & Greenberg, 1990), poorer reactions to child negativity (Mackler et al., 2015), less cognitive readiness to parent (Chang et al., 2004), and more perceived ecological (neighborhood) disorder (Lamis et al., 2014). This latter link is relevant to parenting stress in disadvantaged groups where it can be difficult to parent effectively in neighborhoods that are less safe, contributing to increased parenting stress and more hostile parenting.

Observed Parenting Behavior

Much the same as with parenting beliefs and attitudes, parental self-efficacy can be judged by the quality of the behavior that parents display during interactions with their children. Parental self-efficacy influences the degree to which parents feel capable of managing developmentally salient processes with their children in support of the child's emerging competence, which can obviously be represented in the quality and consistency of the behavior displayed in parents' interactions with their children. Indeed, parent self-efficacy is heavily influenced by parents' experiences with their children and the quality of the parent–child relationship that exists.

A wide range of parenting behaviors has been studied in relation to parenting stress. Chief among these have been parental affect (positivity and negativity), sensitivity, involvement, and intrusiveness. In general, greater parenting stress is associated with more negative parenting behavior, and this is true across developmental periods of interest (Gerstein & Poehlmann-Tynan, 2015; Harden, Denmark, Holmes, & Duchene, 2014; Mills-Koonce et al., 2011). However, such findings are not ubiquitous, and there are indications that some indices of parenting stress are associated more with less positive parental behavior than they are with more negative parenting behavior (Crnic et al., 2005; Jackson & Huang, 2000; Spinelli et al., 2013). For example, in our research, parenting daily hassles were strongly predictive of less maternal positivity and less dyadic pleasure in interactions with five-year-old children but did not predict more maternal negativity or greater dyadic conflict. It may be that these more normative daily hassles may operate to suppress parental positivity than increase parental negativity, although that remains to be further explored across child ages and samples.

Parenting behavior is often conceptualized as a mediator that serves to connect parental experience of stress with some untoward or adverse outcome, usually something associated with problematic competence in the child. This is sensible, as it is difficult to make the conceptual argument that parents' experience of parenting stress directly affects some child specific competence. It is easier to make an argument for a direct effect on the parent such that their psychological well-being, their satisfaction with parenting, or the quality of their behavioral interactions might all be directly affected by the experience of stress associated with parenting.

Indeed, multiple studies have attempted to explore the nature of the mediated pathways linking parenting stress with some important child outcome, surmising that the effect of parenting stress on poor child outcomes is mediated through the effect that parenting stress has on parenting behavior. This describes a process by which the experience of parenting stress influences the nature of parent behavior, likely creating greater negativity, more intrusiveness, less positivity, and/or less sensitivity. In turn, those less optimal parenting behaviors lead to more problematic development in the child. Despite the compelling conceptual argument for such pathways, the evidence in support of such indirect influences is not uniformly compelling (Anthony et al., 2005; Crnic et al., 2005; Mackler et al., 2015). Identifying salient pathways of influence between stress and parenting behavior in the service of child and family competencies merits much further attention given its conceptual coherence.

Coparenting Processes

Recently, attention has begun to develop toward more systemic influences in families, and work on parenting stress has begun to follow. In particular, attention to coparenting processes, as well as marital relationships, has engendered some interest. Coparenting involves the way parents coordinate their parenting, support or undermine each other, and manage conflict regarding childrearing (Minuchin, Rosman, & Baker, 1978). Coparenting processes have been shown to be especially salient to parental adjustment, parenting processes, and child developmental and behavioral competencies (Feinberg, Kan, & Hetherington, 2007; Gable, Crnic, & Belsky, 1994). Further, coparenting has been found to both mediate and moderate the influence of individual parent characteristics, couple relationship quality, and parenting stress on various parenting and child adjustment factors (Feinberg, 2003).

Coparenting provides a prime context for exploring the ways in which parenting stress may affect systemic processes in families. And unlike more individual parenting processes, the connections between parenting stress and coparenting might take various forms, both positive and negative. Parenting stress might undermine parents' abilities to work together, but it is also possible that a parent under stress might also rely on their partner to help encourage a consistent and coherent parenting framework. In the latter case, parenting stress might facilitate more cooperative or compensatory processes between parents. To date, evidence is most suggestive that when mothers' and fathers' combined parenting stress is low, parents are better able to coparent effectively (Feinberg, Jones, Kan, & Goslin, 2010), and coparenting intervention effects are better sustained when mothers and fathers experience less parenting stress.

Several recent longitudinal studies also indicate some important connections between parenting stress and coparenting processes. Using longitudinal survey data to study supportive coparenting processes, Schoppe-Sullivan, Settle, Lee, and Kamp Dush (2016) explored several connective pathways between coparenting and parenting stress. Their findings suggested that fathers' (but not mothers') perceptions of supportive coparenting at three months postpartum mediated the associations between their own (fathers') anxious adult attachment during the third trimester of pregnancy and their parenting stress six months later. Additional tests of moderation revealed that mothers' perceptions of greater supportive coparenting were associated with lower parenting stress only when their parenting self-efficacy was low, but fathers' perceptions of greater supportive coparenting were associated with greater parenting satisfaction only when their parenting self-efficacy was high. This is a prime example of the complex and nuanced relations between parenting stress and parenting processes that emerge when multidimensional longitudinal models are employed. Similar evidence can be found in work by Delvecchio et al. (2015), who reported that levels of family maladjustment and parenting stress were mediated by the quality of the coparenting alliance.

Coparenting offers a window into understanding systemic effects of parenting stress, and to a certain extent, coparenting may reflect on the marital relationship. Surprisingly, there has been precious little study of parenting stress and marital relationship quality, or the bidirectional pathways that might detail relations between parenting stress, marital quality, and parenting efficacy. Over and above the effects of general social support, a positive marital relationship may act as a buffer in the face of high parenting stress (Gerstein et al., 2009; Robinson & Neece, 2015), may predict levels of parenting stress (Williford, Calkins, & Keane 2007), or may be influenced by parenting stress.

Certainly, the construct of "marital quality" has been conceptualized in a number of different ways across studies, highlighting its diverse role in understanding parenting more generally, and parenting stress, more specifically. Despite the likely bidirectionality in relations between parenting stress and marital quality, most studies have examined these factors independently as predictors of parenting behaviors (e.g., Ponnet et al., 2013) or have considered marital quality as a moderating variable. Future directions should continue to consider the pathways of influence that illuminate the mechanisms by which parenting stress and marital quality work together to influence parenting.

Research indicates that poor parent–child relations have been linked to hostile marital relationships (Katz & Gottman, 1996), which may be especially salient for fathers who (more so than mothers) are found to withdraw from their children and/or respond in coercive ways as a result of marital conflict (Crockenberg & Covey, 1991). Given that mothers more often take on the primary caregiving role, it may be easier for mothers to separate marital conflict from the role as a mother whereas for fathers, this "spillover" into the father–child relationship is harder to avoid. Interestingly, however, specific dimensions of hostile mother–father interactions (which could involve coparenting) may be more predictive of parenting than broad measures of marital quality. It has been noted that marital hostility is associated with fathers' negative parenting behaviors only when this hostility occurred during marital conflict resolutions. For mothers, behaviors suggestive of child rejection were a result of withdrawn behavior of fathers during marital conflict (Katz & Gottman, 1996). From a family-systems perspective, efficacy in the parenting role can be influenced by interactions with others, especially individuals that share a close relationship (Merrifield & Gamble, 2013). Consistent with a "spillover" hypothesis, partners that feel unsuccessful in their marital relationship may also distrust their own efficacy in the parenting role.

Spillover is a within-person phenomenon whereby functioning in one psychological domain affects or becomes associated with functioning in another, different domain such as the connections between fathers' marital functioning and father–child relationship factors described above. In contrast, "crossover effects" between parents are more systemic processes that could and should be much more emphasized with respect to parenting stress. Crossover occurs when an individual's functioning in one domain affects or is associated with another individual's functioning in one or more relevant domains. In the case of parenting stress, it may well be that one parent's experience crosses over to have a direct influence on the partner's perceived stress or functioning in other parenting domains. One investigation by Putnick et al. (2010) highlights the potential importance of such crossover effects involving parenting stress. In their study of parents of young adolescents, Putnick et al. (2010) showed that mothers parenting stress has relatively minor influence on fathers' parenting stress, as maternal distress (the PSI subscale) at child age 10 had a small but meaningful effect on father distress at child age 14. In contrast, fathers' stress at child age 10 had consistently broader and larger relations to mothers' parenting stress at child age 14, with links to both maternal distress and child difficult behavior (although not dysfunctional interaction). In each case, higher stress experienced by one parent at child age 10 was predictive of higher parenting stress in the other parent at child age 14. Unfortunately, crossover effects within time periods were not assessed, as it would be important to demonstrate that one parent's stress can influence the others' experience of stress in the moment as well as years later. Identification of concurrent crossover effects creates some methodological challenges, and such research efforts remain for future studies. Nevertheless, crossover effects involving parenting stress have also been found in families of children with intellectual disabilities (see also Neece and Chan, Chap. 5 this volume), as Gerstein et al. (2009) reported that both mothers' and fathers' well-being and marital satisfaction influenced the others' experience of parenting stress, and a positive father–child relationship helped to prevent rising parenting stress in mothers. It is this increasing attention to complex pathways of influence in longitudinal research that is providing more nuanced understandings of stress processes in families.

Mother Father Differences

The attention to coparenting processes highlights the importance of considering the potential differences between mothers and fathers with respect to parenting stress. Despite the emerging interest in coparenting, and the fact that "mothering" is no longer synonymous with "parenting" (Pleck, 2012), it is still the case that a disproportionate number of studies have examined parenting stress with respect to mothers only. Fathers, however, may differentially experience parenting stress, or the effects of the stress experienced may have different implications for fathers than it does for mothers. Some recent studies have included direct analyses of fathers' parenting stress, comparing and contrasting the parenting experience for mothers and fathers. Some of those findings have been described briefly in previous sections, but the issues are addressed more fully below.

Although fathers' parenting stress is now more prominently examined in research studies (Deater-Deckard, 2004), the evidence in support of differences or similarities is equivocal. Some studies find evidence of differences in the absolute levels of parenting stress between mothers and fathers (Delvecchio et al., 2015; Fang, Wang, & Xing, 2012; Skreden et al., 2012), while others do not (Crnic & Booth, 1991; Deater-Deckard & Scarr; 1996; Putnick et al., 2010; Solmeyer & Feinberg, 2011). When differences are found, it is typically mothers that report higher parenting stress. Nevertheless, the field seems no closer to resolving whether mother–father differences exist in the experience of parenting stress than it was a decade ago (Deater-Deckard, 2004). Sampling differences, the changing and evolving role of fathers, and varying conceptualizations of parenting stress are all likely contributors to the mixed findings that have emerged to date. Nevertheless, attempts to simply identify whether or not mothers and fathers differ in their reports of parenting stress are likely to be less meaningful than attempting to identify the conditions or contexts under which similarities and differences emerge.

Findings in studies of the relation between parenting stress and parenting self-efficacy between mothers and fathers have also been inconsistent, with some research identifying negative associations in mothers only (Reece & Harkless, 1998), and other studies finding these associations in fathers (Sevigny & Loutzenhiser, 2010). There are a number of explanations for these discrepancies, most of which have not been empirically tested. These include spillover of work-related stress to parenting stress, differences in working mothers and fathers as compared to stay-at-home parents, and developmental status of children, age of parents, etc. In order to better understand how parenting stress operates in mothers and fathers across various samples, these explanatory factors variables should be accounted for, or directly explored, in future studies.

The differential implications of parenting stress for parenting efficacy and the parent–child relationship have also been explored for mothers and fathers. Findings suggest that although mother–child and father–child relationships are unique, the effects of parenting stress on these relationships are not clearly understood. One suggestion is that father–child relationships are more vulnerable to parental stress than are mother–child relationships (Cummings et al., 2004). Opposing this suggestion however, Ponnet et al. (2013) found that associations between stress and parent–child relationships were equally strong for mothers and fathers. With respect to connections between parenting stress and specific parenting behaviors (e.g., engagement and warmth), contrasting relations are apparent. In studies of mothers, stress in the parenting role was associated with harsher, less responsive parenting behaviors, and less engagement with children, overall (e.g., Almeida, Wethington, & Chandler, 1999). Although the same is likely true for fathers, it has been demonstrated in only a few studies (e.g., Bronte-Tinkew, Horowitz, & Carrano, 2010). Importantly, Bronte-Tinkew et al. (2010) controlled for levels of maternal stress in their study, highlighting father's experience of parenting stress as important, above and beyond mother's experience. Continued examination of the complex interplay between parents' experience of stress (crossover) within and across time and how such processes uniquely contribute to parenting and the parent–child relationship quality should prove important.

Given that fathers are increasingly more involved in the parenting of their children (Lamb, 2010) and are even provided parental leave in many states during the transition to parenthood, the effect of parenting stress for fathers will likely continue to evolve. Currently, inconsistencies are abundant, and a clear picture of mother–father differences in parenting stress, as well as their implications for parental efficacy, has not yet emerged.

Summary

The connections between parenting stress and parental efficacy are at once both straightforward and complex. There is consistent indication that parenting stress is associated with less parental efficacy, lower well-being, less positive interactive behavior, and less positive parenting and coparenting relations. However, the mediating and moderating mechanisms that underlie the connections between these factors are many and operate across pathways of influence that require attention to multidimensional perspectives on family functioning. Parenting stress may be a frequently studied determinant of parenting, and one for which there is a vast literature to digest and multiple methods to integrate, but our understanding remains far too basic to capture the complexity of the transactional processes that connect it to parental self-efficacy and family well-being.

Addressing the developmental and systemic complexities of parenting stress is the next major challenge for the field. Adopting more developmental and systemic perspectives for our work will encourage model building that conceptualizes parenting stress as "whole family" in its function and implication, and will better identify the stress processes that may differentiate developmental periods, care providers, and the multiple ways in parenting self-efficacy might be understood. Variations in measurement can be construed as a methodological challenge, or as a potential strength. Integrating divergent measurement models can be valuable in building frameworks that expand our understanding of parenting stress. No one approach is likely to capture the diversity of stressful processes relevant to parenting, but more multidimensional approaches can better illuminate the nature of this ubiquitous parental experience.

References

Abidin, R. R. (1992). The determinants of parenting behavior. *Journal of Clinical Child Psychology, 21,* 407–412.

Abidin, R. R. (1995). *The parenting stress index professional manual.* Lutz, FL: Psychological Assessment Resources.

Almeida, D. M., Wethington, E., & Chandler, A. L. (1999). Daily transmission of tensions between marital dyads and parent–child dyads. *Journal of Marriage and the Family, 61*(1), 49-61. doi:http://dx.doi.org.ezproxy1.lib.asu.edu/10.2307/353882

Anthony, L. G., Anthony, B. J., Glanville, D. N., Naiman, D. Q., Waanders, C., & Shaffer, S. (2005). The relationships between parenting stress, parenting behaviour and preschoolers' social competence and behaviour problems in the classroom. *Infant and Child Development, 14* (2), 133–154. doi:10.1002/icd.385

Bandura, A. (1977). *Self-efficacy: The exercise of control.* New York, NY: W. H. Freeman.

Baumrind, D. (1991). The influence of parenting style on adolescent competence and substance use. *The Journal of Early Adolescence, 11,* 56–95.

Bronte-Tinkew, J., Horowitz, A., & Carrano, J. (2010). Aggravation and stress in parenting: Associations with coparenting and father engagement among resident fathers. *Journal of Family Issues, 31*(4), 525–555. doi:10.1177/0192513X09340147

Caldwell, B., & Bradley, R. (1984). *Home Observation for Measurement of the Environment.* Little Rock, AR.

Cassells, R.C. & Evans, G.W. (Chapter 2, this volume). Ethnic variation in poverty and parenting stress. In K. Deater-Deckard & R. Panneton (Eds.), *Parental Stress and Child Development: Adaptive and Maladaptive Outcomes.* NY: Springer.

Chang, Y., Fine, M. A., Ispa, J., Thornburg, K. R., Sharp, E., & Wolfenstein, M. (2004). Understanding parenting stress among young, low-income, african-american, first-time mothers. *Early Education and Development, 15*(3), 265–282. doi:10.1207/s15566935eed1503_2

Cheah, C. S. L., Leung, C. Y. Y., Tahseen, M., & Schultz, D. (2009). Authoritative parenting among immigrant Chinese mothers of preschoolers. *Journal of Family Psychology, 23*(3), 311–320. doi:10.1037/a0015076

Crockenberg, S., & Covey, S. L. (1991). Marital Conflict and Externalizing Behavior in Children. In D. Cicchetti, & S. L. Toth (Eds.), *Rochester symposium on developmental psychopathology, 3*, (pp. 235–260). Rochester, NY: University of Rochester Press.

Crnic, K. A., & Greenberg, M. T. (1990). Minor parenting stresses with young children. *Child Development, 61*, 1628–1637.

Crnic, K.A. & Booth, C. (1991). Mother and father perceptions of parenting daily hassles across early childhood. *Journal of Marriage and the Family, 53*, 1042–1050.

Crnic, K. A., & Low, C. (2002). Everyday stresses and parenting. In M. Bornstein (Ed.), *Handbook of Parenting* (2nd ed., Vol. 4, pp. 243–268) Hillsdale, NJ: Erlbaum.

Crnic, K., Gaze, C., & Hoffman, C. (2005). Cumulative parenting stress across the preschool period: Relations to maternal parenting and child behavior at age five. *Infant and Child Development, 14*, 117–132.

Cummings, E. M., Goeke-Morey, M., & Raymond, J. (2004). Fathers in Family Context: Effects of marital quality and marital conflict. In M. E. Lamb (Ed.), *The role of the father in child development*, (4th ed., pp. 196–221). Hoboken, NJ: John Wiley & Sons Inc.

Deater-Deckard, K. (1998). Parenting stress and child adjustment: Some old hypotheses and new questions. *Clinical Psychology: Science and Practice, 5*(3), 314–332.

Deater-Deckard, K. (2004). *Parenting stress*. New Haven, CT: Yale University Press.

Deater-Deckard, K., & Scarr, S. (1996). Parenting stress among dual-earner mothers and fathers: Are there gender differences? *Journal of Family Psychology, 10*(1), 45–59. doi:10.1037/0893-3200.10.1.45

Deater-Deckard, K., Pinkerton, R., & Scarr, S. (1996). Child care quality and children's behavioral adjustment: A four-year longitudinal study. *Child Psychology & Psychiatry & Allied Disciplines, 37*(8), 937–948.

Deater-Deckard, K., Smith, J., Ivy, L., & Petril, S. A. (2005). Differential perceptions of and feelings about sibling children: Implications for research on parenting stress. *Infant and Child Development, 14*(2), 211–225. doi:10.1002/icd.389

Delvecchio, E., Sciandra, A., Finos, L., Mazzeschi, C., & Di Riso, D. (2015). The role of co-parenting alliance as a mediator between trait anxiety, family system maladjustment, and parenting stress in a sample of non-clinical italian parents. *Frontiers in Psychology, 6*, 1–8.

Dohrenwend, B. P., & Shrout, P. E. (1985). "Hassles" in the conceptualization and measurement of life stress variables. *American Psychologist, 40*(7), 780–785. doi:http://dx.doi.org.ezproxy1.lib.asu.edu/10.1037/0003-066X.40.7.780

Dunninga, M. J., & Giallo, R. (2012). Fatigue, parenting stress, self-efficacy and satisfaction in mothers of infants and young children. *Journal of Reproductive and Infant Psychology, 30*(2), 145–159. doi:10.1080/02646838.2012.693910

Fang, H., Wang, M., & Xing, X. (2012). Relationship between parenting stress and harsh discipline in preschoolers' parents. *Chinese Journal of Clinical Psychology, 20*(6), 835–838.

Feinberg, M. E. (2003). The internal structure and ecological context of coparenting: A framework for research and intervention. *Parenting: Science and Practice, 3*(2), 95–131. doi:http://dx.doi.org.ezproxy1.lib.asu.edu/10.1207/S15327922PAR0302_01

Feinberg, M. E., Kan, M. L., & Hetherington, E. M. (2007). The longitudinal influence of coparenting conflict on parental negativity and adolescent maladjustment. *Journal of Marriage and Family, 69*(3), 687–702. doi:http://dx.doi.org.ezproxy1.lib.asu.edu/10.1111/j.1741-3737.2007.00400.x

Feinberg, M. E., Jones, D. E., Kan, M. L., & Goslin, M. C. (2010). Effects of family foundations on parents and children: 3.5 years after baseline. *Journal of Family Psychology, 24*(5), 532–542. doi:10.1037/a0020837

Gable, S., Crnic, K., & Belsky, J. (1994). Coparenting within the family system: Influences on children's development. *Family Relations, 43*, 380–386.

Gerstein, E., Crnic, K., Blacher, J., & Baker, B. (2009). Resilience and the course of daily parenting stress in families of young children with intellectual disabilities. *Journal of Intellectual Disabilities Research, 53*, 981–997.

Gerstein, E. D., & Poehlmann-Tynan, J. (2015). Transactional processes in children born preterm: Influences of mother–child interactions and parenting stress. *Journal of Family Psychology, 29* (5), 777–787. doi:10.1037/fam0000119

Glatz, T., & Buchanan, C. M. (2015). Change and predictors of change in parental self-efficacy from early to middle adolescence. *Developmental Psychology, 51*(10), 1367–1379. doi:10.1037/dev0000035

Gray, P. H., Edwards, D. M., O'Callaghan, M. J., & Cuskelly, M. (2012). Parenting stress in mothers of preterm infants during early infancy. *Early Human Development, 88,* 45–49.

Harden, B. J., Denmark, N., Holmes, A., & Duchene, M. (2014). Detached parenting and toddler problem behavior in early head start families. *Infant Mental Health Journal, 35*(6), 529–543. doi:10.1002/imhj.21476

Jackson, A. P., & Huang, C. C. (2000). Parenting stress and behavior among single mothers of preschoolers: The mediating role of self-efficacy. *Journal of Social Service Research, 26* (4), 29–42. doi:http://dx.doi.org.ezproxy1.lib.asu.edu/10.1300/J079v26n04_02

Jones, T. L., & Prinz, R. J. (2005). Potential roles of parental self-efficacy in parent and child adjustment: A review. *Clinical Psychology Review, 25*(3), 341–363. doi:10.1016/j.cpr.2004.12.004

Katz, L. F., & Gottman, J. M. (1996). Spillover effects of marital conflict: In search of parenting and coparenting mechanisms. In J. P. McHale, & P. A. Cowan (Eds.), *Understanding how family-level dynamics affect children's development: Studies of two-parent families* (pp. 57–76, 112 Pages). San Francisco, CA: Jossey-Bass.

Lamb, M. E., (2010). How do fathers influence children's development? Let me count the ways. *The role of the father in child development* (5th ed., pp. 1–26) Hoboken, NJ: Wiley.

Lamis, D. A., Wilson, C. K., Tarantino, N., Lansford, J. E., & Kaslow, N. J. (2014). Neighborhood disorder, spiritual well-being, and parenting stress in african american women. *Journal of Family Psychology, 28*(6), 769–778. doi:10.1037/a0036373

Leahy-Warren, P., & McCarthy, G. (2011). Maternal parental self-efficacy in the postpartum period. *Midwifery, 27,* 802–810. doi:10.1016/j.midw.2010.07.008

Mackler, J. S., Kelleher, R. T., Shanahan, L., Calkins, S. D., Keane, S. P., & O'Brien, M. (2015). Parenting stress, parental reactions, and externalizing behavior from ages 4 to 10. *Journal of Marriage and Family, 77*(2), 388–406. doi:10.1111/jomf.12163

McQullian, M.E. & Bates, J.E. (Chapter 4, this volume). Parental stress and child development. In K. Deater-Deckard & R. Pannenton (Eds.), *Parental Stress and Child Development: Adaptive and Maladaptive Outcomes.* NY: Springer.

Merrifield, K. A., & Gamble, W. C. (2013). Associations among marital qualities, supportive and undermining coparenting, and parenting self-efficacy: Testing spillover and stress-buffering processes. *Journal of Family Issues, 34*(4), 510–533. doi:10.1177/0192513X12445561

Mills-Koonce, W., Appleyard, K., Barnett, M., Deng, M., Putallaz, M., & Cox, M. (2011). Adult attachment style and stress as risk factors for early maternal sensitivity and negativity. *Infant Mental Health Journal, 32*(3), 277–285. doi:10.1002/imhj.20296

Minuchin, S., Rosman, B.L., & Baker, L. (1978) *Psychosomatic Families: Anorexia Nervosa in Context.* Cambridge, MA: Harvard University Press.

Neece, C.L. & Chan, N. (Chapter 5, this volume). The stress of parenting children with developmental disabilities. In K. Deater-Deckard & R. Panneton (Eds.), *Parental Stress and Child Development: Adaptive and Maladaptive Outcomes.* NY: Springer.

Nygren, M., Carstensen, J., Ludvigsson, J., & Frostell, A. S. (2012). Adult attachment and parenting stress among parents of toddlers. *Journal of Reproductive and Infant Psychology, 30* (3), 289–302. doi:10.1080/02646838.2012.717264

O'Neil, J., Wilson, M. N., Shaw, D. S., & Dishion, T. J. (2009). The relationship between parental efficacy and depressive symptoms in a diverse sample of low income mothers. *Journal of Child and Family Studies, 18*(6), 643–652. doi:10.1007/s10826-009-9265-y

Östberg, M., Hagekull, B., & Wettergren, S. (1997). A measure of parental stress in mothers with small children: Dimensionality, stability and validity. *Scandinavian Journal of Psychology, 38*(3), 199–208.

Pleck, J. H. (2012). Integrating father involvement in parenting research. *Parenting: Science and Practice, 12*(2-3), 243–253. doi:10.1080/15295192.2012.683365

Ponnet, K., Mortelmans, D., Wouters, E., Van Leeuwen, K., Bastaits, K., & Pasteels, I. (2013). Parenting stress and marital relationship as determinants of mothers' and fathers' parenting. *Personal Relationships, 20*(2), 259–276. doi:10.1111/j.1475-6811.2012.01404.x

Pripp, A. H., Skreden, M., Skari, H., Malt, U., & Emblem, R. (2010). Underlying correlation structures of parental stress, general health and anxiety. *Scandinavian Journal of Psychology, 51,* 473–479.

Putnick, D. L., Bornstein, M. H., Hendricks, C., Painter, K. M., Suwalsky, J. T. D., & Collins, W. A. (2010). Stability, continuity, and similarity of parenting stress in european american mothers and fathers across their child's transition to adolescence. *Parenting: Science and Practice, 10* (1), 60–77. doi:10.1080/15295190903014638

Reece, S.M. & Harkless, G. (1998). Self-Efficacy, Stress, and Parental Adaptation: Applications to the Care of Childbearing Families. *Journal of Family Nursing, 4*(2), 198–215. doi:10.1177/107484079800400206

Reitman, D., Currier, R. O., & Stickle, T. R. (2002). A critical evaluation of the parenting stress index-short form (PSI-SF) in a head start population. *Journal of Clinical Child and Adolescent Psychology, 31*(3), 384–392. doi:10.1207/153744202760082649

Robinson, M., & Neece, C. L. (2015). Marital satisfaction, parental stress, and child behavior problems among parents of young children with developmental delays. *Journal of Mental Health Research in Intellectual Disabilities, 8*(1), 23–46. doi:http://dx.doi.org.ezproxy1.lib.asu.edu/10.1080/19315864.2014.994247

Scheel, M. J., & Rieckmann, T. (1998). An empirically derived description of self-efficacy and empowerment for parents of children identified as psychologically disordered. *American Journal of Family Therapy, 26*(1), 15–27.

Schoppe-Sullivan, S., Settle, T., Lee, J., & Kamp Dush, C. M. (2016). Supportive coparenting relationships as a haven of psychological safety at the transition to parenthood. *Research in Human Development, 13*(1), 32–48. doi:10.1080/15427609.2016.1141281

Sevigny, P. R., & Loutzenhiser, L. (2010). Predictors of parenting self-efficacy in mothers and fathers of toddlers. *Child: Care, Health and Development, 36*(2), 179–189. doi:10.1111/j.1365-2214.2009.00980.x

Shea, S. E., & Coyne, L. W. (2011). Maternal dysphoric mood, stress, and parenting practices in mothers of head start preschoolers: The role of experiential avoidance. *Child & Family Behavior Therapy, 33*(3), 231–247. doi:10.1080/07317107.2011.596004

Shumow, L., & Lomax, R. (2002). Parental efficacy: Predictor of parenting behavior and adolescent outcomes. *Parenting, Science and Practice, 2,* 127–150. doi:10.1207/S15327922PAR0202_03

Skreden, M., Skari, H., Malt, U. F., Pripp, A. H., Björk, M. D., Faugli, A., et al. (2012). Parenting stress and emotional wellbeing in mothers and fathers of preschool children. *Scandinavian Journal of Public Health, 40*(7), 596–604. doi:10.1177/1403494812460347

Solmeyer, A. R., & Feinberg, M. E. (2011). Mother and father adjustment during early parenthood: The roles of infant temperament and coparenting relationship quality. *Infant Behavior & Development, 34*(4), 504–514. doi:10.1016/j.infbeh.2011.07.006

Spinelli, M., Poehlmann, J., & Bolt, D. (2013). Predictors of parenting stress trajectories in premature infant–mother dyads. *Journal of Family Psychology, 27*(6), 873–883. doi:10.1037/a0034652

Teti, D. M., & Gelfand, D. M. (1991). Behavioral competence among mothers of infants in the first year: The mediational role of maternal self-efficacy. *Child Development, 62,* 918–929. doi:10.2307/1131143

Thomason, E., Volling, B. L., Flynn, H. A., McDonough, S. C., Marcus, S. M., Lopez, J. F., et al. (2014). Parenting stress and depressive symptoms in postpartum mothers: Bidirectional or unidirectional effects? *Infant Behavior & Development, 37*(3), 406–415. doi:10.1016/j.infbeh.2014.05.009

Weaver, C. M., Shaw, D. S., Dishion, T. J., & Wilson, M. N. (2008). Parenting self-efficacy and problem behavior in children at high risk for early conduct problems: The mediating role of maternal depression. *Infant Behavior & Development, 31*(4), 594–605. doi: http://dx.doi.org.ezproxy1.lib.asu.edu/10.1016/j.infbeh.2008.07.006

Williford, A. P., Calkins, S. D., & Keane, S. P. (2007). Predicting change in parenting stress across early childhood: Child and maternal factors. *Journal of Abnormal Child Psychology, 35*(2), 251–263. doi:10.1007/s10802-006-9082-3

Chapter 12
The Role of Parental Emotion Regulation in Parent Emotion Socialization: Implications for Intervention

Sophie Havighurst and Christiane Kehoe

Parenting is demanding, challenging, and emotionally taxing leaving parents vulnerable to feeling stressed and reactive. Parents are regularly faced with the complex task of remaining calm in the face of a distressed or dysregulated child, while at the same time trying to regulate the child's emotion, problem solve, and/or engage in limit setting (Rutherford, Wallace, Laurent, & Mayes, 2015). If parents face additional stresses (e.g., mental health difficulties, relationship difficulties, financial, or work-related stresses), their own emotions can overwhelm them, making it difficult to respond to their children calmly and in emotionally supportive ways. Further, juggling these demands may be particularly challenging when children are highly emotionally dysregulated (see Chap. 11 by Crnic & Ross for further discussion), heightening the need for parents to manage their own emotions while at the same time teaching their children to understand and regulate their emotions. Substantial evidence has demonstrated that parenting programs can improve the functioning of parents and children, although for parents with difficulties regulating their own emotions, the benefits of such programs have been found to be much weaker (Maliken & Katz, 2013). Efforts to improve parent emotion regulation may, therefore, enhance the impact of parenting interventions or improve the benefits for those who might struggle with high levels of stress and be less receptive to learning new parenting skills.

In this chapter, we explore how parents' capacities to cope with stress and manage their own emotions affect their ability to respond in emotionally supportive and helpful ways with their children. We review the literature about what is known

S. Havighurst (✉) · C. Kehoe
Department of Psychiatry, Mindful: Centre for Training and Research in Developmental Health, University of Melbourne,
Building C, 50 Flemington Street, Flemington, Melbourne, VI 3031, Australia
e-mail: sophie.h@unimelb.edu.au

C. Kehoe
e-mail: ckehoe@unimelb.edu.au

K. Deater-Deckard and R. Panneton (eds.), *Parental Stress and Early Child Development*, DOI 10.1007/978-3-319-55376-4_12

about the relationship between stress, parent emotion regulation, parent mental health difficulties, and parent emotion socialization (i.e., parental modeling of emotional expression, reactions to, and coaching children about emotions). We then outline how we have targeted parents' capacity to respond to stress and learn effective emotion regulation in our Tuning in to Kids (TIK) and Tuning in to Teens (TINT) parenting programs (thereafter referred to as TIK). TIK teaches parents emotion coaching where parents scaffold children's learning about emotions within a supportive, emotionally accepting relationship (Gottman & DeClaire, 1997). In order to teach parents emotion coaching, we have dedicated significant efforts to helping parents regulate their own emotions that occur either in response to their own life stressors or the challenges of parenting. While describing how we have targeted parent emotion regulation, we also propose some theoretical mechanisms by which learning and change might be occurring. Finally, we reexamine some of our previously published intervention efficacy studies of TIK and TINT to look at the influence of parent emotion regulation on intervention outcomes. In doing this, we aim to extend what is known about how parent emotion regulation impacts parent emotion socialization through the lens of a parenting program.

The Role of Parent Emotion Regulation in Emotion Socialization

Emotion socialization theory (Eisenberg, Cumberland, & Spinrad, 1998; Halberstadt, Denham, & Dunsmore, 2001; Katz, Maliken, & Stettler, 2012; Morris, Silk, Steinberg, Myers, & Robinson, 2007) argues that parent emotion regulation is related to the development of children's emotion competence via a number of mechanisms, including that parents model adaptive emotion regulation and are then able to respond supportively when children are emotional. Supportive responding involves parents' ability to recognize their child's emotions, respond by acknowledging and validating their child's emotional experience, talk about emotions, and assist their child to understand and regulate their emotions (i.e., emotion coaching). These aspects of emotion socialization are associated with children having better emotion competence, social functioning, behavior, and academic functioning (Eisenberg et al., 1998; Katz et al., 2012; Morris et al., 2011; Perlman, Camras, & Pelphrey, 2008; Wong, McElwain, & Halberstadt, 2009). Conversely, when parents are unsupportive or emotionally dismissive in response to emotions, their children are more likely to have poorer emotional competence and higher levels of internalizing and externalizing behavior difficulties (Garner, Dunsmore, & Southam-Gerrow, 2008; Raver & Spagnola, 2002; Shipman et al., 2007; Suveg et al., 2008). During times of stress, parents' and children's physiological and psychological reactions can trigger strong emotional responses which may be attenuated or exacerbated by parents' emotion socialization responses (Buck, 1984; Gottman, Katz, & Hooven, 1997).

When parents experience mental health difficulties, sadness or loneliness, fatigue and sleep deprivation, illness, child behavior problems, or other stressful life events, their ability to regulate their own and their child's emotions is readily compromised (Maliken & Katz, 2013; Williford, Calkins, & Keane, 2007). Indeed, parental emotional dysregulation and psychopathology have been consistently linked with unsupportive parenting practices and behavioral and emotional difficulties in children (Zahn-Waxler, Duggal, & Gruber, 2002). Parents with heightened stress sensitivity due to genetic factors, growing up in a stressful environment, or pre-existing mental health difficulties may be particularly at risk of excessive reactivity when faced with parenting stress (Laurent, 2014; Platt, Williams, Ginsburg, Williams, & Ginsburg, 2016). For example, Platt et al. (2016) found that current levels of parenting stress, parent–child dysfunctional interactions, and parents who engaged in 'anxious rearing,' mediated the relationship between stressful life events and child anxiety. A recent study (Breaux, Harvey, & Lugo-Candelas, 2015) that examined the relation between parents' psychopathology symptoms and emotion socialization behaviors found higher levels of psychopathology were related to more unsupportive reactions to children's negative affect. Similarly, when mothers with clinical levels of depression or anxiety have been compared to normal controls, they have been found to have fewer and less effective emotion regulation strategies and greater difficulties in communication and affective involvement (Hughes & Gullone, 2008; Psychogiou & Parry, 2014). Limited self-awareness and regulation of emotion are thought to underlie many forms of psychopathology (Aldao, Nolen-Hoeksema, & Schweizer, 2010), and difficulties with attentional/behavioral regulation in parents can increase their tendency to engage in unsupportive or harsh parenting behaviors (Dix & Meuniera, 2009; Maliken & Katz, 2013). In turn, when either the parent or the child has difficulties with self-regulation and parents responses are unsupportive or harsh, emotions are likely to escalate for both the parent and the child (see Chap. 8 by Finegood & Blair): Yet, it is especially during periods of heightened stress that parents need to be able to regulate their own emotions and use supportive responses to buffer children from the negative impact of stress (Platt et al., 2016).

To date, only a few studies have directly investigated parental difficulties in emotion regulation as a mediator or predictor of parent outcomes in order to understand how stress, emotion dysregulation, and parenting of children's emotions interact (Buck, 1984; Kehoe, Havighurst, & Harley, 2014a, 2015; Mazursky-Horowitz et al., 2015). During periods of stress, difficulties in emotion regulation may make it harder for parents to engage in supportive emotion socialization practices for several reasons. When parents with poor emotion regulation experience high levels of negative affect either in response to stressors, their own mental health difficulties, or due to their child's emotional dysregulation, they may feel overwhelmed or 'flooded,' increasing their likelihood of withdrawal or expression of negative emotions in a dysregulated manner, resulting in neglecting, reactive or hostile discipline practices (Bariola, Gullone, & Hughes, 2011; Katz & Gottman, 1991; Lorber, Mitnick, & Slep, 2015; Mence et al., 2014). For example, Lorber et al. (2015) found that mothers of toddlers who felt flooded by their child's behavior during discipline encounters experienced more negative emotion, showed increased heart rate reactivity and vagal withdrawal (viewed as poor emotion regulation), and this was related to parents' over-reactive and harsh discipline responses. Jackson and Arlegui (2016) found that heightened negative affect hinders the ability of a person to detect someone else's mood change. In addition, parents who report limited access to emotion regulation strategies have reported impulse control difficulties, lower acceptance of emotions (Gratz & Roemer, 2004), and increased likelihood of engaging in punishing or neglecting responses to their child's emotion expression (Buckholdt, Parra, & Jobe-Shields, 2010).

Excessive down-regulation or not showing emotion (i.e., suppression) has also been found to contribute to problems in parenting. Suppression of negative emotions has been found to be related to lower parental positive expressiveness (Hughes & Gullone, 2010), lower use of supportive strategies (problem focused, encouraging of emotion expression, greater positive expressivity), and greater likelihood that the parent would engage in unsupportive parenting (matching the child's distress, negative expressiveness) (Meyer, Raikes, Virmani, Waters, & Thompson, 2014). Maladaptive emotion regulation such as suppression of emotions tends to increase and prolong negative emotion arousal (Gross & John, 2003). In turn, heightened emotional dysregulation (or suppression) in the parent may make it difficult for them to access strategies to constructively manage feelings when solving emotional problems (Maliken & Katz, 2013), and may result in parents' escalating children's negative emotions (Burke, Pardini, & Loeber, 2008; Sheeber et al., 2011), or harsh over-reactive parenting (Lorber & O'Leary, 2005). In one of our recent studies with parents of preadolescents, parents' self-reported difficulties in emotion awareness and regulation were related to parents' greater use of emotion dismissing strategies with their child (parent and youth-reported), such as responding by overriding, punishing, or matching (i.e., become angry when the child is angry; Kehoe, Havighurst, & Harley, 2014b). Other studies have found similar results. For example, parents' lower use of cognitive reappraisal strategies (considered maladaptive) has been associated with higher parental negative expressiveness (Hughes & Gullone, 2010), and parents who express higher levels of negative affect have been found to be less likely to respond supportively to their adolescents' expression of negative emotions (Stocker, Richmond, Rhoades, & Kiang, 2007). Other studies conducted with adults have also found suppressing emotions to be related to poorer outcomes in adults, such as greater anxiety, impaired memory, poorer immune system functioning, and psychological stress (Gross, 2002; Gross & John, 2003; Lynch, Robins, Morse, & Krause, 2001).

Parent emotion awareness also plays an important role in parent's emotion regulation and emotion socialization responses. When parents have deficits in awareness of their own or others emotions, this may impact how they cope with stress and their responsiveness to their children further exacerbating the negative emotions occurring in a situation (Gohm & Clore, 2002; Halberstadt et al., 2001). If parents are unable to recognize emotions (especially lower intensity emotions), their ability to regulate emotions is likely to be compromised, with lower awareness or clarity with emotions having been found to be related to difficulties in emotion regulation (Gratz & Roemer, 2004). Further, parents who have difficulties identifying emotions in themselves or who are less accepting of their own emotions may be less likely to engage in supportive emotion socialization practices, which requires talking about feelings (Salovey, Mayer, Goldman, Turvey, & Palfai, 1995; Yap, Allen, Leve, & Katz, 2008). When emotions are identified at a lower intensity, it is easier for parents to implement emotion regulation strategies (Linehan, Bohus, & Thomas, 2007) and more likely that they will be better equipped to deal with the source of stress (Gohm & Clore, 2002). Finally, it is also possible that when parents are emotionally overwhelmed during high levels of stress, their emotion awareness and ability to engage in perspective taking are compromised due to limited access to executive functions (Suchy, 2011).

These findings suggest that prevention and intervention programs for parents who experience difficulties with emotion awareness and regulation or mental health difficulties may be enhanced by incorporating a focus on how parents manage their own emotions in addition to strategies for parenting. Parental difficulties in emotion regulation have been found to have a negative impact on intervention effectiveness as well as influencing program attendance (Assemany & McIntosh, 2002; Maliken & Katz, 2013). For example, the presence of parental anxiety or depression has been found to limit the effectiveness of treatment on child/youth anxiety outcomes (Cobham, Dadds, & Spence, 1998; Garber et al., 2009; Kendall, Gosch, Hudson, Flannery-Schroeder, & Suveg, 2008). When parents feel overwhelmed by their own difficulties, they may not feel up to attending a session, or when they do attend may find it harder to focus on learning new skills. Poorer session attendance may result in parents missing important information or lacking confidence to implement the skills. The presence of higher levels of depression, anxiety, and/or stress has been found to be related to lower attendance and higher dropout rates in parenting programs, and interferes with skill acquisition as well as skill implementation (Maliken & Katz, 2013; Zubrick et al., 2005). Treatment of these mental health conditions and/or targeting parent emotion awareness and regulation may assist with program attendance and acquisition of new parenting skills.

Given that parent mental health difficulties are a risk factor for maladaptive parenting, a more parsimonious (or 'transdiagnostic') approach to treatment or prevention by targeting common higher order factors (e.g., managing stress and emotion regulation) that underlie emotional disorders and maladaptive parenting would seem to be important (Aldao et al., 2010; Weersing, Rozenman, Maher-Bridge, & Campo, 2012). When parents are able to acquire skills that enable them to increase their awareness and regulation of emotions and implement strategies to manage stress, they are likely to be in a better position to both learn and implement supportive parenting practices. This approach has been taken in a number of interventions including our own work.

Interventions Targeting Parent Emotion Regulation

Published accounts of interventions that target parent emotion regulation and the way parents manage stress in order to improve parenting are limited. A review by Katz et al. (2012) highlighted that the translation of emotion socialization theory from research into practice is in its infancy, with very few parenting interventions specifically targeting all aspects of emotion socialization. A number of interventions for parents are, however, beginning to include components that focus on teaching parents skills in emotional regulation. These can be grouped into three approaches: (1) behavioral parenting programs where the main focus is on teaching behavior management strategies but with added components that target aspects of parent emotion regulation; (2) mindfulness-based interventions that assist parents to manage stress by teaching the principles of mindfulness, such as present-moment awareness, nonjudgment, and compassion to reduce emotional reactivity and improve emotion regulation; and (3) emotion-focused programs which teach parents skills required for adaptive emotion socialization and include components targeting parent emotion awareness and regulation.

Behavioral parenting programs such as Triple P (Sanders & Markie-Dadds, 1996) or The Incredible Years (Webster-Stratton & Reid, 2007) primarily focus on teaching parenting skills to manage children's behaviors and less on teaching parents how to recognize, understand, and manage their own or their child's emotions. These programs have been found effective in improving parent mental health as well as parenting discipline practices and involvement (Furlong et al., 2012). However, up to one-third of families who attend behavioral parenting programs do not benefit (Brestan & Eyberg, 1998; Taylor & Biglan, 1998). This may be because of other stressors occurring for parents (e.g., low income, single parenting, marital conflict, parent emotion regulation difficulties, high levels of stressful life events) that make it difficult for parents to learn the new skills. Behavioral programs have also been found to be less effective when there are parent–child attachment-related difficulties (Maliken & Katz, 2013; Scott & Dadds, 2009; Webster-Stratton & Hammond, 1990) and are less effective with older children and adolescents (e.g., Burke, Brennan, & Cann, 2012; Ralph & Sanders, 2006). It is therefore important, and in keeping with a transdiagnostic approach, to target broader factors such as the way parents manage their own and their child's emotions as a way of reducing the effects of stress and assist in building parenting skills.

To date, only a handful of studies have been conducted that have investigated the effects of adding parent emotion regulation components to behavioral parenting programs (e.g., Lenze, Pautsch, & Luby, 2011; Luby, Lenze, & Tillman, 2012; Sanders, Markie-Dadds, Tully, & Bor, 2000). For example, Sanders and colleagues (2000) investigated the value of including strategies to help reduce marital conflict (i.e., communication skills) and stress-coping skills as additional components to a behavioral parenting program. These additional components resulted in reduced observed negative child behaviors compared to teaching standard behavioral management skills alone; however, these differences were no longer present at 1-year follow-up. Other studies that were reviewed have only had very small sample sizes, and so, it is not yet clear whether there are benefits of adding parent emotion regulation components to a behavioral parenting program.

Mindfulness parenting interventions target how the parent responds to stress by improving emotion regulation skills and managing reactivity (e.g., Coatsworth, Duncan, Greenberg, & Nix, 2010). Duncan, Coatsworth, and Greenberg 2009) proposed five dimensions of mindful parenting which are thought to foster specific parenting skills and promote more responsive parenting: (a) listening with full attention (which assists the parent in accurately perceiving the child's verbal and behavioral expressions); (b) nonjudgmental acceptance of self and child (reduces unrealistic expectations of self and the child and increases parenting self-efficacy); (c) emotional awareness of self and child (increases responsiveness to the child's emotions and reduces parental negative emotions); (d) self-regulation in the parenting relationship (better emotion regulation and less over-reactive automatic discipline); and (e) compassion for self and child (fosters less self-blame and positive affection, reduces negative affect). In addition, the process of 'decentering' (i.e., pausing before reacting and noting that feelings are just feelings) is thought to facilitate parents' ability to endure strong emotions that are so often elicited during parent–child interactions and when encountering stress (Duncan et al., 2009). These components of parenting are very similar to key elements of emotion socialization. Parenting interventions that have incorporated mindfulness have been found to improve parenting and the parent–child relationship (Altmaier & Maloney, 2007; Benn, Akiva, Arel, & Roeser, 2012), as well as reducing youth externalizing difficulties (Bögels, Hoogstad, van Dun, de Schutter, & Restifo, 2008). A study with at-risk youth (aged 10–14 years) provided preliminary evidence that teaching children and parents mindfulness (e.g., awareness and acceptance of emotions) was effective in increasing parents' emotion awareness and regulation as well as enhancing parent–youth relationships (Coatsworth et al., 2010).

There are a handful of emotion-focused programs that directly focus on parent emotion regulation as well as teaching emotion coaching parenting. Short and colleagues (2014) conducted a pilot study of an emotion-focused intervention delivered to incarcerated mothers prior to reunification with their children after prison. Of the 47 parents who all attended a behavioral parenting program, 29 received an additional Emotions Program while 18 did not. The Emotions Program (15 $\times$ 2 h sessions over 8 weeks) was based on Dialectical Behavior Therapy (Linehan et al., 2007) and the Tuning in to Kids parenting program (Havighurst & Harley, 2007), with nine sessions focused on teaching mothers' emotion regulation and six sessions targeting emotion coaching skills. The Emotions Program was found to be related to significantly less criminal behavior post-release compared to those mothers who did not attend the program. However, mothers in both conditions showed improvements in emotion regulation, emotion socialization, and mental health. Moretti and Obsuth (2009) published outcomes of a 10-session attachment-based parenting intervention which included a focus on parent emotion regulation and empathy as well as improving the parent–youth relationship. In a sample of parents of adolescents (aged 12–16 years) at risk of aggressive behavior, outcomes were significant reductions in parent-reported youth internalizing and externalizing behavior difficulties as well as improved affect regulation in youth.

Our own Tuning in to Kids (TIK) parenting program aims to improve the emotion socialization of children and also targets parent emotion awareness, regulation and stress management as key parts of the intervention (Havighurst & Harley, 2007). TIK teaches parents emotion coaching skills; that is how to recognize, understand, and manage their own and their children's emotions. The emotion coaching style was identified by Gottman, Katz and Hooven (1996) and includes five steps (Gottman & DeClaire, 1997). When children experience emotions, parents: (1) notice the emotion, (2) see this as an opportunity for intimacy and teaching; (3) communicate an understanding and acceptance of the emotion; (4) assist the child to use words to describe how they feel; and (5) if necessary, assist with problem solving and/or set limits around behavior (Gottman & DeClaire, 1997). The program focuses on increasing skills required for each of the five steps, including understanding where beliefs about emotions come from (e.g., family of origin experience) and how these experiences influence attitudes and responses to emotions. TIK aims to prevent problems developing in children, promote emotional competence (in parents and children), and when present, reduce and treat problems with children's emotional and behavioral functioning. TIK is a six-session group program that is extended over a longer duration for parents with more complex needs. The program, first developed for parents of preschoolers, has been adapted and extended for fathers as well as for parents of toddlers/primary aged children/adolescents, and for parents of children who have experienced trauma or have difficulties with anxiety and behavior problems. The TIK program and its variants (e.g., Tuning in to Teens) have been evaluated in a series of randomized controlled trials, demonstrating the program's positive impact on parenting as well as on child emotional competence and other social and behavioral outcomes. To date, these studies have shown the program to be beneficial for reducing parent's emotion dismissing, increasing empathy and emotion coaching, improving parenting confidence, improving children's emotion competencies, and reducing child/adolescent internalizing and externalizing behavior problems (Duncombe et al., 2014; Havighurst et al., 2015; Havighurst, Kehoe, & Harley, 2015; Havighurst et al., 2013; Havighurst, Wilson, Harley, Prior, & Kehoe, 2010; Kehoe et al., 2014b; Lauw, Havighurst, Wilson, Harley, & Northam, 2014; Wilson, Havighurst, & Harley, 2012, 2014; Wilson, Havighurst, Kehoe, & Harley, 2016). Importantly, the extension of this work to other independent research groups will help to validate the effectiveness of TIK and Tuning in to Teens across cultures and for more varied populations. Current trials are underway in Norway, Germany, Iran and the USA.

Components of TIK that Target Parent Emotion Regulation

We now turn to describe the Tuning in to Kids approach in more detail in order to demonstrate how specific emotion-related parenting skills are targeted and how these may be particularly important for parents when their capacity to regulate emotions is compromised, such as during times of stress. Throughout the TIK program we consider that there is a parallel process between parents developing their own emotion regulation and teaching their children about emotions. We use four main approaches for improving parent's ability to manage emotions effectively, including:

1. Teaching parents emotion awareness
2. Examining the influence of parents' family of origin on their emotion competence and their meta-emotion philosophy (beliefs and reactions to emotions)
3. Building parents' emotional self-care, and
4. Teaching parents' emotion regulation skills.

In our experience of running many parenting groups using the TIK suite of programs, all four of these components are important to target in order to change how parents regulate their emotions which in turn impacts their parenting around emotions with their children. Further, different strategies work for different parents, and we have found having a selection of approaches that dovetail toward a similar common theme (regulating emotions) is important. Psycho-education and exercises about parent's own emotion regulation are delivered in a nonthreatening way in order to reduce possible parental defensiveness. We found in the early stages of developing TIK that it was possible to 'scare parents off' if they thought, 'this is all about me!', and so while we gently introduce the idea that parents' emotions shape children's emotional learning, we mainly begin to target parents' emotion awareness/regulation from session 2 of the program onward. The following outlines the different exercises that we use in TIK to build parent emotion regulation along with proposed mechanisms via which these skills and intervention processes may work.

Parent Emotion Awareness. Emotion awareness and understanding provides the foundation for healthy regulation of emotions and includes the capacity to notice and accurately identify one's own and other's emotions (Halberstadt et al., 2001). In TIK, there is a focus on building parents' and children's emotion awareness in order to facilitate emotion understanding and regulation. Learning is scaffolded in a step-by-step approach across the six sessions, beginning with asking parents to notice emotions in their child (homework in session 1) and then in session 2 to attempt to label these emotions via reflecting the feeling to the child (I wonder if you are a little sad right now?). Session 2 of the program also more formally builds emotion awareness for parents in a warm-up exercise called 'The Bear Stickers' where parents choose a sticker to represent an emotion they have had throughout the week. They are then asked (as a whole group or in a discussion with one other parent participant) to name the emotion, describe what led to them feeling this way, locate where they feel this emotion in their body, consider the thoughts that accompanied the emotion and (in some variants of the program) consider how they felt about having this emotion (meta-emotion beliefs). This exercise is typically very illuminating with many parents having difficulty labeling their own emotions. Reasons for this may be because they are not accustomed to sharing this information, because they have poor emotion awareness and have never paid attention to their own emotions in a conscious way, may find it difficult to locate emotions in their body, or may have never considered how they think/feel about having emotions. This exercise provides a framework for future discussions about emotion awareness in the program as well as providing parents with a new template for self-reflection about emotions and a technique for how emotions might be explored with their child.

Considerable attention is paid in the program to increasing parents' awareness of their child's emotions with reciprocal benefits for the parents' own emotional learning. Parental awareness of their child's anger, sadness, and fear has been found to decline from preschool to early adolescence (Stettler & Katz, 2014). Many parents struggle to identify their child's emotions, remaining focused on misbehaviors or their own overwhelmed feelings. Sometimes children have to really escalate their emotions for their parent to notice. The TIK program attempts to help parents recognize emotions via noticing facial expressions, body language, and tone of voice and identifying a time when their child is more likely to want to talk about their emotions (such as while driving in the car or at bed time). Through this learning many parents report that the skills are mutually beneficial for them.

Additionally, in session 3 TIK uses an activity called '*The emotion detective*,' which involves giving parents a list of common child (or adolescent) scenarios/situations and asking them to find a similar adult equivalent and to identify how they would feel in this situation. This assists parents to 'step into their child's shoes' and encourages perspective taking as well as awareness of emotions that the child might be experiencing. Helping parents to engage in perspective taking may not only help to identify their child's feeling but also assist the parent to remain less reactive (Webb, Miles, & Sheeran, 2012) and respond more supportively, thereby inherently being emotionally regulating. In turn, having feelings validated may help to lower the intensity and duration of the child's emotional experiences. Together, this allows the child to process emotions by focusing on their feelings rather than internalizing or engaging in dysregulated behaviors, while also reducing parenting stress and the experience of negative emotions for the parent (Gottman et al., 1997; Schutte et al., 2001; Shenk & Fruzzetti, 2011).

Finally, to further build parent (and child) emotion awareness we use emotion faces posters (which include an emotion face plus an emotion label underneath), ask parents to talk with their children about emotions, and encourage parents to read emotion-focused books to their children. In addition, a list of 100 emotion words under the headings of happy, sad, angry, and scared is given to parents to encourage them to use a wider emotion vocabulary. Many parents who attend our programs will say that they do not know the meaning of some of the emotion words on our feeling faces posters or emotions lists and this often becomes a focus of teaching by program facilitators. Increasing children's emotion vocabulary has been found to assist them with emotion regulation (Saarni, 1999), and we believe it also assists parents with the same skills.

We hypothesize that helping parents to become aware of and name emotions (step 1 and step 4 of emotion coaching) provides parents with an anchor for present-moment awareness, like the focusing on breath does in a mindfulness meditation (Hill & Updegraff, 2012). This allows parents to shift to thinking about how they or their child are feeling, rather than suppressing emotions or becoming reactive. Often parents report being calmer by just trying to recognize emotions. The focus on awareness of emotions also allows parents to be more present during interactions and enhances empathic responding, facilitating greater intimacy and connection (Block-Lerner, Adair, Plumb, Rhatigan, & Orsillo, 2007; Yap, Allen, & Ladouceur, 2008) consistent with mindfulness parenting interventions (Duncan et al., 2009). By increasing awareness of emotions and attention to the child's emotional response, ineffective patterns of interactions that have become automatized (i.e., are largely unconscious) can be recognized and changed (Bargh & Ferguson, 2000; Dumas, 2005). Awareness of one's own parenting behavior and altering automatic responses are also key components of other effective parenting interventions such as Triple P (Sanders et al., 2000) and the Incredible Years (Webster-Stratton & Reid, 2007).

Family of Origin and Meta-Emotion Philosophy

Responding to challenging behaviors and intense emotions in one's children can lead to strong feelings in parents (e.g., powerlessness, guilt, helplessness, anger, rage, sadness, embarrassment, shame) and may remind them of their family of origin and past experiences (see Chapter 10 by Mileva-Seitz & Fleming for discussion on the intergenerational effects of parenting). We primarily learn about emotions from those with whom we have close relationships (such as siblings or peers) and/or who play a caregiving role in childhood—experiences which shape our attitudes and reactions to emotions (Dunn, Brown, & Beardsall, 1991). Identification of the messages parents received about emotions during their childhood (e.g., anger must not be expressed; crying and showing sadness is weak; it is silly to worry) will influence their capacity to remain calm and responsive when faced with the stress of parenting and strong emotions in themselves or their children. Therefore, a critical way in which we address parents' capacity to regulate emotions that arise during parent–child interactions is by exploring their experiences in their own family of origin with emotions in order to understand how these have shaped their beliefs and reactions to emotions in themselves and others. This is also known as Meta-Emotion Philosophy (Gottman et al., 1997).

There is now substantial evidence linking the intergenerational transmission of attachment patterns to parents' capacity to regulate emotions and subsequently to their emotional responsiveness to their children (e.g., Beijersbergen, Juffer,

Bakermans-Kranenburg, & van IJzendoorn, 2012; Kim, Capaldi, Pears, Kerr, & Owen, 2009; Schore & Schore, 2008). Schore (2008) highlights that early attachment relationships provide the basis for adaptive (and maladaptive) regulation of emotion, and shapes the way the brain processes emotions in future relationships. Other research has also highlighted that parents' family of origin emotional expressiveness influences parents' current emotional expressiveness and emotion-scaffolding behaviors (Baker & Crnic, 2005): parents who experienced more negative emotional expressivity in their family of origin were less likely to engage in emotion-scaffolding behaviors with their toddlers. In our TIK groups, many parents will say that avoidant, minimizing, or punitive responses to emotions in their family of origin were not helpful and continue to cause them stress or difficulty in the present day, both as an individual and as a parent.

Exploration of family of origin experiences, memories, and meta-emotion occurs slowly and carefully in TIK, allowing parents the option to opt out or not to speak when group or pair discussions focus on these topics. The depth of exploration of family of origin and meta-emotion philosophy is determined by the facilitator's assessment of how capable the group is in talking about this topic as well as the facilitator's skill and competence (i.e., less experienced facilitators might not go into this in much depth; experienced therapists delivering the program in clinical settings might explore this at length across an extended eight-session version of the program). This process of exploring beliefs about emotions and a person's history with respect to emotions is (in our experience) critical to assisting parents to learn emotion coaching. It increases awareness and insight and reduces parental reactivity (both in how they respond to stress and in parenting), creating the calm and focus necessary for a parent to adopt a child-centered approach when responding to emotions in the child. Others have also found this process to be important for change (e.g., Greenberg & Pascual-Leone, 2006; Lane, Ryan, Nadel, & Greenberg, 2015). To alter intergenerational patterns of emotionally rejecting parenting it is necessary to develop connected relationships, learn emotional and cognitive regulation skills, and experience a process of working through past experiences (Leerkes & Crockenberg, 2006).

There are a number of reasons why addressing family of origin experiences and resultant meta-emotion beliefs may be helpful. Parents' histories with emotions are likely to impact their reactions to emotions by triggering past memories and engaging unhelpful beliefs or schema (Young, Klosko, & Weishaar, 2006). For example, if a parent has experienced rejection as a child, when similar emotions are triggered during interactions with their own child (as they so often can be with an autonomy-seeking toddler or an individuating teen), parents may feel very hurt by their own child's need for autonomy (perceived as rejection) and may be more likely to experience heightened negative affect and beliefs that activate harsh, rejecting responses or withdrawal. This process of asking parents to reflect on and consider their family of origin surrounding emotional experiences is akin to the processes involved in schema-focused or emotion-focused psychotherapy where changes are thought to occur by accessing past experiences and evoking the emotions consistent with these memories in order to work through and alter automatic dysfunctional patterns of thinking, feeling, behaving, and interacting (Greenberg & Safran, 1989). Through this therapeutic process, intense automatic reactions are reduced because the emotion no longer activates the (often unconsciously) remembered past emotional experience. Reflection on past (emotional) familial experiences is also a core component of psychoanalytic psychotherapy and is seen as integral to reducing the influence of defenses (Freud, 1896). As a brief six- to eight-session group program TIK does not have sufficient time or an established agenda for this degree of therapeutic work. However, the group process often enables parents to reflect, consider, and access past formative experiences with emotions in order to separate out what is current and what is past as well as to provide them with new scripts/reappraisals for responding to emotions in themselves and their children. Parents' emotion regulation improves as a consequence of this by reducing automatic responses of anger or distress that may occur when their children are emotional or they are experiencing stress in their lives.

Emotional Self-Care. Parenting is often a highly stressful experience and occurs simultaneously alongside many other personal, relational, professional, and public demands (see Chap. 3 by Nomaguchi & Milkie). It is, therefore, critical for parents to develop skills in managing stress. Self-care refers to behaviors that maintain and promote physical and emotional well-being, including factors such as sleep, exercise, use of social support, emotion regulation strategies, and mindfulness practices (Myers et al., 2012; Quick, Wright, Adkins, Nelson, & Quick, 2013; Salmon 2001). As such, self-care activities can include a daily mediation practice, regular time for exercise, slow breathing, yoga, taking a hot bath, or just sitting down for a cup of tea. The regular practice of self-care helps to reduce stress as well as to prevent more reactive parenting; others have also found self-care strategies useful in mental health and parenting interventions (e.g., Linehan et al., 2007; Salmon 2001). In TIK, parents are asked to notice when they feel their emotions rising. Regularly tuning into lower intensity emotion arousal, such as mild frustration or stress, and considering emotional self-care at this time allows the parent to be calmer and enable them to be more aware of and able to assist their child. Parents often do not recognize the importance of self-care and report feeling guilty and selfish about taking this time. Others are impeded from using self-care because of limited resources. By exploring barriers to engaging in self-care, these beliefs can be addressed and parents can learn that looking after one's own emotional well-being is an important proactive emotion regulation strategy to help manage the stress of parenting enabling the parent to be more emotionally responsive.

Emotion Regulation Skills. The development of skills in regulating emotions and managing stress is highly important for mental health and parenting (Aldao et al., 2010). We have found that if parents report that they are overwhelmed by stress and have limited access to emotion regulation strategies, they typically struggle to use emotion coaching successfully. The last sections of our chapter have highlighted that TIK recognizes that in order to be able to engage in empathic responding (which lies at the heart of emotion coaching), parents require good emotion awareness. If emotions are not able to be recognized, parents may miss the opportunity to respond. On the other hand, if a parent's own emotional experience during an interaction with their child is strong and they are unable to regulate their heightened negative arousal and/or distress, they are more likely to respond in a self-focused rather than child-focused manner (Eisenberg, 2000). Therefore, key components of TIK are becoming aware of one's own emotion regulation patterns and learning emotion regulation skills.

In TIK, we teach three main ways of regulating emotions that fall into the categories of pausing, calming, or releasing. In addition, we teach strategies which parents can use in advance (i.e., self-care) and 'in the moment,' with a specific focus on regulating anger, anxiety, and stress. 'Building in a pause' for parents is one of the simplest 'in the moment' techniques for parents to learn and is critical for reducing emotion reactivity. Parents are taught that during moments of 'emotional flooding' it is difficult to access cognitive strategies, and therefore, pausing can be more effective. Methods for building in a pause include running their hands under cold water, taking 10 slow deep breaths, stepping out of the room, paying attention to their senses (smell, colors, textures), having a sip of cold water, visualizing a red traffic light, or telling oneself to 'STOP.' The concept of 'building in a pause' helps parents to break from automatic reactions and engage in more child-centered parenting and is consistent with mindfulness techniques (Duncan et al., 2009; Linehan et al., 2007). Calming strategies may include parents breathing slowly, having some quiet time in their room, having a bath or a shower, or talking to someone who they find calming. These strategies are also consistent with anxiety management techniques used in cognitive behavioral therapy (Beck, Rush, Shaw, & Emery, 1979; Hawton, Salkovskis, Kirk, & Clark, 1989). Emotional release activities include exercise, tensing and releasing different muscle groups, having a good cry, twisting a towel, or weeding the garden. These strategies are explored with parents to find those that uniquely fit with the parents' preferred way of calming or releasing the physical aspects of emotions. Parents are also encouraged to use the calming and releasing activities preventatively as part of their self-care. Stress-releasing activities, such as tense and release exercises that enable a person to let go of physical tension and strong emotions occurring as part of the fight or flight response are also an effective component of cognitive behavioral therapy (Beck et al., 1979; Hawton et al., 1989).

Mindfulness techniques are taught in facilitator-led meditation/relaxation, and internet links are provided to a range of resources that can assist parents to learn new skills for calming their reactivity in advance (e.g., self-care). Parents are encouraged to use these 'in the moment' strategies when they are stressed and need to down-regulate their own emotional intensity (e.g., progressive muscle relaxation, breathing). Some of these techniques have also been found important in other emotion regulation-focused interventions for adults (e.g., mindfulness; Duncan et al., 2009; Linehan et al., 2007) and for children (e.g., the PAThS program; Greenberg, Kusche, Cook, & Quamma, 1995).

Lastly, we have found that teaching parents the five steps of emotion coaching outlined by Gottman and DeClaire (1997) helps them regulate their own emotions because they shift to a more child-centered approach to parenting where they go through five practical steps to approach the emotions that their child is experiencing. Instead of thinking 'Oh, he is such a difficult child!', 'She is so out of control!', "I can't stand this!', 'Why does he have to ruin everything!' (which contributes to parents' emotions escalating), we encourage parents to view the emotional moment as an opportunity for connection and teaching. This is a form of cognitive reappraisal (Gross & Thompson, 2007), whereby the parent no longer sees the child's emotions as overwhelming and as something to overcome or avoid, but instead sees that their child is struggling and develops some confidence as they work through each emotion coaching step. For example, 'What is he/she feeling?', 'Can I teach him/her?', 'Can I label the emotion?', 'Can I empathize?', 'Can I breathe slowly and slow down my reactions until my child calms': then, 'what might we do to work through this situation?' Helping parents dynamically adjust their responses in emotional moments enhances their ability to manage parenting stress, regulates their own emotions, and gives them tangible skills for responding to their child.

Does Parent Emotion Regulation Influence the Outcomes of Tuning into Kids/Teens?

In order to further examine the role of parent emotion regulation and coping with stress on parenting around children's emotions, we reexamined some of our own data to see whether the TIK program was moderated by parent psychological distress or poor emotion regulation at baseline. In our first TIK efficacy trial we considered whether parents' baseline difficulties in awareness and regulation, parents' psychological distress, or parents baseline negative expressiveness moderated changes in parents' emotion dismissing, emotion coaching, or empathy at six-month follow-up (Havighurst et al., 2010). With the exception of parents' negative expressiveness, none of our other moderator analyses were statistically significant, suggesting that all intervention parents reported improvements in emotion socialization regardless of baseline functioning. Interestingly, parents' baseline negative expressiveness did moderate the effect of TIK on parents' emotion coaching at six-month follow-up ($P = .012$). Specifically, although all intervention parents showed significant improvements on emotion coaching, intervention parents with low negative expressiveness showed significantly greater improvements. It may be that low-level negative expressiveness in this sample was representative of a group of parents who were not aware of their emotions, or felt uncomfortable showing them. Learning skills in awareness and understanding of emotions may have enabled these families to be less dismissive of their own child's emotion experience. Alternately, parents who were less negatively expressive may have been better able to learn the emotion coaching skills because they were not flooded by their own emotions.

For our study where TIK was delivered as part of a multi-systemic intervention to families where the 5–9 year old child was identified at risk for conduct disorder, i.e., top 7–8% of child behavior problems, we considered parents' psychological distress (measured via DASS, a screening measure for stress, anxiety and depression; Lovibond & Lovibond, 1995) and parents' baseline negative expressiveness as moderators of program effects on parents' emotion dismissing, emotion coaching, or empathy (Havighurst et al., 2015). None of the three-way interactions were significant, indicating that the changes held for all intervention participants, regardless of baseline severity of parents psychological functioning. With this at-risk sample, TIK was also compared with a behavioral parenting program (Duncombe et al., 2014). In this study, TIK was found to be more effective in reducing child behavior problems than the behavioral parenting program for parents who had higher levels of emotional difficulties themselves. We hypothesized that this was because the program had a focus on emotion regulation for the parent providing an important set of skills for those parents who had poorer mental health.

We also investigated whether the impact of Tuning in to Teens (TINT) was moderated by parents' baseline level of internalizing difficulties and problems with awareness and regulation of emotion (Kehoe, 2014; Kehoe et al., 2014b). Again, none of the moderator analyses were significant, indicating that regardless of baseline severity, a greater decrease in emotion dismissing and youth functioning (internalizing and externalizing difficulties) was reported by intervention parents and preadolescents, when compared to control participants.

These findings suggest that the positive outcomes from TIK and TINT are found with parents regardless of parents' emotion regulation—both those low and high in emotion regulation prior to the intervention equally show improvements. One study suggests that parents with greater psychological difficulties may make greater progress in TIK than when using a behavioral parenting program perhaps because of the additional focus in TIK on parent emotion regulation helping parents to manage their own response to parenting stress as well as their own mental health.

Conclusion

Parents' ability to manage stress and regulate their emotions has been found to be related to their capacity to respond to their children's emotions. A review of the literature found that better parent emotion regulation has been found to be associated with more favorable emotion coaching and supportive response to children's emotion socialization. The TIK parenting program which targets parent emotion socialization and parent's own emotion regulation has a considerable focus on building emotion regulation through increasing emotion awareness, exploring family of origin and meta-emotion philosophy, increasing parent emotion self-care, and teaching specific emotion regulation skills, especially for managing anger, anxiety, and stress. These all play an important role in assisting parents to understand and regulate their own emotions thereby reducing the stress of parenting, contributing to a calmer family emotion climate, and enabling them to use the five steps of emotion coaching with their children. This transdiagnostic approach to intervention, which assists parents in their capacity to cope and improves parenting (and dually influences child outcomes), allows exploration of how parenting stress, emotion regulation, and child functioning are connected. This also allows greater consideration of how parenting interventions need to go beyond just a focus on how they respond to the child but also to engage parents in learning and applying skills in how they manage stress and their own emotional functioning. This combination is likely to produce the most powerful intervention outcomes.

References

Aldao, A., Nolen-Hoeksema, S., & Schweizer, S. (2010). Emotion-regulation strategies across psychopathology: A meta-analytic review. *Clinical Psychology Review, 30,* 217–237. doi:10.1016/j.cpr.2009.11.004

Altmaier, E., & Maloney, R. (2007). An initial evaluation of a mindful parenting program. *Journal of Clinical Psychology, 63*(12), 1231–1238. doi:10.1002/jclp.20395

Assemany, A. E., & McIntosh, D. E. (2002). Negative treatment outcomes of behavioral parent training programs. *Psychology in the Schools, 39*(2), 209–219. doi:10.1002/pits.10032

Baker, J. K., & Crnic, K. A. (2005). The relation between mothers' reports of family-of-origin expressiveness and their emotion-related parenting. *Parenting: Science and Practice, 5*(4), 333–346. doi:10.1207/s15327922par0504_2

Bargh, J. A., & Ferguson, M. J. (2000). Beyond behaviourism: On the automaticity of higher mental processes. *Psychological Bulletin, 126*(6), 925–945. doi:10.1037//0033-2909.126.6.925

Bariola, E., Gullone, E., & Hughes, E. (2011). Child and adolescent emotion regulation: The role of parental emotion regulation and expression. *Clinical Child and Family Psychology Review,* 1–15. doi:10.1007/s10567-011-0092-5

Beck, A. T., Rush, A. J., Shaw, B. F., & Emery, G. (1979). *Cognitive therapy of depression.* New York: Guildford Press.

Beijersbergen, M. D., Juffer, F., Bakermans-Kranenburg, M. J., & van IJzendoorn, M. H. (2012). Remaining or becoming secure: Parental sensitive support predicts attachment continuity from infancy to adolescence in a longitudinal adoption study. *Developmental Psychology, 48*(5), 1277–1282. doi:10.1037/a0027442

Benn, R., Akiva, T., Arel, S., & Roeser, R. W. (2012). Mindfulness training effects for parents and educators of children with special needs. *Developmental Psychology, 48*(5), 1476–1487. doi:10.1037/a0027537

Block-Lerner, J., Adair, C., Plumb, J. C., Rhatigan, D. L., & Orsillo, S. M. (2007). The case for mindfulness-based approaches in the cultivation of empathy: Does nonjudgmental, present-moment awareness increase capacity for perspective-taking and empathic concern? *Journal of Marital and Family Therapy, 33*(4), 501–516. doi:10.1111/j.1752-0606.2007.00034.x

Bögels, S., Hoogstad, B., van Dun, L., de Schutter, S., & Restifo, K. (2008). Mindfulness training for adolescents with externalizing disorders and their parents. *Behavioural and Cognitive Psychotherapy, 36*(02), 193–209. doi:10.1017/S1352465808004190

Breaux, R. P., Harvey, E. A., & Lugo-Candelas, C. I. (2015). The role of parent psychopathology in emotion socialization. *Journal of Abnormal Child Psychology,* 1–13. doi:10.1007/s10802-015-0062-3

Brestan, E. V., & Eyberg, S. M. (1998). Effective psychosocial treatments of conduct-disordered children and adolescents: 29 years, 82 studies, and 5272 kids. *Journal of Clinical Child Psychology, 27,* 180–189. doi:10.1207/s15374424jccp2702_5

Buck, R. (1984). *The communication of emotion.* New York: Guilford.

Buckholdt, K. E., Parra, G. R., & Jobe-Shields, L. (2010). Emotion dysregulation as a mechanism through which parental magnification of sadness increases risk for binge eating and limited control of eating behaviors. *Eating Behaviors, 11,* 122–126. doi:10.1016/j.eatbeh.2009.10.003

Burke, K., Brennan, L., & Cann, W. (2012). Promoting protective factors for young adolescents: ABCD parenting young adolescents program randomized controlled trial. *Journal of Adolescence, 35*(5), 1315–1328. doi:10.1016/j.adolescence.2012.05.002

Burke, J. D., Pardini, D. A., & Loeber, R. (2008). Reciprocal relationships between parenting behavior and disruptive psychopathology from childhood through adolescence. *Journal of Abnormal Child Psychology, 36*(5), 679–692. doi:10.1007/s10802-008-9219-7

Coatsworth, J. D., Duncan, L. G., Greenberg, M. T., & Nix, R. L. (2010). Changing parent's mindfulness, child management skills and relationship quality with their youth: Results from a randomized pilot intervention trial. *Journal of Child and Family Studies, 19*(2), 203–217. doi:10.1007/s10826-009-9304-8

Cobham, V. E., Dadds, M. R., & Spence, S. H. (1998). The role of parental anxiety in the treatment of childhood anxiety. *Journal of Consulting and Clinical Psychology, 66*(6), 893–905. doi:10.1037/0022-006X.66.6.893

Dix, T., & Meuniera, L. N. (2009). Depressive symptoms and parenting competence: An analysis of 13 regulatory processes. *Developmental Review, 29*(1), 45–68. doi:10.1016/j.dr.2008.11.002

Dumas, J. E. (2005). Mindfulness-based parent training: Strategies to lessen the grip of automaticity in families with disruptive children. *Journal of Clinical Child and Adolescent Psychology, 34*(4), 779–791. doi:10.1207/s15374424jccp3404_20

Duncan, L. G., Coatsworth, J. D., & Greenberg, M. T. (2009). A model of mindful parenting: Implications for parent-child relationships and prevention research. *Clinical Child and Family Psychology Review, 12*(3), 255–270. doi:10.1007/s10567-009-0046-3

Duncombe, M. E., Havighurst, S. S., Kehoe, C. E., Holland, K. M., Frankling, E., & Stargatt, R. (2014). Comparing an emotion- and a behavior-focused parenting program as part of a multi-systemic intervention for child conduct problems. *Journal of Clinical Child and Adolescent Psychology*. doi:10.1080/15374416.2014.963855

Dunn, J., Brown, J., & Beardsall, L. (1991). Family talk about feeling states and children's later understanding of others' emotions. *Developmental Psychology, 27*(3), 448–455. doi:10.1037/0012-1649.27.3.448

Eisenberg, N. (2000). *Empathy and sympathy*. New York: Guilford Press.

Eisenberg, N., Cumberland, A., & Spinrad, T. L. (1998). Parental socialization of emotion. *Psychological Inquiry, 9*(4), 241–273. doi:10.1207/s15327965pli0904_1

Freud, S. (1896). *The Aetiology of Hysteria, Standard Edition, vol. 7*: Hogarth Press.

Furlong, M., McGilloway, S., Bywater, T., Hutchings, J., Smith, S. M., & Donnelly, M. (2012). Behavioural and cognitive-behavioural group-based parenting programmes for early-onset conduct problems in children aged 3–12 years. *Cochrane database of systematic reviews*. doi:10.1002/14651858.CD008225.pub2

Garber, J., Clarke, G. N., Weersing, V. R., Beardslee, W. R., Brent, D. A., Gladstone, T. R. G., … & Iyengar, S. (2009). Prevention of depression in at-risk adolescents: A randomized controlled trial. *JAMA, The Journal of the American Medical Association* (21), 2215–2224. doi:10.1001/jama.2009.788

Garner, P. W., Dunsmore, J. C., & Southam-Gerrow, M. (2008). Mother-child conversations about emotions: Linkages to child aggression and prosocial behavior. *Social Development, 17*(2), 259–277. doi:10.1111/j.1467-9507.2007.00424.x

Gohm, C. L., & Clore, G. L. (2002). Four latent traits of emotional experience and their involvement in well-being, coping, and attributional style. *Cognition and Emotion, 16*(4), 495–518. doi:10.1080/02699930143000374

Gottman, J. M., & DeClaire, J. (1997). *The heart of parenting: How to raise an emotionally intelligent child*. London: Bloomsbury.

Gottman, J. M., Katz, L. F., & Hooven, C. (1996). Parental meta-emotion philosophy and the emotional life of families: Theoretical models and preliminary data. *Journal of Family Psychology, 10,* 243–268. doi:10.1037/0893-3200.10.3.243

Gottman, J. M., Katz, L. F., & Hooven, C. (1997). *Meta-emotion: How families communicate emotionally*. Mahway, New Jersey: Lawrence Erlbaum Assoc.

Gratz, K. L., & Roemer, L. (2004). Multidimensional assessment of emotion regulation and dysregulation: Development, factor structure, and initial validation of the Difficulties in Emotion Regulation Scale. *Journal of Psychopathology and Behavioral Assessment, 26*(1), 41–54. doi:10.1023/B:JOBA.0000007455.08539.94

Greenberg, M. T., Kusche, C. A., Cook, E. T., & Quamma, J. P. (1995). Promoting emotional competence in school-aged children: The effects of the paths curriculum. *Development and Psychopathology, 7,* 117–136. doi:10.1017/S0954579400006374

Greenberg, L. S., & Pascual-Leone, A. (2006). Emotion in psychotherapy: A practice-friendly research review. *Journal of Clinical Psychology, 62*(5), 611–630. doi:10.1002/jclp.20252

Greenberg, L. S., & Safran, J. D. (1989). Emotion in psychotherapy. *American Psychologist, 44* (1), 19–29. doi:10.1037/0003-066X.44.1.19

Gross, J. J. (2002). Emotion regulation: Affective, cognitive, and social consequences. *Psychophysiology, 39*(3), 281–291. doi:10.1017/S0048577201393198

Gross, J. J., & John, O. P. (2003). Individual differences in two emotion regulation processes: Implications for affect, relationships, and well-being. *Journal of Personality and Social Psychology* (2), 348–362. doi:10.1037/0022-3514.85.2.348

Gross, J. J., & Thompson, R. A. (2007). Emotion regulation: Conceptual foundations. In J. J. Gross (Ed.), *Handbook of emotion regulation* (pp. 3–24). New York: Guilford Press.

Halberstadt, A. G., Denham, S. A., & Dunsmore, J. C. (2001). Affective social competence. *Social Development, 10*(1), 79–119. doi:10.1111/1467-9507.00150

Havighurst, S. S., Duncombe, M. E., Frankling, E. J., Holland, K. A., Kehoe, C. E., & Stargatt, R. (2015a). An emotion-focused early intervention for children with emerging conduct problems. *Journal of Abnormal Child Psychology, 43*(4), 749–760. doi:10.1007/s10802-014-9944-z

Havighurst, S. S., & Harley, A. (2007). *Tuning in to kids: Emotionally intelligent parenting program manual.* Melbourne: University of Melbourne.

Havighurst, S. S., Kehoe, C. E., & Harley, A. E. (2015b). Tuning in to teens: Improving parental responses to anger and reducing youth externalizing behavior problems. *Journal of Adolescence, 42,* 148–158. doi:10.1016/j.adolescence.2015.04.005

Havighurst, S. S., Wilson, K. R., Harley, A. E., Kehoe, C. E., Efron, D., & Prior, M. R. (2013). "Tuning in to Kids": Reducing young children's behavior problems using an emotion coaching parenting program. *Child Psychiatry and Human Development, 44*(2), 247–264. doi:10.1007/s10578-012-0322-1

Havighurst, S. S., Wilson, K. R., Harley, A. E., Prior, M. R., & Kehoe, C. E. (2010). Tuning in to Kids: Improving emotion socialization practices in parents of preschool children—Findings from a community trial. *Journal of Child Psychology and Psychiatry, 51*(12), 1342–1350. doi:10.1111/j.1469-7610.2010.02303.x

Hawton, K., Salkovskis, P. M., Kirk, J., & Clark, D. M. (1989). *Cognitive behaviour therapy for psychiatric problems: A practical guide.* Oxford, England: Oxford University Press.

Hill, C. L. M., & Updegraff, J. A. (2012). Mindfulness and its relationship to emotional regulation. *Emotion, 12*(1), 81–90. doi:10.1037/a0026355

Hughes, E. K., & Gullone, E. (2008). Internalizing symptoms and disorders in families of adolescents: A review of family systems literature. *Clinical Psychology Review, 28,* 92–117. doi:10.1016/j.cpr.2007.04.002

Hughes, E. K., & Gullone, E. (2010). Parent emotion socialisation practices and their associations with personality and emotion regulation. *Personality and Individual Differences, 49*(7), 694–699. doi:10.1016/j.paid.2010.05.042

Jackson, M. C., & Arlegui-Prieto, M. (2016). Variation in normal mood state influences sensitivity to dynamic changes in emotional expression. *Emotion, 16*(2), 145–149. doi:10.1037/emo0000126

Katz, L. F., & Gottman, J. M. (1991). 'Marital discord and child outcomes: A social psychophysiological approach'. In Garber, J. & Dodge, K.A. (eds.) The Development of Emotion Regulation and Dysregulation:. Cambridge: Cambridge University Press (pp. 129–156). doi:10.1017/CBO9780511663963.008

Katz, L. F., Maliken, A. C., & Stettler, N. M. (2012). Parental meta-emotion philosophy: A review of research and theoretical framework. *Child Development Perspectives, 6*(4), 417–422. doi:10.1111/j.1750-8606.2012.00244.x

Kehoe, C. E. (2014). *Tuning in to Teens: Examining the efficacy of an emotion-focused parenting intervention in reducing pre-adolescents' internalising difficulties.* (Doctor of Philosophy Unpublished thesis), The University of Melbourne, Melbourne. Retrieved from http://hdl.handle.net/11343/43025

Kehoe, C. E., Havighurst, S. S., & Harley, A. E. (2014a). Examining the efficacy of an emotion-focused parenting intervention in reducing pre-adolescents' internalising and externalising problems. In *Paper presented at the 28th International Congress of Applied Psychology Paris.*

Kehoe, C. E., Havighurst, S. S., & Harley, A. E. (2014b). Tuning in to Teens: Improving parent emotion socialization to reduce youth internalizing difficulties. *Social Development, 23*(2), 413–431. doi:10.1111/sode.12060

Kehoe, C. E., Havighurst, S. S., & Harley, A. E. (2015). Somatic complaints in early adolescence: The role of parents' emotion socialization. *Journal of Early Adolescence, 35*(7), 966–989. doi:10.1177/0272431614547052

Kendall, P. C., Gosch, E., Hudson, J. L., Flannery-Schroeder, E., & Suveg, C. (2008). Cognitive-behavioral therapy for anxiety disordered youth: A randomized clinical trial evaluating child and family modalities. *Journal of Consulting and Clinical Psychology* (2), 282–297. doi:10.1037/0022-006X.76.2.282

Kim, H. K., Capaldi, D. M., Pears, K. C., Kerr, D. C. R., & Owen, L. D. (2009). Intergenerational transmission of internalising and externalising behaviours across three generations: Gender-specific pathways. *Criminal Behaviour and Mental Health, 19*(2), 125–141. doi:10.1002/cbm.708

Lane, R. D., Ryan, L., Nadel, L., & Greenberg, L. (2015). Memory reconsolidation, emotional arousal, and the process of change in psychotherapy: New insights from brain science. *Behavioral and Brain Sciences, 38*. doi:10.1017/S0140525X14000041

Laurent, H. K. (2014). Clarifying the contours of emotion regulation: Insights from parent- child stress research. *Child Development Perspectives, 8*(1), 30–35. doi:10.1111/cdep.12058

Lauw, M. S. M., Havighurst, S. S., Wilson, K. R., Harley, A. E., & Northam, E. A. (2014). Improving parenting of toddlers' emotions using an emotion coaching parenting program: A pilot study of tuning into toddlers. *Journal of Community Psychology, 42*(2), 169–175. doi:10.1002/jcop.21602

Leerkes, E. M., & Crockenberg, S. C. (2006). Antecedents of mothers' emotional and cognitive responses to infant distress: The role of family, mother, and infant characteristics. *Infant Mental Health Journal, 27*(4), 405–428. doi:10.1002/imhj.20099

Lenze, S. N., Pautsch, J., & Luby, J. (2011). Parent-child interaction therapy emotion development: A novel treatment for depression in preschool children. *Depression and Anxiety, 28*(2), 153–159. doi:10.1002/da.20770

Linehan, M. M., Bohus, M., & Thomas, R. L. (Eds.). (2007). *Dialectical behavior therapy for pervasive emotion dysregulation: Theoretical and practical underpinnings*. NY: Guilford Press.

Lorber, M. F., Mitnick, D. M., & Slep, A. M. S. (2015). Parents' experience of flooding in discipline encounters: Associations with discipline and interplay with related factors. *Journal of Family Psychology. Advance online publication.* doi:10.1037/fam0000176

Lorber, M. F., & O'Leary, S. G. (2005). Mediated paths to overactive discipline: mothers' experienced emotion, appraisals, and physiological responses. *Journal of Consulting and Clinical Psychology, 73*(5), 972–982. doi:10.1037/0022-006X.73.5.972

Lovibond, P. F., & Lovibond, S. H. (1995). The structure of negative emotional states: Comparison of the Depression Anxiety Stress Scales (DASS) with the beck depression and anxiety inventories. *Behavior Research Therapy, 33,* 335–343. doi:10.1016/0005-7967(94)00075-U

Luby, J., Lenze, S., & Tillman, R. (2012). A novel early intervention for preschool depression: Findings from a pilot randomized controlled trial. *Journal of Child Psychology and Psychiatry and Allied Disciplines, 53*(3), 313–322. doi:10.1111/j.1469-7610.2011.02483.x

Lynch, T. R., Robins, C. J., Morse, J. Q., & Krause, E. D. (2001). A mediational model relating affect intensity, emotion inhibition, and psychological distress. *Behavior Therapy, 32*(3), 519–536. doi:10.1016/S0005-7894(01)80034-4

Maliken, A. C., & Katz, L. F. (2013). Exploring the impact of parental psychopathology and emotion regulation on evidence-based parenting interventions: A transdiagnostic approach to improving treatment effectiveness. *Clinical Child and Family Psychology Review, 16*(2), 173–186. doi:10.1007/s10567-013-0132-4

Mazursky-Horowitz, H., Felton, J. W., MacPherson, L., Ehrlich, K. B., Cassidy, J., Lejuez, C. W., et al. (2015). Maternal emotion regulation mediates the association between adult attention-deficit/hyperactivity disorder symptoms and parenting. *Journal of Abnormal Child Psychology, 43,* 121–131. doi:10.1007/s10802-014-9894-5

Mence, M., Hawes, D. J., Wedgwood, L., Morgan, S., Barnett, B., Kohlhoff, J., & Hunt, C. (2014). Emotional flooding and hostile discipline in the families of toddlers with disruptive behavior problems. *Journal Of Family Psychology: JFP: Journal Of The Division Of Family Psychology Of The American Psychological Association (Division 43), 28*(1), 12–21. doi:10.1037/a0035352

Meyer, S., Raikes, H. A., Virmani, E. A., Waters, S., & Thompson, R. A. (2014). Parent emotion representations and the socialization of emotion regulation in the family. *International Journal of Behavioral Development, 38*(2), 164–173. doi:10.1177/0165025413519014

Moretti, M. M., & Obsuth, I. (2009). Effectiveness of an attachment-focused manualized intervention for parents of teens at risk for aggressive behaviour: The connect program. *Journal of Adolescence, 32*(6), 1347–1357. doi:10.1016/j.adolescence.2009.07.013

Morris, A. S., Silk, J. S., Morris, M. D. S., Steinberg, L., Aucoin, K. J., & Keyes, A. W. (2011). The influence of mother–child emotion regulation strategies on children's expression of anger and sadness. *Developmental Psychology, 47*(1), 213–225. doi:10.1037/a0021021

Morris, A. S., Silk, J. S., Steinberg, L., Myers, S. S., & Robinson, L. R. (2007). The role of the family context in the development of emotion regulation. *Social Development, 16*(2), 361–388. doi:10.1111/j.1467-9507.2007.00389.x

Myers, S. B., Sweeney, A. C., Popick, V., Wesley, K., Bordfeld, A., & Fingerhut, R. (2012). Self-care practices and perceived stress levels among psychology graduate students. *Training and Education in Professional Psychology, 6*(1), 55–66. doi:10.1037/a0026534

Perlman, S. B., Camras, L. A., & Pelphrey, K. A. (2008). Physiology and functioning: Parents' vagal tone, emotion socialization, and children's emotion knowledge. *Journal of Experimental Child Psychology, 100*(4), 308–315. doi:10.1016/j.jecp.2008.03.007

Platt, R., Williams, S., Ginsburg, G., Williams, S. R., & Ginsburg, G. S. (2016). Stressful life events and child anxiety: Examining parent and child mediators. *Child Psychiatry and Human Development, 47*(1), 23–34. doi:10.1007/s10578-015-0540-4

Psychogiou, L., & Parry, E. (2014). Why do depressed individuals have difficulties in their parenting role? *Psychological Medicine, 44*(7), 1345–1347. doi:10.1017/S0033291713001931

Quick, J. C., Wright, T. A., Adkins, J. A., Nelson, D. L., & Quick, J. D. (2013). Preventive stress management: Principles, theory, and practice *Preventive stress management in organizations* (2nd ed.). (pp. 103–113). Washington, DC, US: American Psychological Association.

Ralph, A., & Sanders, M. R. (2006). The 'teen Triple P' positive parenting program: A preliminary evaluation. *Youth Studies Australia, 25*(2), 41–48.

Raver, C. C., & Spagnola, M. (2002). "When my mommy was angry, I was speechless": Children's preceptions of maternal emotional expressiveness within the context of economic hardship. *Marriage and Family Review, 34,* 63–88. doi:10.1300/J002v34n01_04

Rutherford, H. J. V., Wallace, N. S., Laurent, H. K., & Mayes, L. C. (2015). Emotion regulation in parenthood. *Developmental Review, 36,* 1–14. doi:10.1016/j.dr.2014.12.008

Saarni, C. (1999). *The development of emotional competence*. New York: Guilford Press.

Salmon, P. (2001). Effects of physical exercise on anxiety, depression, and sensitivity to stress: A unifying theory. *Clinical Psychology Review, 21,* 33–61. doi:10.1016/S0272-7358(99)00032-X

Salovey, P., Mayer, J. D., Goldman, S. L., Turvey, C., & Palfai, T. P. (1995). Emotional attention, clarity, and repair: Exploring emotional intelligence using the trait meta-mood scale. In J. W. Pennebaker (Ed.), *Emotion disclosure and health*. Washington, DC: American Psychological Association.

Sanders, M. R., & Markie-Dadds, C. (1996). Triple P: A multilevel family intervention program for children with disruptive behaviour disorders. In T. Cotton & H. Jackson (Eds.), *Early intervention and prevention in mental health* (pp. 59–85). Melbourne, Australia: Australian Psychological Society.

Sanders, M. R., Markie-Dadds, C., Tully, L. A., & Bor, W. (2000). The Triple P-positive parenting program: A comparison of enhanced, standard, and self-directed behavioral family intervention for parents of children with early onset conduct problems. *Journal of Consulting and Clinical Psychology, 68*(4), 624–640. doi:10.1037/0022-006X.68.4.624

Schore, J. R., & Schore, A. N. (2008). Modern attachment theory: The central role of affect regulation in development and treatment. *Clinical Social Work Journal, 36*(1), 9–20. doi:10.1007/s10615-007-0111-7

Schutte, N. S., Malouff, J. M., Bobik, C., Coston, T. D., Greeson, C., Jedlicka, C., … & Wendorf, G. (2001). Emotional intelligence and interpersonal relations. *The Journal of Social Psychology, 141*(4), 523–536. doi:10.1080/00224540109600569

Scott, S., & Dadds, M. R. (2009). Practitioner review: When parent training doesn't work: theory-driven clinical strategies. *Journal of Child Psychology and Psychiatry and Allied Disciplines, 50*(12), 1441–1450. doi:10.1111/j.1469-7610.2009.02161.x

Sheeber, L. B., Kuppens, P., Shortt, J. W., Katz, L. F., Davis, B., & Allen, N. B. (2011). Depression is associated with the escalation of adolescents' dysphoric behavior during interactions with parents. *Emotion, 12*(5), 913–918. doi:10.1037/a0025784

Shenk, C. E., & Fruzzetti, A. E. (2011). The impact of validating and invalidating responses on emotional reactivity. *Journal of Social and Clinical Psychology, 30*(2), 163–183. doi:10.1521/jscp.2011.30.2.163

Shipman, K. L., Schneider, R., Fitzgerald, M. M., Sims, C., Swisher, L., & Edwards, A. (2007). Maternal emotion socialization in maltreating and non-maltreating families: Implications for children's emotion regulation. *Social Development, 16*(2), 268–285. doi:10.1111/j.1467-9507.2007.00384.x

Shortt, J. W., Eddy, J. M., Sheeber, L., & Davis, B. (2014). Project home: A pilot evaluation of an emotion-focused intervention for mothers reuniting with children after prison. *Psychological Services, 11*(1), 1–9. doi:10.1037/a0034323

Stettler, N., & Katz, L. F. (2014). Changes in parents' meta-emotion philosophy from preschool to early adolescence. *Parenting: Science and Practice, 14*(3/4), 162–174. doi:10.1080/15295192.2014.945584

Stocker, C. M., Richmond, M. K., Rhoades, G. K., & Kiang, L. (2007). Family emotional processes and adolescents' adjustment. *Social Development, 16*(2), 310–325. doi:10.1111/j.1467-9507.2007.00386.x

Suchy, Y. (2011). *Clinical neuropsychology of emotion*. New York, US: The Guilford Press.

Suveg, C., Sood, E., Barmish, A., Tiwari, S., Hudson, J. L., & Kendall, P. C. (2008). "I'd rather not talk about it": Emotion parenting in families of children with an anxiety disorder. *Journal of Family Psychology, 22*(6), 875–884. doi:10.1037/a0012861

Taylor, T. K., & Biglan, A. (1998). Behavioral family interventions for improving child-rearing: A review of the literature for clinicians and policy makers. *Clinical Child and Family Psychology Review, 1*(1), 41–60. doi:10.1023/A:1021848315541

Webb, T. L., Miles, E., & Sheeran, P. (2012). Dealing with feeling: A meta-analysis of the effectiveness of strategies derived from the process model of emotion regulation. *Psychological Bulletin, 138*(4), 775–808. doi:10.1037/a0027600

Webster-Stratton, C., & Hammond, M. (1990). Predictors of treatment outcome in parent training for families with conduct problem children. *Behavior Therapy, 21,* 319–337. doi:10.1016/S0005-7894(05)80334-X

Webster-Stratton, C., & Reid, M. J. (2007). Incredible years parents and teachers training series: A head start partnership to promote social competence and prevent conduct problems. In P. Tolan, J. Szapocznik, & S. Sambrano (Eds.), *Preventing youth substance abuse: Science-based programs for children and adolescents.* (pp. 67–88): American Psychological Association.

Weersing, V. R., Rozenman, M. S., Maher-Bridge, M., & Campo, J. V. (2012). Anxiety, depression, and somatic distress: Developing a transdiagnostic internalizing toolbox for pediatric practice. *Cognitive and Behavioral Practice, 19*(1), 68–82. doi:10.1016/j.cbpra.2011.06.002

Williford, A. P., Calkins, S. D., & Keane, S. P. (2007). Predicting change in parenting stress across early childhood: Child and maternal factors. *Journal of Abnormal Child Psychology, 35*(2), 251–263. doi:10.1007/s10802-006-9082-3

Wilson, K. R., Havighurst, S. S., & Harley, A. E. (2012). Tuning in to Kids: An effectiveness trial of a parenting program targeting emotion socialization of preschoolers. *Journal of Family Psychology, 26*(1), 56–65. doi:10.1037/a0026480

Wilson, K. R., Havighurst, S. S., & Harley, A. E. (2014). Dads tuning in to kids: Piloting a new parenting program targeting fathers' emotion coaching skills. *Journal of Community Psychology, 42*(2), 162–168. doi:10.1002/jcop.21601

Wilson, K. R., Havighurst, S. S., Kehoe, C. E., & Harley, A. E. (2016). Dads tuning in to kids: Preliminary evaluation of a fathers' parenting program. *Family Relations, 65*(4), 535–549. doi:10.1111/fare.12216

Wong, M. S., McElwain, N. L., & Halberstadt, A. G. (2009). Parent, family, and child characteristics: Associations with mother- and father-reported emotion socialization practices. *23*(4), 452–463 doi:10.1037/a0015552

Yap, M. B. H., Allen, N. B., & Ladouceur, C. D. (2008a). Maternal socialization of positive affect: The impact of invalidation on adolescent emotion regulation and depressive symptomatology. *Child Development, 79*(5), 1415–1431. doi:10.1111/j.1467-8624.2008.01196.x

Yap, M. B. H., Allen, N. B., Leve, C., & Katz, L. F. (2008b). Maternal meta-emotion philosophy and socialization of adolescent affect: The moderating role of adolescent temperament. *Journal of Family Psychology, 22*(5), 688–700. doi:10.1037/a0013104

Young, J. E., Klosko, J. S., & Weishaar, M. E. (2006). *Schema Therapy: A practitioner's guide*: New York : Guilford Publications, 2006.

Zahn-Waxler, C., Duggal, S., & Gruber, R. (2002). Parental psychopathology. In M. H. Bornstein (Ed.), *Handbook of parenting* (pp. 295–327). Mahwah, NJ: Lawrence Erlbaum Associates.

Zubrick, S. R., Ward, K. A., Silburn, S. R., Lawrence, D., Williams, A. A., Blair, E., … & Sanders, M. R. (2005). Prevention of child behaviour problems through universal implementation of a group behavioural family intervention. *Prevention Science, 6*(4), 287–304. doi:10.1007/s11121-005-0013-2

Index

K. Deater-Deckard and R. Panneton (eds.), *Parental Stress and Early Child Development*, DOI 10.1007/978-3-319-55376-4

Printed by Printforce, the Netherlands